P9-DUF-790

The opinions are in on
SECOND OPINION
by
Dr. Isadore Rosenfeld

"Although this book is entitled *Second Opinion*, it contains much more than a consideration of why, when, and how valuable is another opinion. It is, indeed, a pragmatic, instructive, and highly readable book for the average layman who desires authentic information about medical and health matters. In a wide-ranging discussion of medical illnesses from asthma to angina, from cataracts to cancer, and from cholesterol to contraception, Dr. Rosenfeld has provided a no-nonsense presentation of current authentic medical information that will permit the layman to understand better the judgments rendered by the physician and to determine whether a second opinion is desirable."

—Michael E. DeBakey, M.D.
The Methodist Hospital, Houston

"This is one of the best-written books for the lay public that I have read on medical treatment. . . . The information is current and highly accurate. I will strongly recommend this book to my patients and friends."

—Antonio M. Gotto, Jr., M.D.
Chairman, Department of Medicine
Baylor College of Medicine

"*Second Opinion* is an easy-to-read, enjoyable account of the latest advances in medical treatment, a book which finally makes it possible for the layman really to understand why, when, and where to ask for a consultation. . . ."

—Mary Lasker

SECOND OPINION

Isadore Rosenfeld, M.D.

Revised and Updated

BANTAM BOOKS
TORONTO · NEW YORK · LONDON · SYDNEY

SECOND OPINION

*A Bantam Book / published by arrangement with
The Linden Press*

PRINTING HISTORY

Lindèn Press edition published March 1981
Literary Guild Full Selection April 1981
Serialized in *Self Magazine, Vogue, Cosmopolitan, Bestways,
Your Good Health Review and Digest* and *New York Times Special
Feature Syndication* February through April 1981.
Bantam edition / June 1982

Cover photo by Alex Gotfryd.

ISBN 0-553-20562-5

Published simultaneously in the United States and Canada

Bantam Books are published by Bantam Books, Inc. Its trademark, consisting of the words "Bantam Books" and the por-
trayal of a rooster, is Registered in U.S. Patent and Trademark
Office and in other countries, Marca Registrada. Bantam
Books, Inc., 666 Fifth Avenue, New York, New York 10103.

PRINTED IN THE UNITED STATES OF AMERICA

0 9 8 7 6 5 4 3 2 1

In memory of my father,
whom I miss so much,
and my wonderful mother,
with deepest love and gratitude.

Acknowledgments

I very much appreciate the kindness of my various colleagues, who reviewed the chapters dealing with their particular areas of expertise, and gave me the benefit of an invaluable second opinion on what I had written.

THYROID, Drs. Eugene Cohen and David Becker

CATARACTS, Dr. Robert Coles

DIABETES AND HYPOGLYCEMIA, Drs. Thomas Roberts and Eugene Cohen

EAR, NOSE AND THROAT, Dr. Wilbur J. Gould

ASTHMA, Dr. James P. Smith

DERMATOLOGY, Dr. Richard Gibbs

SEXUALLY TRANSMITTED DISEASES, Drs. Richard Roberts and Lewis Drusin

CARDIOVASCULAR DISEASES, Dr. Michael J. Wolk

VASCULAR DISEASES, Dr. Jerrold Lieberman

NEUROLOGICAL DISORDERS, Dr. Frank Petito

GYNECOLOGICAL DISEASES, Dr. Myron Buchman

UROLOGICAL DISORDERS, Drs. Russell Lavengood and Jon Reckler

GASTROINTESTINAL DISORDERS, Dr. Howard Goldin

ARTHRITIS, Dr. Charles Christian

CANCER, Drs. William Cahan and Morton Coleman

Contents

SECOND
OPINION

Preface

Even If You Love Your Doctor

In my first book, *The Complete Medical Exam*, I took you step by step through the ideal physical examination or checkup. In this volume I deal with *treatment*—the natural sequel to diagnosis. And the basic message I want to convey is that there is usually more than one way to skin a cat in medicine; that for every ailment there is almost always more than one form of therapy. You *do* have alternatives in the way your medical problems can be handled, and in these pages, you will find them.

This book was written for *patients*—to tell you why, when (and sometimes where) to ask for a second medical opinion. No matter how devoted you are to your doctor or how much you dislike antagonizing him, you owe it to yourself to consult with another expert when you are ill and not responding to treatment, or when you are presented with a diagnosis or prognosis that may drastically alter the course of your life, or when a major operation is recommended.

No Rare Diseases Here

A word about what you will find in this book and how it is organized. I have tried to keep the information practical and written in layman's language, not technical jargon. In selecting the subject matter, I have called upon my own experience, reviewed the latest literature dealing with each topic and asked appropriate specialists to double-check the accuracy of the final manuscript. Because of the rapid developments in medicine, there may already be changes in some of the treatments that I have recommended or described.

1

But these are relatively few and minor, in view of the fact that I have completely revised the contents and brought them up to date for this paperback edition.

Although comprehensive, this is not a complete medical text. I have not included discussions of exotic or rare diseases. But you will find advice about treatment of such disorders as asthma, overweight, hepatitis, impotence, heart trouble, blood pressure, stroke, difficult pregnancy, ulcer or circulatory problems—to name but a few of the more common troubles you are likely to encounter.

You Usually Have Several Options (About Which You May Not Be Told)

Your doctor usually has several alternatives at his disposal to treat most conditions. One may be better, more convenient or more appropriate for you than another. You should know—or be made aware of—all these options when you are sick, and you should be able to discuss them freely with your physician. Unfortunately, either because they are too busy, or don't believe that it's really any of your business, some doctors don't tell you that you have any choice at all, or what it is. That attitude is not in your best interest, nor is it likely to result in optimal medical care for you.

I have listed your options in the management of every disorder discussed, with enough information about each of them so that you can help judge what is best for you when a decision has to be made. The preferences that I express are not necessarily better for you than those your own doctor recommends. However, they reflect my own experience and, perhaps, a different point of view of which you should at least be aware.

When you have finished reading this book, or those pages in which you are specifically interested, you will understand why your doctor has made a particular recommendation, for example, to operate or not to operate, to give anticoagulants (blood thinners) or to withhold them, to use antibiotics or to avoid them, and so on. As a result, you will be more confident about that advice and less likely to worry when one of your friends tells you that his physician prescribed totally different treatment for the same ailment. If your doctor's suggestions leave you puzzled or uneasy, you will be able to discuss intelligently with him whatever reservations you have about the therapy he suggests and to decide whether you want to consult another physician.

One Opinion May Be Enough (or All You Are Able to Get)

I'm not for a moment suggesting that a second opinion is *always* necessary. You needn't see another doctor for something trivial like a cold, muscle spasm or a mild tension headache. As a matter of fact, you may not want a consultation even when you are seriously sick, as long as the diagnosis is obvious, the treatment seems straightforward and, most important, you are getting better. Finally, a life-threatening emergency may not allow the luxury of time for another opinion. When you are in shock from hemorrhage, and the bleeding must be stopped immediately, you can't wait for a consultant to get dressed and come over "in the fullness of time."

When the Verdict Surprises You

But for the many situations or diseases that may require major surgery (malfunctioning heart valves, coronary artery obstruction, aneurysms), that may be out of control despite treatment (diabetes, chronic backache due to a disc somewhere in your spine), that may impair the quality of your life (arthritis, impotence, infertility, stroke, serious emotional disorders) or that may affect its duration (cancer, advanced arteriosclerosis), you should ask for another opinion. For example, you consult your doctor for what you always thought was a little "indigestion" and he ends up telling you something that worries and alarms you, like "your electrocardiogram is very abnormal. You may need cardiac surgery. You'll have to come to the hospital for an angiogram." Or, after a routine checkup, you hear "I'm sorry, but there is a suspicious lump in your breast which may be malignant. We'd better get a biopsy."

You suddenly find yourself on the conveyor belt of medicine, carried along into a future over which you no longer have any control. Your life is threatened and your key

concern now is "What are my options?" That question is what
this book is all about.

Examples of Important Alternatives. Would You Recognize Them?

You probably wouldn't need much persuading to ask for a
second opinion if you were very sick and not responding to
treatment, or if your doctor gave you some dramatically bad
news that, if true, might completely change the course of
your life. But would you know enough to ask for a second
opinion in the following hypothetical situations, every one of
which, as you will learn in these pages, has important alternatives in diagnosis, therapy or outlook?

You have cramps in your leg at night and your feet are
always cold. You're told that it must be due to poor circulation. (page 209)

One night, you are awakened by chest pressure that
frightens you. It disappears in a few minutes. Your ECG the
next day is normal. You are reassured that you do not have
heart disease, because "angina is always effort-induced and
never comes on at rest." (page 148)

You develop a lump in the thyroid gland. Your doctor
advises its removal, because "no lump anywhere should ever
be left alone." (page 41)

A lump has been found in your breast. The surgeon asks
for your permission in advance to do whatever is necessary at
the time of the biopsy, depending on what he finds. (page
351)

In the course of a routine check of your vision, your eye
doctor finds that you have cataracts. Although your vision
isn't all that bad, he recommends their removal. (page 49)

Your chronic fatigue and lassitude are said to result from
low blood pressure, for which you're given treatment. (page
199)

After suffering for years from hemorrhoids you finally
decide to do something about them. An operation is advised.
(page 326)

You had a mild heart attack about three months ago, and you are recovering very well. But suddenly you develop abdominal pain and gas after eating "rich foods." A gallbladder X ray is done, and you are advised to have surgery as soon as possible. (page 303)

You are found by X ray to have a duodenal ulcer. It responds to treatment with antacids and Tagamet, and you have no more symptoms. Although you are feeling well, a few weeks later you are advised to have another X ray to see whether the ulcer has healed. (page 282)

You are thirty-eight years old, have wanted a child for many years, and have only now become pregnant. Plans are made for your delivery, and there is no mention of having an amniocentesis. (page 268)

You leave the hospital after your heart attack, and you ask your doctor several specific questions about sex and other activities. He tells you to "take it easy" for a while and then "play it by ear." (pages 173–75)

You're a traveling salesman and recently had a sexual encounter with an attractive woman whom you met in the hotel lobby. A few days later, you develop a watery penile discharge. You are told that it must be gonorrhea, and a culture to confirm the diagnosis is not necessary. (page 111)

You have had psoriasis for many years, and it is getting worse. Your family doctor tells you to resign yourself to the fact that there is no effective treatment for this skin disease. (page 92)

You have had angina for years, and have adjusted your life style so that you manage pretty well. Nevertheless, you are advised to have bypass surgery to prevent your having a heart attack and to ensure a longer life. (page 161)

One of your testes has never descended into the scrotum. You are told that you need do nothing about it, since one testis is all you need. (page 243)

You have always tired more easily than most of your friends, and you finally consult a doctor about it. After a routine physical exam, he finds nothing wrong but prescribes some thyroid pills anyway to "pep you up." (page 33)

Your parents both died in their eighties from "old age." You have never had an important ache or pain, but your cholesterol level is 260 mgm percent. You are advised to protect yourself by following a strict low-cholesterol diet. (page 138)

You have noticed a reddish-black "mole" on your skin. Your family doctor says he doesn't think it is anything to worry about, but he would like to check it again in about two months. (page 99)

You have chronic asthma, which becomes worse whenever you spend any time at home with your cat. You are advised to be desensitized to the animal, and that it is not necessary to give her away. (page 83)

You are a sixty-eight-year-old man and have developed myasthenia gravis. Your eye muscles are getting weaker, and you now have some difficulty swallowing. You are advised to have your thymus gland removed. (page 235)

You have poor arterial circulation in the legs and, despite giving up cigarettes and following all the doctor's orders, the pain has begun to cripple you. You are told that there is no alternative to surgery. (page 208)

Your enlarged prostate was removed some time ago. You also have high blood pressure. You now find you have trouble ejaculating normally. Both you and your urologist assume that it is the result of your operation. (page 321)

You experience a discomfort in your chest after eating, and you tell your doctor about it. A thorough physical exam shows you to be in excellent health, with normal ECG and chest X ray. You both conclude that it must be indigestion. (page 283)

You have arthritis involving several joints. Aspirin eases the pain, but you still feel miserable. You are told that there is no cure for arthritis and that you must learn to live with your symptoms. (page 373)

You have been told that too much cholesterol is an important cause of heart disease, and so you decide to eliminate milk and other dairy products from your children's diet, as well as your own. (page 138)

You are scheduled to have your cataract removed by the new technique of phako-emulsification. You are sixty-eight years old, and are told that you will be given spectacles after surgery because the intraocular lens is still experimental and hazardous. (page 52)

You have been reading about the dangers of untreated hypertension, so you have your doctor check it. He assures you that it is only mildly elevated, and that such slight hypertension doesn't really need any treatment. (page 136)

After taking four tablets of Inderal a day for several months, you find that, although it did help your angina, it interfered too much with your sex life. Your doctor admits that this is entirely possible, and he has you stop the drug abruptly for a few months to see what happens. (page 155)

You're nine weeks pregnant and want an abortion. Your gynecologist plans to do it in his office using the traditional "scraping" technique. (page 262)

Biopsy of a lump in your breast reveals it to be malignant. You're told the safest approach is to have a radical mastectomy. (page 351)

You develop pain in the calves of your legs after walking briskly for five or six blocks. When you stop, the pain goes away. Examination reveals some narrowing of the arteries in the legs. You are advised to have an operation at your earliest convenience. (pages 203–4)

You find that estrogens are of great help in controlling your hot flushes due to the menopause. But you have been advised to stop taking these hormones, because they can cause cancer of the uterus. (page 359)

You are a woman in your thirties and are aware that everyone considers you a "complainer." Among your problems are migraine headaches, vague chest pains and an irregular heartbeat. Your doctor has never come up with any important abnormalities, and your chest X ray and ECG are also normal. He suggests that you see a psychologist or psychiatrist. (pages 125–26)

You have had cataracts for years, but now your vision is really bad, so you decide to have surgery. Your opthalmologist tells you that none of the newer procedures for removing them have really been proved safe and effective and that he will use traditional surgical methods. (page 50)

You are a twenty-six-year-old homosexual male and are found to have gonorrhea of the anus. Your doctor agrees to treat you with tetracycline because (a) it is just as effective as penicillin in this disease, and (b) you don't like shots. (page 114)

You are forty-eight years old and have some benign lumps in the breast. An aunt died of breast cancer some years ago. You are advised against annual mammography because (a) it is unnecessary, and (b) it exposes you to the danger of radiation. (page 351)

You have a chronic sinusitis, which is being treated with frequent irrigation and drainage. (page 73)

You have a goiter that is not particularly attractive cosmetically but is giving you no problems. Your doctor recommends that it be removed anyway. (page 40)

You have valvular disease of your heart due to old rheumatic fever. The pills and injections that formerly worked quite well are not nearly as effective any more. You are advised to have valve replacement in the nearest hospital, where they do "quite a few" of these procedures, and where it would be very convenient for your family and friends to visit. (page 124)

You have been treated for rheumatic heart disease for several years, and now you have become pregnant for the first time. You are advised to have an abortion to avoid undue strain on your heart. (page 124)

You are in your middle twenties and are found to have an overactive thyroid gland. Treatment with antithyroid medication has not been successful. Surgical removal of the gland is recommended, and you are referred to a good general surgeon. (page 36)

Despite your conscientious adherence to a rigid low-fat diet, you continue to suffer from gallbladder attacks. You have been advised to have surgery, but you don't like operations. You are delighted to hear that gallstones can now be dissolved with medication, and you decide to go that route. (page 303)

You are in your early sixties and have a hernia and a little "prostate trouble." Arrangements are made to repair the hernia. (page 321)

Your doctor detects an aneurysm of the aorta when he examines your abdomen. Special tests reveal it to exceed 5.8 cm. in size. You are advised to come back every six months for re-evaluation. (page 218)

You have high blood pressure, and despite losing weight, exercising and cutting down on your salt intake, the readings don't get any better. You are prescribed medication that kills your sex drive and leaves you tired to boot. When you complain about the treatment, you are told that it is the lesser of two evils, since untreated hypertension will give you a stroke. (page 136)

You are almost sixty years old, a diabetic and overweight. You can't seem to lower your blood-sugar levels, no matter how good you are about your diet. You also don't feel too well, and you have some vaginal itching. You are told the antidiabetic pills are dangerous and that you must have insulin. (page 61)

You are getting a little deaf and find it especially hard to make out women's voices in a crowded room. You are advised to go to a hearing-aid store to be fitted for a hearing aid. (page 77)

Your six-year-old child had a sore throat several times last year and has just had another. You are advised to have her tonsils and adenoids removed. (page 76)

You are a seventy-year-old woman with palpitations and some shortness of breath, but you have never had chest pain. Your doctor tells you that it must be due to "heart trouble," in view of your age. (page 119)

You are a sixty-five-year-old man and have to get up two or three times a night to empty your bladder. You suddenly develop a stuffy, running nose and are given nasal deconges-tants. (pages 73–74)

You have an enlarged prostate which, according to your urologist, will require early surgical removal. In the mean-time, you develop an ulcer and are given antispasmodics to reduce your gastric discomfort. (page 288)

In the course of an upper G.I. series done to see whether you have an ulcer, the radiologist has come up with a surprise finding of gallstones. You're told they should be removed surgically as soon as possible. (page 303)

You are a great lover and have no problem with sexual desire or ability to have an erection. You therefore conclude that the cause of your barren marriage is your wife's infertility. (page 240)

You develop swelling and pain in your right leg. It's also warm to the touch. Your doctor examines the leg, says he *thinks* you have phlebitis and recommends anticoagulation. (pages 203–4)

You became diabetic in your late forties. Although your blood sugar is always somewhat higher than it should be despite your diet, you feel perfectly well. You are told that that means you probably will need insulin. (page 61)

You are chronically nervous and tired. Your doctor cannot find a physical basis for your complaints. You finally consult a diet specialist, who diagnoses hypoglycemia. (page 67)

You have been diagnosed as having a gastric (stomach) ulcer. Medication results in control of your symptoms. A few weeks later, you report the good news to your doctor, who discharges you as cured. (page 287)

You have finally decided to go ahead with a much-needed prostatectomy. Your urologist recommends complete removal rather than "shaving it" through the penis. (page 321)

You are twenty-three years old, single, and would like to go to nursing school. But you have chest pain and palpitations, and you wonder if you are strong enough. Your doctor tells you that he hears an innocent heart murmur, which has nothing to do with your symptoms. (page 119)

You are a thirty-year-old woman and have been diabetic since childhood. You become pregnant and want very much to have the baby, but you are told that the risks to you and the infant are too great. (pages 62–63)

You are a middle-aged man. In the past few months, you have had to get up two or three times a night to empty your bladder. You now have to "go" more frequently during the day. The lack of sleep has begun to wear you out. Your doctor tells you that the prostate is not big enough yet to warrant its removal. (page 321)

Your child snores and is a mouth-breather. You are advised to have his adenoids removed. (page 76)

Your ulcer is not responding to medical treatment, so you are advised to have psychotherapy. (page 289)

You are infertile because your sperm are "inadequate." A routine physical exam reveals you to be otherwise healthy. You are told that there is nothing more to be done, since sick sperm cannot make babies. (page 240)

It is vital to your health that you never become pregnant again. You agree to sterilization and are advised to have a hysterectomy. (page 277)

You call your doctor at 3 A.M. because you have an oppressive feeling in your chest and are sweating. He comes to the house, records an ECG, and tells you that it is a mild heart attack, and that you would be more comfortable at home than in the hospital. (page 119)

In the course of a routine exam, you are advised to have a cardiac pacemaker put in, because, even though you have never had any symptoms, your slow heart rate, together with other ECG abnormalities, makes you vulnerable to cardiac arrest. (page 179)

You have had hemorrhoids for years, and Preparation "H" is all you have ever needed. You suddenly notice much more bright-red blood in your stool, but are reassured that it is all coming from your hemorrhoids. (page 326)

Doctors have for years been unable to cure your impotence. You have read about penile prosthetic devices, but since they don't use them at your hospital, you suspect that they are only a gimmick, and that no reputable urologist would have anything to do with that sort of thing. (page 240)

You find that a cortisone ointment for which you used to require a doctor's prescription helps your psoriasis rash. This drug is now available "over the counter," thanks to a recent government deregulation. So, you apply it as much and as often as you like, since if it is available without a prescription, it must be completely safe. (page 93)

Your teen-age daughter has a bad case of acne. She is told to give up all the "junk foods" that she has been eating, because acne and pimples are caused by a bad diet. (page 97)

Because you smoke too much, you have been going for a chest X ray every year. Now you read that the American Cancer Society says that it is no longer necessary as long as you feel well. You plan to follow that advice. (page 347)

You are told you have cancer of the ovary and that it is too late for surgery because the malignancy has already spread. (page 360)

You are found to have a small malignancy of the bowel. The surgery is successful, and the tumor is entirely removed. You are told that follow-up chemotherapy is unnecessary. (page 360)

You have noted some recurrent vaginal bleeding. A careful exam fails to reveal the cause, so your doctor recommends that you may as well have your uterus removed to "be done with it." (page 359)

You have attacks of transient double vision. You are advised to have an arteriogram to visualize the circulation in the brain. (page 160)

You are only fifty-three years old, and have become impotent. A routine physical exam reveals no abnormalities, and you are advised to have psychotherapy. (page 240)

You have "diverticulitis," with periodic lower abdominal cramping, pain and fever. You are given a strict, low-residue diet to follow. (page 312)

You have a "spastic colon," with recurrent diarrhea, especially when you are nervous. You are told that your best bet is to see a psychiatrist. (page 318)

You have either ulcerative colitis or Crohn's disease. Your life has been complicated by severe bowel symptoms, pain and misery. You are advised to have the diseased portion of the bowel surgically removed. (page 315)

You develop pain and swelling of the big toe. It turns out to be gout. In addition to medication, you are given a strict diet, eliminating all the rich foods that cause gout. (page 384)

You have a "chronic" bad back. A complete workup shows it to be due to a disc, and surgery is recommended. (page 389)

So here are just 82 pieces of advice or information frequently given to patients by their doctor, a friend, or the media. They cover the gamut of almost every area of health and disease. In every instance the "fact" is either wrong, outdated or debatable—and the following pages tell you why. This is only a representative sampling of the hundreds of other options you have in the spectrum of disease prevention and management covered in this text.

You will note a page number beside each "situation" referred to above. That reference deals with the particular question at hand, but as you peruse these pages, you may well find the same problem referred to or approached from a different perspective in a different area.

1

A Second Opinion—Why, When and How

The kind of medical advice you may opt to question is not necessarily limited to a critical situation. Second thoughts about a diagnosis or treatment may stem from a variety of sources—as the following cases illustrate.

Four Opinions for a Common Cold

Suppose you are coughing, ache all over and feel pretty awful. You know that it's just "a virus," "the flu," "the grippe" or "a bad cold," but because your chest hurts when you cough, you're worried—you may have "walking pneumonia." And so you go to the doctor. He examines you, and then insists on a chest X ray (which you'd rather not have because of the hazards of radiation) just to be sure. "It's only a cold," he tells you. "Here's a prescription for twenty antibiotic pills. Take four a day for five days."

On your way home you meet a friend who, you're sure, would just love to hear all about your illness. You describe your symptoms in detail. You remind him that you never get just a mild cold like everyone else—yours always seem to border on pneumonia. This one is so bad, you tell him, the doctor even prescribed twenty antibiotic capsules. Your friend looks at the prescription. (This is the beginning of a second opinion.) "Wow, that's the stuff that almost killed me last year. I heard somewhere they're planning to withdraw it from the

14

market. Take my advice and double-check on it." You're now somewhat less confident about your doctor and his treatment.

Your Wife the Specialist

You arrive home coughing and sneezing and show the prescription to your wife. (You are into your third opinion now.) She happens to know a great deal about medicine, and she tells you that you are and always have been a hypochondriac, that all anyone needs for a "plain cold" is chicken soup, fluids, a few aspirin tablets and lots of extra Vitamin C (of which you have been taking five a day for as long as you can remember). She shows you a clipping she saved (she follows the medical literature avidly) which reports recent experiments proving that vapors from chicken soup really have a beneficial effect on the lining of the nasal and bronchial tubes. In her considered and final opinion, the antibiotic is certainly not necessary. Besides which, *her* doctor never prescribes an antibiotic for a simple cold.

Now you're torn. Everyone knows who actually wears the pants in the family, but maybe in this instance, your wife is right. You sneak upstairs and phone "Doc" at the drugstore. (Now you are soliciting your fourth opinion.) He reassures you this particular drug is not about to be withdrawn from the market as your friend suggested. It is perfectly safe, and he sends it right over before you can change your mind.

Chicken Soup and Antibiotics

It's time to eat. You have as much of a meal as your appetite permits. It includes the chicken soup, lots of tea with lemon, and ginger ale for dessert—all of which were prescribed by your wife. But you keep looking at that twelve-dollar bottle of capsules sitting there, waiting to be opened. It would be a waste to return them, since it's "Doc's" policy never to take back any medicine—opened or not. You consider all the pros and cons, and finally, apprehensively, you take one. You wait around, look at your tongue in the mirror once or twice, expecting the worst—a terrible rash, hives, wheezing or diarrhea. Six hours later you find that it did you no harm, and so you take another. But just to be on the safe side, you also swallow two aspirins and go to bed.

In the morning, after a surprisingly good sleep, you

wake up feeling much better. At this point, you have to decide about the eighteen remaining, expensive antibiotic capsules. Chances are that you will do one of the following: (a) Stop the antibiotics because you believe the two you took have already cured you. (You will, of course, continue for several days heavy on the chicken soup, honey, garlic, Vitamin C, mustard plasters on the chest, and gallons of hot tea with lemon.) (b) You will take more of the antibiotics but certainly not four a day, as prescribed—maybe only one or two for another forty-eight hours; four a day was probably too many for you anyway. (c) You'll actually finish the antibiotic capsules exactly as the doctor instructed you to. If you do that, you are in the minority.

Note that whichever course you follow was determined by four opinions—and for nothing more serious than a common cold.

Your Neighbor the Diagnostician

Have you ever had the following experience? You develop a pain in the calf of your leg. You look at it, then touch it. It is slightly reddened and tender. You hurry over to the doctor because you are afraid there may be something wrong with your circulation. On your way to his office, you are suddenly aware of a surprising number of amputees on the street. The doctor examines you and says you have a mild phlebitis (inflammation of the veins). He tells you not to worry, to go home, rest in bed with your leg elevated on pillows and to apply warm, moist heat to the tender area. As you get off the bus, you meet your next-door neighbor mowing the lawn. He asks why you're limping. So you tell him your troubles. It turns out he had "exactly the same thing" last year. (Second opinion developing.) But *his* doctor, who is also his friend (they play golf together every Wednesday afternoon), took better care of him than yours did of you. He rushed him directly to the hospital, ordered many tests, and prescribed anticoagulants (blood thinners) to prevent a blood clot from traveling to his lungs (embolism). "But, did you actually have phlebitis?" you ask desperately. "Or was it something worse?" "What could be worse? Of course, it was phlebitis—and in the left [or right] leg too, just like you." Now you are really worried.

After a conference with your mother (the third opinion) and several phone calls later to knowledgeable people, all of whom have had vein trouble at one time or another, you get so many conflicting opinions you decide to see another doctor. (Second medical, ninth opinion in all). Your neighbor was right. This new doctor sends you to the hospital forthwith, where your leg is kept elevated and moist heat is applied—but no one gives you the anticoagulants you expected. For this, you might just as well have stayed home. Your postphlebitic friend visits you, proud and gratified that his intervention resulted in your hospitalization. But he is appalled that you are not having your blood thinned as he did. He convinces you to get yet another opinion (your third medical consultation so far) about the anticoagulants. Thank goodness you did, because this latest doctor, in fact, recommends that blood thinners be started immediately. In a few days, you come home—cured. You are told to continue the anticoagulants for several more weeks, just in case.

All's well that ends well, but now you are convinced that some doctors don't know their business—and one of them happens to be yours. You blanch at the thought of what might have happened if you hadn't by chance met your neighbor that day.

Life Without a Gallbladder?

This last example may also ring a bell. You have noticed recently that an hour or two after eating fatty or fried foods, you experience an uncomfortable fullness in your "stomach" and are getting rid of enormous amounts of gas one way or another. The discomfort actually borders on pain. You finally consult the really good doctor who gave you the anticoagulants for the phlebitis. He listens to your symptoms, examines you and orders a gallbladder X ray. The verdict? Bad news—gallstones. "What do I do now, Doctor?" "We'd better make arrangements to have that gallbladder removed." "The whole gallbladder? Why not just the stones?" you ask innocently, wondering how one can live without a gallbladder. "Don't be ridiculous. We don't take the stones out and leave the gallbladder," he "answers," obviously irritated by your stupidity. (Well, that will teach you to ask him medical questions in the future.) You are now intimidated, but still curious; why "not just the stones"? So you leave his office, all set to have the operation he suggested. You now have visions of yourself in the operating room with the anesthesia mask over your face (you've always had a secret fear of blurting out something embarrassing as they put you to sleep). And you think of all the pain, the tubes in your nose and needles in your veins, the stitches, the scars, the works—if you ever wake up, that is.

Uncle Phil to the Rescue

When you finally get home, everyone can see that something terrible has happened to you—even though you're very brave and say nothing. You simply ask whether Aunt Milly didn't die from a gallbladder operation. One thing leads to another. You break down and tell the family the bad news. Luckily, Uncle Philip is there for dinner. He is the family medical expert, because he once thought of becoming a doctor himself. (He actually ended up as a shoe salesman but never lost his interest in medicine.) "A gallbladder operation? That's ridiculous. No one gets operated for gallstones anymore. Don't you know there are pills you can take to dissolve them?" (A semiprofessional second opinion, but a strong one.) You wonder why your doctor didn't tell you about this great advance. Is it possible that Uncle Phil knows more than someone with an M.D. degree?

You go to bed disquieted, and toss and turn all night. The few winks of sleep you get are filled with nightmares— your surgeon is an imposter; the orderly taking care of you after the operation is a homicidal maniac; worst of all, your hospital insurance has expired and the bill amounts to $10,000.

Good News: The Doctor's Out

In the morning, you call your physician and are relieved when his secretary tells you he is not in. You are embarrassed to admit that you checked on him with Uncle Phil, and you certainly don't want him to know that you are planning to get another opinion. You leave a message for the doctor to hold off with the arrangements for surgery for the time being. You concoct some story about getting your affairs in order, and you say you will get back to him in a few days. Then you arrange to see a consultant (second medical opinion). He listens to your story and asks to see the gallbladder X rays taken yesterday. Since you were too timid to request them from the first doctor, they have to be taken again. This second physician, obviously more experienced, looks at the new films, confirms the presence of the stones, tells you that an operation is definitely not necessary at this time and prescribes a low-fat diet. He also advises you to forget about Uncle Phil's new medicine, the one that dissolves gallstones, because it hasn't been around very long, doesn't work in every case, and may give you side effects worse than the operation itself. You can't get over your good luck in finding this great doctor.

Whom Can You Trust?

If you were the same person who in succession had the cold, phlebitis, and gallstones, you would really be disillusioned, wouldn't you? Whom can you trust when you get sick? It seems that every doctor you see offers different advice each time something goes wrong. As you read on, you will come to understand that the various doctors you consulted for each of the problems may *all* have been correct. As a matter of fact, so was Uncle Phil. But which advice you follow is in the final analysis essentially up to you. The important point is that you know what your options are.

Judgment, Experience and Personal Preference

The doctor who prescribed antibiotics for your cold may have been concerned that at your age, and with your particular susceptibility, you might become dangerously ill if your cold were to be complicated by pneumonia; so he suggested the antibiotics as a preventive. A second physician might have waited twenty-four or forty-eight hours to see if you could shake the infection yourself, avoiding the unnecessary use of a medication that could produce its own side effects—a perfectly legitimate difference of opinion.

The doctor who did not prescribe blood thinners for your phlebitis may have felt that because the particular veins involved were superficial you were not likely to suffer a blood clot to the lungs—that the risk of the anticoagulants causing an internal hemorrhage was greater than the danger of a potential embolism (especially if you happen to have high blood pressure). The second doctor probably agreed, because he sent you to the hospital, where you could be watched for evidence of the kind of phlebitis that might cause embolism, but he didn't give you anticoagulants either. The last physician decided to take no chances with the embolism and gave you anticoagulants. All three were right, each in his own way.

The doctor who recommended surgery for your gallstones may have felt that you would ultimately need the operation anyway, and he preferred to do it now, when you were younger, otherwise healthy and better able to tolerate it than you might be in the future. (He should have answered your question "Why not remove just the stones?" by telling you that a gallbladder with stones in it is diseased and will simply keep making more until it is removed.) The physician who suggested that you wait with the operation preferred to give you the benefit of the doubt, hoping that you would fall into the substantial category of patients in whom symptoms clear up and never recur. Each of these points of view is perfectly legitimate. Which one you choose to follow depends on a host of personal considerations.

Second Opinions That Made a Difference

The hypothetical cases described above should not leave you with the impression that alternative treatment approaches for any given disease are always only a matter of preference (yours or the doctor's), and that it makes no real difference in the long run how your case is managed. One opinion may be wrong, in which event, the correct second one can, in fact, mean the difference between success and failure—even life and death. The following examples illustrate that point.

An "Obvious" Case of Coronary Artery Disease

Some years ago, a colleague asked me to see a fifty-seven-year-old man in whom the diagnosis was not clear and the results of treatment unsatisfactory. The patient's major complaint was that he tired very easily and became unduly short of breath when walking quickly or climbing stairs. I listened to the description of the symptoms and examined the man very carefully, but I could not find very much wrong. The electrocardiogram, however, was definitely abnormal. I concluded, as the family doctor had, that the patient had mild coronary disease. There wasn't much more I could do but make some minor changes in the dosage of the medications prescribed. I also suggested how he might modify his life style so as to live more comfortably with his illness.

The patient accepted my findings and recommendations with some disappointment. After a few weeks, when it was clear that he was no better, *he* asked for a *third* opinion. The case was reviewed by another cardiologist, who did not agree with the diagnosis of coronary-artery disease. He suggested instead that the patient had constrictive pericarditis—that is, formation of a thick, fibrous band around the heart. This is usually the result of a viral infection or an inflammation of the pericardium, the normally thin envelope of tissue enveloping the heart. This constriction prevents the heart from expanding fully, thus causing a decrease in its output of blood. The symptoms and electrocardiographic abnormalities of which the patient complained were due to this diminished cardiac efficiency. A simple operative procedure released the band around the heart and the man returned almost immediately to a normal, active life.

What lesson is to be learned from this particular case? First, that if you are feeling poorly and one consultant can't help you, don't stop there. You must continue to look for help until you find it especially when the diagnosis is vague. This man surely would have deteriorated slowly and insidiously, if the right diagnosis had not been made and the proper treatment instituted. He knew enough to ask for another opinion, and his doctors cooperated willingly—two important ingredients for effective medical care.

Think (and Ask) Twice Before You Retire

Several years ago a forty-six-year-old man came to me for a "heart checkup." A year or so earlier, in the course of a routine examination, he was shocked to hear that his electrocardiogram was abnormal. What's more, he was assured that sometime in the past he must have suffered a heart attack. The news stunned and puzzled him, because he simply could not recall any symptoms that even remotely suggested heart trouble. Because the ECG was "diagnostic," it was concluded that his heart attack must have been "silent," as happens in about 25 percent of cases. Since he was relatively young and the electrocardiogram very abnormal, his doctor advised him to "take it easy." (That was twenty years ago, when we had a very different understanding and outlook on heart disease.) When the patient asked for more specific advice, like should he retire, the answer was "yes, if you can afford it." Fearful of the next heart attack (to which he was obviously vulnerable) and in order to prevent it, he decided to sell his factory. He ended up, however, retiring not only from business, but from life itself. He began to spend his time just sitting at home, feeling sorry for himself. He walked, talked and acted like an old man. He even became impotent because of his fear of dying during sexual intercourse.

He came to see me not because he doubted the diagnosis, but to be reassured that in the interval since his last examination he had not sustained another heart seizure without knowing it. (His own doctor, to whom he normally would have gone, had retired from practice.)

In listening to his history, I could not elicit any symptoms to suggest there was anything wrong with his heart. He had no chest pain or pressure, no unusual shortness of breath and no palpitations. Then I recorded an electrocardiogram. Now it was my turn to be surprised. I found no evidence whatsoever of any previous heart attack. What I did see was a pattern called WPW (named after the cardiologists who first described it—Wolff, Parkinson and White). This is a variation in the form of the tracing which makes it *look* abnormal but which, in fact, in no way indicates cardiac damage. It is an electrical artifact, a freak of nature, a variant—something that you are born with and does not as a rule shorten the life span. The bad news this man had been given twenty years earlier was based on an incorrect interpretation of the electrocardiogram. If he had sought a second opinion at that time, he would have been spared all his sorrow and suffering.

Remember that as newer diagnostic medical techniques become available—echocardiograms, CT scanners, nuclear imaging and the like—more and more doctors may be using them before they are really expert in their interpretation. Undergoing a sophisticated, expensive new test is no guarantee that the result you get will be accurate. All the more reason to think of asking for another opinion, especially when the news is unexpected or bad.

A "Hopeless" Case with a Happy Ending

Let me tell you about one more experience to make my point. The wife of one of my doctor friends developed severe headaches and attacks of double vision. She consulted a senior neurologist, who, after thorough testing, discovered a brain tumor. The patient asked for and was told the diagnosis. She was advised that surgery was not possible, and her only alternative was radiation which would shrink the tumor somewhat and alleviate the headaches, but would not cure her. This gallant lady settled her affairs and prepared to live out her last few months in the greatest possible comfort. Her husband, the doctor, knew better than to "shop around" for another opinion. This was, after all, an open-and-shut case confirmed by an eminent brain specialist. But the patient was persuaded by a non-medical friend to see someone else. Reluctantly she consulted an equally prestigious neurosurgeon, who agreed with the diagnosis, but not with the treatment or outlook. He felt confident that the tumor could be completely removed. With nothing to lose, my friend underwent surgery, and it was entirely successful. The tumor was a large one, pressing on her brain. After its removal, her symptoms disappeared and she returned to a normal life in a few weeks. That was fifteen years ago.

2

Patient Care Versus Doctor Ego

The System and the Individual Patient

We are justifiably proud of the excellent doctors, hospitals and medical care available in the United States. These stem from our research capacity, technological skill and system of medical education. But high national standards are not always reflected in the kind of care an individual patient receives from any one doctor for a specific illness. Correct diagnosis and treatment depend on *your* physician's awareness of the latest medical findings relevant to *your* specific problem.

Every physician has a hard time keeping up with all there is to know—that's why we specialize and perhaps *overspecialize*. Furthermore, doctors are busy, are chronically overworked and usually have too many sick patients to look after. There simply isn't the time to attend all the important conferences where critical new information about the management of your particular disease may be disseminated. And reading the medical literature conscientiously at home may not be enough either. The lapse between the time an important discovery is made and when it is reported in the professional journals is often as long as a year or more. It is entirely possible that some other doctor has the answer to your problem, and can make life a lot easier (and longer) for you. So, when you are in a difficult medical situation never hesitate to ask for the extra input of a second opinion.

All Men (and Doctors) Are Not Created Equal

You may occasionally find yourself in a critical medical situation in which the proper decision requires not only up-to-date knowledge and technology, but particularly good judgment and experience as well. A famous surgeon once said he could teach any student *how* to perform an operation in weeks—to learn *when* to do it usually takes years. There is a wide spectrum of such skill, training, judgment and experience within the medical profession. Most patients either are not aware of this reality or fail to act on it. Unless they do, accepting the first decision that comes along as final and binding may sometimes result in tragedy.

Loyalty or the Fear of Retribution?

Why, then, despite the fact that some physicians know more than others, or have better training, judgment and experience, do so many patients still hesitate to ask for a second opinion when it is really needed? Fear. They pretend that it is because of affection or personal loyalty to the doctor. "I wouldn't want to offend (insult, hurt, anger) him," is how they rationalize it—and what they probably believe. The truth in most cases, is that they don't want to lose his good will. They want to be sure that the next time they are sick, they won't get the cold shoulder instead of immediate attention.

This fear of "retribution" is sometimes, but not always, justified. While many doctors (usually the better ones) welcome requests for consultation and, in fact, often initiate the process themselves (especially when they are faced with a complicated problem or when things aren't going well), others do not. They make it quite clear that a second opinion is unnecessary and that your request is an insult to them. So, in order to avoid an unpleasant confrontation and a compromised relationship with your doctor (with its attendant consequences on your medical care), you may consult someone else surreptitiously.

How many times have I asked patients whether they wished me to send a report to their family doctor, only to be told, "Please don't. I wouldn't want to hurt his feelings." But, somehow or other, he often learns that they have gone elsewhere. Then, he is doubly furious because it was done behind his back. Some doctors are angry even when the patient is candid. I remember one man who, suffering from severe angina pectoris, consulted me after his own cardiologist had recommended an immediate coronary bypass operation. I advised him to try certain medications first. He asked me to convey my opinion and findings to his doctor, which I did. It was all open and aboveboard. A few weeks later, the patient developed severe chest pain during the night and called his physician, who refused to make a house call, on the grounds that "I'm not Dr. Rosenfeld's errand boy." He was offended that this man had asked for and accepted an opinion other than his own. I like to think such "colleagues" represent a minority.

How to Ask for a Second Opinion

What, then, is a patient to do? In my experience, the answer does not lie in timidity or subterfuge. If you are worried about your health, want the option of some other form of treatment, or simply wish to be sure that the diagnosis and management of your problem are correct, get a second opinion, but do it in the following way. First, tell your doctor about it. Don't have him learn at second hand that you have been to someone else. Then ask *him* to recommend the consultant. Patients often come to their doctor requesting that he consult with a certain specialist they have heard about. It is possible, however, that your doctor doesn't think this man is likely to be of help, in which case he won't be happy about conferring with him. So let *him* choose the consultant. Patients are sometimes leery about doing it that way. They believe the second man may be in cahoots with the first and rubber-stamp whatever his friend says. If that's something you are worried about, then by all means, make a clean break with your "past" and start over again elsewhere. Frankly, in my experience, I have rarely encountered a physician who went along with a colleague whom he knew to be wrong.

Despite the foregoing, there will be occasions when *you* should insist on choosing the consultant rather than having your doctor do it. If you live in a small community, or one in which medical opinion is "homogeneous" about how to treat your particular problem and you know that there exists an entirely different school of thought about it, don't hesitate to make your own arrangements. A good example is cancer of the breast. As you will see later in these pages, there is a legitimate and very important debate about how best to treat a localized malignant breast lump. Some specialists still insist on aggressive surgery, others prefer a more limited operation, and there are even those who recommend radiation without any cutting at all. The matter remains in flux. Data supporting each technique are still being accumulated. If *all* the doctors in your area are agreed on one approach, go elsewhere so that you can at least hear the other side of the story. You deserve to know what choices you have.

If your request for another opinion is turned down just because your physician objects on *principle* to having someone else in, it is time to change doctors. *In the final analysis, what medicine is all about is patient care, not doctor ego.* Should you decide to switch, be candid about it. Ask to have your complete record forwarded to your new doctor so that you won't need to repeat all the tests that you have already been through. Doctors must comply with such requests; it is required by law.

When Two Doctors Disagree

You may now wonder, "What do I do if the second opinion differs from the first? When do I ask for a third opinion? Whose advice do I finally take?" Those are difficult questions to answer in the abstract. If you can't choose between two divergent recommendations, and don't know instinctively which is the better for you, then you will need to consult a final arbiter. It's a nuisance, of course, but far better than having treatment that is unnecessary or wrong. And you may never be sure who was "right" in the final analysis. But simply having been made aware that an important difference of opinion does exist gives you an option, and *you* may end up having to make the final decision. That's sometimes the best way.

A word of caution at this point. Just as there are patients who take several "1-a-day" vitamins every morning, because "if one is good, ten must be better," so there are individuals who are convinced that one can never have enough opinions about an illness. They spend their time and money soliciting as many consultations as they can. They do so, not because of any conflict in the advice they've been given, but because no one has yet told them what they want to hear. Once they get the opinion they were hoping for all along, they discontinue the search.

Holy Surgery

That kind of behavior is not only time consuming and expensive but can also be dangerous. I remember one man who consulted me because of recurring attacks of chest pain, shortness of breath and loss of consciousness. I found that the trouble lay in a severely diseased heart valve that, in my judgment, needed replacement. The patient panicked at this advice and asked to be seen by another cardiologist at my hospital. The consultant agreed with my recommendations. The patient then suggested that perhaps a specialist from another center might have a different viewpoint. In order to satisfy him, I arranged for yet another doctor to review the case. He too concurred in the need for surgery. At this point, my patient, who was deeply religious, called upon his pastor for an opinion. I don't know how the clergy make their decisions in such situations, but he advised this man not to have the operation during the next fourteen days. After that, it would be perfectly safe for him to do so.

I was delighted that the matter was now settled. In order to protect the patient, I kept him in hospital while awaiting surgery. When the two weeks were up, my man changed his mind again and asked to be discharged so that he could think it all over "a little more." He left my care, and finally found a physician who told him the operation was not only too risky but also unnecessary. Six weeks later, the patient died suddenly, as I had feared he might. He was only sixty-eight years old, and his operative risk was less than 5 percent. This man had gone from doctor to doctor until he finally found one who told him not to have an operation—the opinion he was looking for all along.

The purpose of this book, insofar as it educates the lay public, is to strengthen the traditional doctor-patient relationship, which is so essential to good medical care and is the cornerstone of American medicine.

But that relationship must be sound, open and healthy enough to withstand your asking for consultation when necessary.

3

The Thyroid Gland
—Regulating Your Thermostat

The Honest Broker

The thyroid has an extremely important job to do, setting the energy level of the body. It is a straightforward, honest, aboveboard gland. It sits right there in the front of your neck and, as long as it is "well," remains invisible. When something does go wrong, it is generally apparent (unlike other organs or structures that, hidden deep in the brain, chest or abdomen, make it necessary for us to call in the heavy diagnostic artillery when trouble develops). If the gland enlarges, for whatever reason, it is usually obvious. When it becomes inflamed it hurts, and you can easily identify the source of the pain; if it develops a tumor, the lump may be discernible right under your fingers or your doctor's; when it isn't working properly—that is, when it is making too much of its hormone or too little—the thyroid signals both to you and to your doctor that something is awry. Treatment of any malfunction is usually straightforward and successful, and that even includes cancer, which, in the thyroid gland, is uncommon, almost always slow-growing and curable.

But You Have to Listen

So, in every respect—location, appearance and symptoms—the thyroid does not often hide what is going on. But it does ask in return that you pay attention to what it is trying to tell you, and act accordingly. Despite its good intentions, the thyroid's messages are sometimes subtle and therefore either missed or misinterpreted. Treatment of the various diseases that affect it is also occasionally controversial. Under those circumstances, a second opinion may be desirable—as you will see below.

Setting Your Thermostat

Think of the thyroid gland as your body's thermostat, controlling how fast it burns up fuel. The substance it produces, thyroid hormone, circulates throughout the body in the bloodstream. The healthy gland makes just enough to keep you functioning on an even keel. But sometimes it produces too much hormone, in which event your body's "engine" is, revving too fast, too little hormone so it's always cold and stalling.

The amount of hormone produced depends not only on the state of health of the thyroid itself, but on two other glands situated in the brain, called the pituitary and the hypothalamus. The thyroid and these two "associates" are constantly exchanging chemical and nervous signals, so that precisely the right quantity of hormone is manufactured and released into the bloodstream. This level is in large part responsible for your energy, appearance and the pace at which you live.

There are several disorders of the thyroid gland with which you should be familiar. These include *hypothyroidism* (when the gland produces too little hormone); *hyperthyroidism* (when it makes too much); *goiter* (a swelling of the gland that is more commonly found in women and, which if large enough, looks like a bicycle tire encircling the neck); and benign or cancerous *lumps* of the thyroid itself.

When There's Not Enough Hormone

When the thyroid gland is very sluggish and doesn't produce nearly enough hormone, anyone can recognize the resulting symptoms. Such patients may be fat, but then it is not the jolly, lively, full of fun Santa Claus kind of fat with rosy cheeks and a glint in the eye. They are "sick" fat, dull and constipated. The skin is sallow, with a lemon tint, dry, with little or no perspiration. The voice is hoarse and low-pitched and speech is slow. In women the menstrual flow is heavy, and they are apt to have trouble becoming pregnant. The hands and face are puffy, especially around the eyelids. Hypothyroid individuals are apt to be less alert than those around them and are often hard of hearing; they are always tired, and tend to sleep a great deal. They are usually too apathetic to complain, but when they do, it frequently is about the cold weather. They are also often depressed, and for good reason. Life isn't much fun. Such thyroid underfunction occurs in both sexes but is more common in women than men.

Sex Is Okay, But Frankly, They Would Rather Sleep

So much for the picture of classic hypothyroidism (*myxedema*), in which the amount of circulating thyroid hormone is very, very low and has been that way for some time. But people not so obviously deficient, who have only a little less thyroid than they need, are not so easily recognized. In some cases, they go through life undiagnosed and untreated. The skin tends to be dry, despite abundant use of cream and oil; the hair is coarse and comes out in bunches when it is washed and brushed. These individuals are always "tired"; they lack energy, need lots of sleep, dress a little more warmly than everyone else, don't like air-conditioning (but love the hot weather), and dream secretly of moving to a warm climate some day. They would never admit it to anyone, but although they enjoy sex when they get around to it, frankly, both men and women would rather sleep. When the condition is finally diagnosed, the difference a little thyroid pill makes is incredible.

If your doctor suspects, from his examination, that you are hypothyroid, there are laboratory tests he can obtain to confirm his clinical impression. The amount of thyroid hormone circulating in the blood can be measured quite accurately, and in hypothyroidism is lower than it should be. That triggers off a chain of other abnormal tests, because virtually every organ and function of the body, fueled by the thyroid, is operating at reduced capacity—much like a "brown-out" in an energy crisis. So, in long-standing disease we often find evidence of anemia (because the bone marrow is sluggish); the cholesterol is high (because there is not enough thyroid hormone to "burn it off"); the waves or complexes in the electrocardiogram are not as tall, and the heart rate is slow; the chest X ray often demonstrates a swollen heart, with fluid in the pericardial sac that surrounds it; the electroencephalogram (brain-wave test) is abnormal too. When we strike the knees with our little hammer, the jerk response is less brisk. At the ankle, the tendon reflex there is slow to return, a particularly useful test for your doctor to perform.

But Thyroid Hormone Is Not a Vitamin

Mild thyroid deficiency is often overlooked, because its symptoms are "nonspecific" and occur in a host of other, unrelated states, including simple boredom, depression, nutritional anemia and gluttony. So, there is a temptation and tendency to diagnose someone with these complaints as "hypothyroid" without documentation. Thyroid hormone is then prescribed to the naturally fat, slow, cold and dull among us, in order to "perk them up." It rarely does so, unless there is a genuine need for replacement therapy.

I do, however, believe there is a gray area, wherein patients with mild underfunction of the thyroid gland nevertheless have normal laboratory values. If that is what your doctor suspects, he may give you a small dose of thyroid for several weeks or months—just to see if it helps—and sometimes it does. But thyroid hormone is not a harmless vitamin supplement. When taken by the wrong people for the wrong reasons (that is, by those who are not hypothyroid), even ordinary doses are not without danger. Thyroid supplements can make you nervous and irritable, can give you a rapid and sometimes irregular heartbeat, and cause weight loss. If you are elderly and have high blood pressure or some underlying heart condition, unnecessary thyroid hormone prescribed to make you "feel better" can create serious problems. I have seen many patients subjected to all kinds of complicated tests to explain their palpitations, nervousness and weight loss, because they didn't tell the doctor that they were taking "just a little thyroid"—and he didn't think to ask. So it is a good idea, whenever you are prescribed thyroid hormone, to ask for the evidence on which the treatment is based. If that evidence seems vague or casual, ask for a second opinion.

Feedback Signals to the Gland

Extra thyroid hormone taken by mouth for whatever reason results in a higher level in the bloodstream, and the thyroid gland then receives a signal to make less. After all, why should the gland keep working to make its hormone, when you are swallowing in pill form all that the body needs—and more— every morning? But then, having been turned off for a while, the gland, now accustomed to working less hard, becomes sluggish. When that happens, should you abruptly stop taking the extraneous supply, you will be hypothyroid for a while, until normal glandular function is restored.

The Hyperthyroid Gland—Too Many RPMs

When there is too much thyroid hormone in your system because the gland is overproducing it, you will present a typical picture in most cases. You are nervous, can't sit still; are always complaining of the heat, perspiring when everyone else is bundled up; tend to have more frequent bowel movements; continue to lose weight, despite a ravenous appetite, because your body's thermostat is set too high. When you stick out your tongue or outstretch your hands, they have a fine tremor. Your palms are hot and wet. Chances are that palpitations, due to a rapid, sometimes irregular heart action brought you to the doctor. In women, the menstrual flow is very much reduced, and conception may be difficult. And even though the body motor is highly "revved," desire for sex is usually reduced. In fact, I have occasionally seen breast enlargement in men with overactive thyroid glands. And that doesn't bode well for their sexual prowess. Occasionally friends will tell you that your eyes are beginning to bulge and you may notice double vision because your ocular muscles are weakened by the hyperthyroidism.

When the Symptoms Are Subtle

The foregoing is the description of a patient in whom the overactivity of the thyroid gland is obvious. Often, however, as in hypothyroidism, the picture is more subtle, especially in older persons. They may simply be "nervous" or irritable and have unexplained weight loss despite eating well. They may complain of palpitations or develop heart failure. Because they are old, these symptoms may be interpreted as evidence of heart disease. After all, aren't the elderly entitled to a little heart trouble? So the possibility of thyroid overactivity may be overlooked and untreated. If you suddenly and for no discernible reason develop "heart failure," make sure to ask whether your thyroid function has been checked.

The hyperactive thyroid gland is almost always enlarged to some extent, either diffusely or with one or more discrete lumps or nodules in it. Such nodules, when they occur, may function independently of the rest of the thyroid and produce excessive amounts of hormone all by themselves.

When You Just Don't Get Over an Emotional Shock

Hyperthyroidism occurs most frequently in women between the ages of thirty and forty years. We don't understand what causes it—probably some breakdown in the immune-control mechanisms of the body. I have seen it develop in several persons after severe emotional crises. The husband of one of my patients was convicted of tax fraud and sent to jail. Her shame, sadness and guilt were immense. Shortly thereafter, she began to lose weight and suffer palpitations. Everyone told her this was to be expected—a typical reaction to stress. She finally consulted me because she had lost some fifty pounds, and was continuing to do so even after her husband's release from prison. By the time I saw her, the diagnosis was obvious. Other women in my practice became hyperthyroid after the death of a child or a spouse; one elderly lady developed it after she was mugged and robbed. So if you are suddenly "nervous" in response to a crisis, and remain that way even after it is over, see to it that your thyroid function is evaluated before being relegated to the psychiatric category.

Just Following Orders

Doctors do not always agree about the best way to suppress exaggerated thyroid function. Unlike hypothyroidism, where we simply replace the amount of hormone you are lacking, treatment of an overactive gland may present difficulties because the problem is usually not in the thyroid itself. At least in the beginning, the gland appears to be the victim of some disorder in the immune system that stimulates it to make more hormone than it should. Since we don't know how to attack the underlying disorder, we vent our therapeutic fury on the thyroid gland, which is only responding to abnormal signals from some "higher authority."

Although none of the three basic methods of "cooling off" the hyper gland really gets to the root cause, they nevertheless do control the symptoms. But remember, whereas hypothyroidism can easily be treated by an internist, you should consult an endocrinologist or thyroid specialist for the management of hyperthyroidism.

Suppressing the Overactive Gland

One method of treating hyperthyroidism is to give you an antithyroid drug (propylthiouracil) that blocks the formation of the hormone within the thyroid gland. In other words, the gland is no longer able to respond to the sick signal that whips it into frenzied overproduction. But even as we suppress the gland, we may give you some thyroid hormone at the same time, to make sure that you have at least some function.

Antithyroid drugs are probably the most desirable treatment for hyperthyroid women in the childbearing age (usually under thirty) in whom the disease is of recent onset and is mild, and in the gland only slightly enlarged. If you fall into that category and any other form of therapy is suggested, get another opinion. These agents may be expected to effect a cure in about 35 percent of such cases. (The response to this medication is not as good as when the thyroid is very large and of irregular consistency.) While waiting for the action of the drug to take effect, your symptoms, if severe, can be controlled by several other medications, the most effective of which is Inderal (propranolol) or some other beta-blocker. (see page 157)

Antithyroid drug therapy is usually continued for a year. We then stop it and assess your thyroid function, to see whether it will remain normal after the drug is withheld. There is some new evidence that a whole year of treatment may not be necessary, that if the propylthiouracil is stopped as soon as your gland becomes normal—usually after several weeks or months—the cure rate is just as high as if you had continued it for a year. So if you are told to take the drug for a full twelve months, ask whether that time can't be shortened.

In the majority of patients, the gland bounces right back to the overactive state after the propylthiouracil is stopped. Should that happen, you will need treatment either with radioactive iodine or surgery. Both these techniques virtually guarantee a cure, but in so doing, destroy most or all of the thyroid gland permanently—one by radioactivity, the other by the scalpel. You should be aware of the risks and benefits of both methods of treatment.

The Case For and Against Radioactivity

Radioactive-iodine therapy works in the following way. Iodine introduced into the body in whatever form, ends up in the thyroid. So, to get any radioactive material into the hyperthyroid gland in order to destroy it, we render some iodine radioactive and have you drink a measured amount of it. The solution itself is without taste, odor, or color—just like ordinary water. The iodine is absorbed, goes directly to the thyroid, where the radioactivity starts to work on the overactive gland. One drink usually does the trick, but sometimes two or more are needed. This form of treatment is clean, safe and effective. It avoids the need for taking antithyroid drugs (which have only a 35 percent cure under optimal circumstances) three times a day for months. It also spares you the pain, risk and complications of surgery.

When You're Pregnant or Under Thirty

Why not treat every hyperthyroid patient in this way? More and more doctors are actually doing so, with two exceptions—pregnant women and those under thirty. We don't want to give a big dose of radioactivity to an expectant mother, because it crosses the placenta and destroys the thyroid gland of the unborn fetus too. Even if you're not pregnant, but still in the childbearing years, there is at least the theoretical possibility that the radioactivity may alter your genes in some way as to affect a future pregnancy. There is also the matter of potential malignancy occurring later in life. As far as I know, the administration of radioactive iodine has never been proved to cause any kind of cancer. However, the suspicion exists that it can, so in order to be safe, such treatment is usually withheld from young persons of either sex.

The Exact Radioactive Dose—An Estimate

One of the complications of radioactive iodine is that, in attacking the hyperfunctioning gland, it leaves some 40 to 70 percent of patients hypothyroid within ten years. Sensitivity to radioiodine varies from person to person. It is very difficult to calculate the exact amount necessary to control the overactive gland and still not render it underactive. So be prepared to become hypothyroid after being treated this way. If and when that happens, you will need replacement hormone. That simply means taking thyroid supplement for the rest of your life—not a terrible prospect.

The Pros and Cons of Surgery

All of which brings me to the pros and cons of removing the overactive thyroid gland surgically. This procedure is most widely performed in children, in adults under forty years of age, and in pregnant women who have not responded to drug treatment—none of whom should normally receive radioactive iodine for the reasons mentioned above. It is not safe to have the operation while the gland is very "hot," because surgical manipulation at that time can worsen the condition. You will need a few weeks of antithyroid drug therapy first.

Every patient considering thyroid surgery should have a second opinion for a very special reason—one that the surgeon is not likely to discuss with you. Thyroidectomy is not an easy operation. It requires skill and experience to avoid several important possible complications. When I was a medical student and resident, before the widespread use of radioactive iodine for the treatment of hyperthyroidism, surgical residents were doing scores of these procedures every year. By the time they finished their training, they were really skilled at it. However, over 700,000 patients who would otherwise have had their thyroid removed surgically, have since received radioiodine instead. Today, a surgeon-in-training may do two or three thyroidectomies a year, hardly enough to give him the necessary skill. So, be sure to determine how much experience the doctor has had *in this particular operation* before you let him operate. You can do that by asking him directly, or better still, letting your internist find out.

Complications of Thyroid Surgery

The risk of dying from thyroid surgery is really minimal, except when the patient is very sick or old (in which case the radioactive-iodine method is preferable anyway). But surgery may lead to complications short of death. If too much of the gland is removed, you will be left hypothyroid (but less frequently than after radioactive iodine). The incidence is about 15 to 20 percent in the first year and 2 percent every year thereafter. A more important danger is that the surgeon might inadvertently cut a nerve very close to the thyroid gland that supplies the vocal cords. Should that happen, you will be hoarse forever. Also, the four parathyroid glands, which control calcium and bone metabolism, may be removed by mistake, since they are very small and are situated near the thyroid gland. In that event, you will require treatment for underfunction of the parathyroid glands for the rest of your life. Finally, there is the risk of hemorrhage during the operation, because of the many blood vessels in the area. For all these reasons, the operation is considered delicate. Be sure to pick the right surgeon.

When the Eyes Have It

There is one important exception to my earlier statement that any malfunction of the thyroid gland can be treated successfully. About 15 percent of patients with hyperthyroidism have bulging or protruding eyes, a complication that often poses more than just cosmetic problems. When this causes damage to the eyeball or the optic nerve itself—which happens from time to time—vision is affected. Unlike the other symptoms of an overactive thyroid gland, the prominent eyes are caused not by excessive thyroid hormone, but by some other process that is not well understood. So, treating the thyroid gland has no direct effect on the eyes, although they do tend to improve or stabilize somewhat when the hyperthyroidism is controlled.

The Impact of Iodized Salt

Suppose you were born and raised before the days of iodized salt in an area where the soil and consequently the food you ate was deficient in iodine (the Great Lakes in the northern United States, the mountainous areas of the Andes, the Himalayas). Since iodine is the major constituent of thyroid hormone, when the body does not get enough of it, the gland produces less hormone. You would think that would cause it to shrink. The reverse is true. In fact, it gets bigger and bigger as its cells work harder to make as much hormone as they can with less of the raw material (iodine) than they need. The result is a goiter—an enlarged and lumpy thyroid gland that may or may not produce extra hormone. When it does, it's called a "toxic goiter"; when it doesn't, it is "nontoxic."

Who's Got the Goiter?

A goiter may appear during puberty and pregnancy, when the body's demand for thyroid hormone is increased. Certain drugs called goitrogens (examples are lithium, widely used in the treatment of manic-depressive states, and occasionally some of the oral antidiabetic drugs) may also cause goiters.

When to Have the Goiter Removed

Most goiters are nontoxic—that is, they do not make extra hormone and so produce no biological symptoms. But they must nevertheless be carefully watched since a small proportion do gradually become hyperthyroid (for reasons that are not understood). Patients sometimes want the excess goiter tissue removed for cosmetic reasons. Also, the goiter may have to be excised if it becomes so large as to compress nearby structures, causing cough, hoarseness and difficulty in swallowing. But remember, a goiter is rarely malignant, and you should have it operated on only if its appearance disturbs you, or you suffer pressure symptoms from it or possibly because it's toxic. If surgery is recommended for any other reason, ask for a second opinion, from an endocrinologist.

Thyroid Tumors—Bad and Not So Bad

Various kinds of growths or nodules are very common in the thyroid gland, and may be present in 40 percent of Americans. Most are asymptomatic. When a thyroid lump appears, we first want to make certain it is neither frankly malignant nor potentially so. This is done first by a careful history-taking (has the lump been increasing in size over a short period of time—an ominous piece of information; did you sometime in the past receive radiation to your neck for some reason or other—like for treatment of acne—lumps in such patients are more likely to be malignant; do other members of your family have a history of cancer of the thyroid or of any other "hormone-producing" gland—you're more vulnerable to have a malignancy if it runs in the family). An appropriate work-up might include a radioactive scan of the thyroid gland. You drink a *tracer* amount of radioactive iodine, which is picked up by the gland and then outlined when scanned by a geiger counter. If the nodule in question does not absorb radioactivity, we call it "cold"; if it does, it is referred to as "hot." "Hot" nodules are almost never malignant; "cold" nodules may be or become so later on in about 10 percent of cases. "Hot" nodules are treated with thyroid pills or, in some cases, with radioactive iodine.

We now use sonar techniques to help differentiate cancerous from noncancerous "cold" thyroid nodules. Those that appear to be solid when the sound waves are directed at them are more likely to be malignant than those in which the growth is *cystic*—that is, containing pockets of fluid. But this distinction is not always reliable. So to be absolutely certain of the diagnosis, discuss the feasibility of getting a needle aspiration of the lump. This has an accuracy of 85 percent to 90 percent, but must be done by a trained, experienced physician. Together with the history and other tests, it usually provides the final answer. Incidentally, chances of a single nodule being malignant are greater in men than in women or the young. The presence of more than one lump reduces the chance of malignancy. If you are either reassured about a nodule in your gland and told to leave it alone *or* advised to have it surgically removed—without a thorough evaluation, ask for a second opinion from a thyroid specialist.

When to Remove the Cold Nodule

You may be advised to have a cold nodule excised even if all tests are negative, especially if there is a family history of thyroid cancer. But this operation is rarely an emergency, since most thyroid cancers grow very slowly. If, under close observation, the nodule doesn't get any bigger for months or years, many specialists prefer to leave it alone. However, we almost always take it out in the following circumstances: in children; when it appears to be growing rapidly; if the patient has had previous radiation to the head or neck; when the nodule is so big that it causes pressure symptoms; and in men under 40 years of age.

Your Friendly Thyroid Cancer

If you have thyroid cancer, don't panic. First, have the diagnosis evaluated by a thyroid specialist, because such cancer is rare. Then, if it is confirmed, be reassured by the fact that thyroid cancer is an infrequent cause of death in the United States. Years ago patients with such malignancies were subjected to extensive, surgical procedures. A good part of the neck, its muscles, even the jaw, were removed. That is hardly ever done these days. Almost all cases can be cured or controlled by excision of the tumor together with any involved glands in the area. This is followed by suppressive doses of thyroid hormone for life, in order to prevent any recurrence.

I remember a very dramatic case some twenty years ago. The patient was a beautiful woman of twenty-one. In the course of a routine examination, I detected what felt suspiciously like cancer on the side of her neck—a hard, irregular, painless lump stuck to the surrounding tissues. I referred her to a surgeon, who removed the gland. Under the microscope, it was seen to contain highly malignant-looking tissue. When a cancer grows wildly, it distorts the cells from which it originated so that the pathologist may have difficulty deciding whence it came. Hers was such a tumor. A thorough search of the body—the liver, the intestinal tract, the skin, the bone marrow—failed to reveal any malignancy. We suspected that it originated in the adjacent thyroid gland, but were unable to feel anything suspicious in it.

The problem we now faced was how to treat this woman, having removed a gland with a malignancy whose origin we didn't know. Several surgeons recommended a radical dissection operation. This would have meant a horrendous, disfiguring procedure—the removal of most of the jaw, as well as a search for and excision of any involved glands elsewhere in the neck.

We decided to wait for further evidence of tumor spread before doing any operation. It was my own feeling that since the abnormal gland we had excised and examined already represented spread of the tumor, it probably was seeded elsewhere, and extensive surgery now would be too late anyway to make a difference. And so we waited for the next evidence of the cancer's metastasis. Twenty-one years later, we are still waiting, but my patient isn't. She has since had two children and remains totally free of any disease whatsoever. If she had gone to Lourdes, we would now be talking about a miracle. If she had been given Laetrile, it would have represented a "cure."

Although we never did find the source of the malignant lymph gland, I suspect that it was a thyroid cancer which had spread to the one gland and no further. This woman's story represents one of the medical mysteries that we encounter from time to time, but it also attests to the rather benign course of "malignant" thyroid cancer. And, incidentally, we never did anything to the thyroid itself. The gland is still sitting there, with no evidence of any disease whatsoever within it.

KEY FACTS TO REMEMBER

Thyroid gland disorders are very common. Although their diagnosis and treatment are usually straightforward, subtle malfunction may go unrecognized. This is especially true when the gland is *sluggish*. Simple replacement of the deficient thyroid hormone will correct the symptoms of hypothyroidism. However, taking thyroid pills for fatigue and lack of energy when function of the gland is actually normal is of no benefit and not without risk.

Treatment of an *overactive* gland may be complicated, and can be done in one of three different ways—anti-thyroid drugs, radioactive iodine and surgery. Selecting the right one for you is crucial. You should always have a second opinion from an endocrinologist, particularly one specializing in thyroid disease, before the final choice of therapy is made. If the gland is to be removed surgically, make sure of the surgeon's skill in this particular, delicate operation.

Lumps, or *nodules*, of the thyroid gland are of several different kinds. Some are potentially malignant. Always make sure, when told that yours is or is not, that the conclusion is based on an adequate evaluation.

Thyroid cancer is uncommon, usually slow-growing, responds to treatment, and is not often a threat to life. Proper recognition and therapy are, nevertheless, very important. The joint efforts of an endocrinologist and an *oncologist* (cancer specialist) should be obtained if you are given that diagnosis.

4

Cataracts—A Disorder of the Young and the Old

On a Happy Day, You Can See Forever

I remember, many years ago, long before I became a doctor, reading an interview given by Winston Churchill. In it, he marveled at the fact that he was "getting younger," as evidenced by a sudden ability to read fine print without glasses. I couldn't understand this "miracle" at the time, but I felt that it couldn't happen to a nicer person. Then, not long ago, one of my friends, a vigorous man in his early seventies, married a beautiful young woman. Everything appeared to be standing up to the challenges of the age difference between them. One day, in a particularly happy frame of mind, the elderly bridegroom confided to me. "Doctor," he said, "never discourage a spring-winter marriage. It has great advantages for both partners. Many women prefer older men because of their experience, stability and wisdom." (He didn't even mention money.) "As far as I am concerned, it has made me feel years younger. I know you won't believe this, but I'm rejuvenated in every respect."

At this point, I expected a discussion of his born-again sex life; I was surprised when he continued, "The most striking change of all is in my vision. I can now actually read fine print, like the phone book or the stock-market quotations in the newspaper, without wearing my reading glasses." He paused, awaiting my reaction to this incredible news, certain that I would challenge it. I didn't, because although I couldn't vouch for the vigor of some of his other functions, the story of his improved vision came as no surprise. I had learned a great deal since Churchill's announcement years earlier.

This happy phenomenon is not at all, in fact, evidence of rejuvenation. Quite the contrary. The improvement of near vision described by my friend is unfortunately only temporary and usually occurs in elderly persons who were farsighted (presbyopic) to begin with. Often referred to as "second sight," it reflects the development of myopia—shortsightedness—due to early cataract formation. As the cataract forms, the natural lens in the eye becomes more permeable and absorbs water. This thickens it and changes its shape, so that it now bends the rays of light more acutely, making the patient nearsighted (myopic). Because the degree of farsightedness is reduced by this change in refraction, near vision is improved for a while. But you can't have it both ways—it also causes increased blurring of distant vision (something my patient in his euphoria did not notice). After a relatively brief period of stability, eyesight begins to deteriorate as the cataract continues to expand.

Chances Are You'll Have Them Too

Although cataracts affect mostly older people (their removal is the most commonly performed surgical procedure among Medicare patients in the United States), they do occur in younger persons as well. At any given time, there are some three million Americans who have impaired vision due to cataracts. Eye doctors perform almost 500,000 operations every year to extract them. So, there is a good chance that this disorder has either already affected you or will at some time in the future.

Is Your Eye Doctor Up to Date?

If you have a cataract, it is important that you know your treatment options. In recent years, there has been major progress in eye surgery and its postoperative management. It is critical that you be able to judge whether you are being offered the best of the new procedures available because, unfortunately, not every eye specialist is trained to perform some of these more modern techniques. It is entirely possible that a doctor will suggest an older method in the name of conservatism, when the real reason is his lack of skill or experience with the newer approaches.

It's Like Boiling the White of an Egg

Let me review briefly what a cataract is, how it forms and the various methods of dealing with it. The lens within your eye works very much like the one in your camera. It focuses the rays of light that strike it on to the retina behind the eye. Here specialized cells gather this information and transmit it, via the optic nerve, directly to the brain, where the image is interpreted as the object you see. If the area of the brain making this visual interpretation is damaged, you are not able to "see" even if the rest of the visual apparatus— the eye, retina and optic nerve are working perfectly.

The normal lens is clear and transparent, but certain chemicals, diseases, infections and injuries can render it opaque. When that happens, you have a cataract. A good analogy can be made with the white of an egg, which, like your lens, is made of protein. Raw egg white is clear and transparent. After boiling, the protein becomes cloudy. That is what happens to the natural lens of your eye when it develops a cararact; you can no more see through the full-blown, or "ripe," cataract than you can through the white of a boiled egg.

Why Cataracts Develop

As mentioned earlier, this change in the transparency of the lens is not limited to the elderly. Anyone at any age can develop cataracts from a variety of causes—injury, effects of radiation, infections, certain diseases like diabetes mellitus, chronic exposure to infrared rays, or as a result of several different medications, notably cortisone in large amounts. However, three quarters of all cataracts do occur in those over sixty-five years of age. About 20 percent of persons between the ages of forty and sixty-five have them. They may also develop in the newborn and children. I won't discuss the mechanisms of cataract formation in the very young, because that is a complicated process. Suffice it to say that they are usually the result of some toxic effect, nutritional deficiency, injury—or infection in the mother during pregnancy (e.g., German measles). In adults, the most common cause of cataract formation is what we call "senile degeneration."

Whatever the mechanism, a developing cataract will cause the gradual and, usually, painless deterioration of your eyesight. You may find yourself always looking for a better light by which to read, or you may keep cleaning your glasses because they frequently seem to be getting "fogged up." You may feel as if there is a veil covering your eyes, and you try to rub it away. You may notice that driving your car at night has become more difficult because the oncoming headlights cause an uncomfortable glare or halo. (This latter symptom is due to the fact that when the light rays hit the cloudy lens, they are scattered instead of passing right through to the retina as they do when the lens is transparent.)

Seeing Better in the Dark

The extent and kind of visual impairment and its severity really depend on how opaque the lens has become and which portions of it are involved. For example, some patients with cataracts may actually see better in dim than in bright light. This happens when most of the lens is normal except for the central portion directly behind the pupil. Since pupils constrict in bright light, if the clouding of the lens happens to be located mostly behind the pupil, you will have trouble seeing when illumination is good. But when it is dim, the pupils open wider, allowing more light to hit that part of the lens that is unaffected, thus improving your vision.

Poor Vision? Not Necessarily Cataracts

Just because you can't see or read as well as you used to doesn't necessarily mean that you are developing cataracts. More likely, you simply need to have your glasses changed. Occasionally, a gradual decrease in vision is due to glaucoma, which, if untreated, can result in permanent blindness. Or the doctor may come up with other causes for impaired vision, the most important of which is vascular (blood vessel) changes in the eyes. (Keep your fingers crossed against that diagnosis, for which virtually nothing can be done at this time.) Macular degeneration—a change that entails loss of vision in the elderly—is yet another disorder for which there is no effective therapy thus far.

If the ophthalmologist does find evidence of early cataract formation, he will want to re-examine your eyes at regular intervals to see how rapidly it is progressing. Some patients with slow-growing cataracts can avoid surgery for years simply with new glasses from time to time. Unlike glaucoma, there are no drops or medications that can improve failing eyesight due to cataracts. There have been some recent reports suggesting that aspirin started early in life and taken regularly thereafter may help prevent lens clouding later in life. This does not seem like a practical solution, because of the difficulties sometimes caused by chronic use of that drug. Also, L-tryptophan, a naturally-occurring amino acid (protein) promoted as a non-narcotic sleeping aid and obtainable without prescription in health food stores may accelerate cataract formation. It should probably be avoided if you are beginning to develop a cataract. Practically speaking, however, there is essentially nothing that you or your doctor can do to influence the speed with which your cataracts develop.

When to Have Your Cataract Removed

Unlike many situations involving surgery in which you have no say about the timing of the operation, *the decision when to have a cataract removed is almost always up to you*. Cataract surgery is rarely an emergency, except in some instances, when the cataract has completely matured. In this circumstance the eye may become inflamed or develop acute glaucoma, mandating emergency lens removal. But in almost every other instance, you should have the operation when *you* think you need it. Age is not a factor. I have found that patients usually decide to undergo surgery when their life style is compromised because of poor vision. For example, the surgeon who can no longer see well enough to operate, the executive who has trouble making out charts or other data, or the retired person who can no longer watch TV or read.

Your Surgical Options

Let's suppose, then, that you can't see the numbers on the bus or read the menu in a restaurant; changing your eyeglasses doesn't help anymore either. You cannot drive a car with confidence, and driving is essential to your livelihood; it is time to have the cataract out. The operation is simple and safe, and it results in restored vision in about 95 percent of cases. But there are certain facts you must know about the operation and what to expect after it is done.

Cataract surgery basically involves getting rid of the cloudy lens. The capsule that surrounds it may also be removed (intracapsular cataract extraction), or a portion at the very back of the lens may be left behind (extracapsular cataract extraction). Both procedures can be performed under either general or local anesthesia, and will require a two to four day hospital stay.

Another way of removing the cataract is by phako-emulsification. (*Phako* is derived from the Greek word for "lens.") A needle-like ultrasonic probe is inserted through the pupil into the cloudy lens. It vibrates at 40,000 cycles a second, breaking up the lens and emulsifying it into a liquid which is then sucked out by the same needle. The procedure is simple, provided that your doctor knows how to do it. You can usually go home the same or the next day and resume your normal activities. This ultrasonic method can be performed in about 80 percent of cases and is preferred for most patients. In the remaining 20 percent, the lens is so thick that it can't be completely broken up by the sound waves and so must be extracted in toto, the intracapsular way. *Discuss with your doctor how he plans to remove your cataract before it is done.* If he chooses not to use phako-emulsification, find out why. If you are not satisfied with the reason, by all means ask for another opinion.

Whichever technique is used, if you have two dense cataracts, one is taken out at a time, with an interval of months before the other eye is treated. The reason is obvious. You want to be sure the first operation was a success before proceeding with the second. The poorer eye is always done first, leaving you the better one, while the corrected eye is recovering.

Replacing the Lens

Let's assume that you have had the surgery. Now that you have no lens, you are obviously going to need something to focus the rays of light to the back of your eye. At this point you have three basically different options. Choosing the right one is important.

The oldest and, by today's standards, the least desirable lens-replacement technique is to fit you with spectacles. We have all seen such people wearing their heavy, thick eyeglasses, walking about very precariously, holding on for support. With these glasses, the image from the affected eye appears to the brain to be 30 percent larger than it actually is. This degree of distortion results in double vision if only one eye has been fixed, but instability and poor balance even if both eyes have the spectacles.

Contact Lenses—You Need a Steady Hand

Your natural lens can also be replaced by a contact lens which, if you can tolerate it, is preferable to the thick spectacles of yesteryear, because it gives much better vision, with only about 6 percent distortion. However, a contact lens, especially the "hard" variety, can cause pain and irritation, especially in patients with dry eyes or abnormality of the eyelids. Newer long-wearing soft lenses represent a major advance in this field. They can be left in the eye for several weeks or months, then removed, cleaned and replaced. However, "hard" or "soft", the fact that every contact lens does have to be taken out from time to time may constitute a serious drawback, especially for the elderly, whose coordination is less than perfect and whose hands may tremble or are unsteady. But when they can be left in place and tolerated for several months, the doctor can remove them and clean them for the patient.

A word of caution, however, about these extended wear lenses. They are occasionally vulnerable to changes in the environment which cause them to lose some of their water content. This, in turn, may result in damage to the eye because the fit of the lens may become too tight. Among the situations you should be careful about are frequent long flights, (the air in a plane is dry), hair dryers blowing into the eye, or strong winds. Chronic use of antihistamines by persons with allergies can also cause drying out of these extended-wear lenses.

The Intraocular Lens: Why the Controversy?

We come now to the most exciting (and controversial) technique of all—the plastic lens that is inserted in the eye at the time of operation and simply left there. It is not taken out and replaced like a contact. It all sounds very wonderful, and really is, but if it is recommended to you, get a second opinion all the same. Because, despite their many obvious advantages, intraocular lenses were, until quite recently frequently associated with serious complications. Many patients required re-operation, some several times. The artificial lens frequently became infected, irritated and inflamed, and had to be removed, sometimes resulting in the loss of the eye. In short, it could be a mess. These complications were due to a combination of inadequate surgical technique, poor lens design and inferior quality control. Some devices were sold with sharp edges, others fell apart in the eye after they were implanted; a few were contaminated and incompletely sterilized in the manufacturing process. Add to this the fact that there were doctors who, in their rush to complete, took crash courses in how to insert the lens, and you had the perfect setup for the early disastrous results. For this reason, despite the fact that one patient in four undergoing cataract surgery in the United States is given such a lens, the Food and Drug Administration in this country still monitors the results of this procedure very closely. Some eye specialists and consumer groups also continue to view it as controversial.

The "Holiday Inn" Diploma

Despite official conservatism with respect to the intraocular lens, results have improved steadily and impressively over the years. There is now much better quality control in their manufacture. Indeed, the major worry now is not the lens itself, but the skill of the surgeon implanting it—and *that's* why you need a second opinion. Fortunately, fewer doctors are learning to perform the operation at weekend courses in some motel (the "Holiday Inn" diploma). Properly done, the success rate of this operation is now 90 to 95 percent. For this reason, a panel of distinguished eye specialists at the National Eye Institute have concluded (although not unanimously) that intraocular lenses have "significant visual advantages" over the other techniques and their use is "almost as safe as extraction of the cataract alone."

The Battle of Britain and the Lens

Incidentally, how the intraocular lens came about is a particularly fascinating story. During the Battle of Britain, several Allied pilots were injured when bullets shattered their plastic windshields, sending splinters into their eyes. One particularly astute English ophthalmologist noted that these tiny fragments did not seem to irritate the eye, and could often be left alone without causing symptoms. Years later, during a routine cataract operation, one of his assistants commented how wonderful it would be if some way could be devised to replace the natural lens with a translucent, artificial one that the eye would tolerate for long periods of time. The ophthalmologist remembered his wartime observations and set about trying to find such a material. Although his initial results were disastrous, a Dutch eye specialist followed through with the idea and succeeded in creating the prototype of the lens in use today.

Are You a Candidate for the Intraocular Lens?

Intraocular lenses are not suitable for everyone. Here are the current guidelines to which you should refer if you are offered this form of treatment: Think twice about accepting an implanted lens (a) if you are under sixty years of age (because we don't yet know how long the lens will last); (b) if you have only one potentially good eye (if anything goes wrong with the lens, you've had it); (c) if you have eye disease due to diabetes; (d) if you have ever had a detached retina; or (e) if you suffer from glaucoma. There are occasional exceptions to these recommendations, but the final decision requires an expert, and that is whom you should have advising you in this situation.

First Japanese, Then Russian and Now American— But Will It Work?

As long as we're talking about eye operations, here's another one which may be recommended to you—and for which you should definitely get a second opinion. It goes by the name of *radial keratotomy*— something you've probably never heard of before.

This is a surgical treatment for myopia or nearsightedness. The usual way of dealing with this eye disorder is with corrective lenses. However, some thirty years ago a Japanese eye doctor thought that he could correct this condition by operating on the eye, thus sparing people the trouble of wearing glasses. Despite the fact that within ten years of this surgery, almost all of Dr. Sato's patients required corneal transplants to prevent blindness, a Russian ophthalmologist has seized on the basic Japanese idea and devised a new surgical approach. Under local anesthesia, he makes a series of eight to sixteen cuts through the cornea. This flattens the central part of the eyeball, reducing the degree of myopia.

In my opinion, given the experience so far, the concept of an operation on the cornea to eliminate the need for glasses or contact lenses, is unacceptable at this time. This is especially so if the degree of myopia is not great. However, because this procedure caught the public "eye," the National Eye Institute is sponsoring a $2,000,000, five-year clinical study known as PERK (prospective evaluation of radial kerototomy) in eight eye centers across the country. They will be following exact guidelines and surgical techniques to evaluate the procedure objectively. You may call them in Washington if you want to volunteer for this operation. All you have to do is promise to come for follow-up for a specific period of time.

While I am not, at present, enthusiastic about this procedure, if for some reason you feel that glasses or contact lenses are unacceptable to you, enroll in this government-monitored program rather than going to an ophthalmologist who advertises that he performs the operation.

KEY FACTS TO REMEMBER

Over 500,000 cataract operations are performed each year in the United States. There are now several newer and simpler surgical techniques that you should know about. It may be worth your while to get a second opinion from another ophthalmologist as to how your cataract is to be removed.

The timing of cataract surgery should almost always be up to the patient. It is rarely an emergency; it needs to be done only when the patient's vision is so impaired that it interferes with his (or her) life style. But remember, cataract formation is only one cause of deteriorating eyesight.

After the diseased lens of the eye is removed, it must be replaced in some manner—by thick spectacles (the least satisfactory method); by contact lenses (better, but sometimes difficult to put in and take out); or by lenses implanted within the eye at the time of surgery. The latter technique requires special skill and precautions. If you are over sixty years of age and need cataract surgery, ask for a second opinion from an eye doctor whichever lens is offered to you.

5

Diabetes Mellitus—
When Life Is Too Sweet

Despite all the diabetics among us (one out of four
Americans is an actual or potential diabetic, or a "carrier"
—and the incidence is increasing by almost 10 percent every
year), there are still a great many popular and important
misconceptions about this disorder. You should know what
they are, because even if you are not now among the known
ten million Americans who have the disease you may be one
of the many who will develop it in their lifetime, or one of
the four million who has it and doesn't know it.

Diabetes—Fact and Fancy

The first myth about diabetes is that insulin, discovered
in 1921, cures it. While insulin is necessary for the well-being
of many diabetics, especially pregnant women and children,
it is not a cure. We need no better proof than the fact that
diabetes, with its complications, remains the third leading
cause of death in this country (after heart disease and cancer).
It is responsible for about 300,000 deaths each year, reducing
life expectancy among its victims by one-third. The second
mistaken assumption is that diabetes is one disease—that,
like a rose, "diabetes is diabetes is diabetes." "Juvenile" or
insulin-dependent diabetes is a different entity from the
diabetes that has its onset in adult life. As a rule, their

treatment, complications and outlook are different. The third fallacy is that people who like sweets and indulge in them to excess are likely to become diabetic. What you eat has nothing to do with *causing* the disease—the wrong food can only make it worse once you already have it. Finally, there are still those who believe that everyone with diabetes is condemned forever to a stark, sparse, boring diet and destined to take insulin for life. The truth is that most diabetics may now eat virtually what they wish, provided they avoid sugar—and only one in ten adults with the disorder ever needs insulin.

What is Diabetes?

The diabetic state results from the fact that there is not enough insulin available to "burn away" the sugar in your blood. That is actually an oversimplification, because in some diabetics (notably those who are overweight) the insulin supply is plentiful, but for some reason, it doesn't seem to work on the sugar as it should.

Most people learn that they are diabetic when the doctor finds "too much" sugar in their blood. That news may come as a big shock, especially if, as happens so often, it is discovered in the course of a routine examination and there have been no symptoms whatsoever. Or you may suddenly develop the classic symptoms of the disease—excessive thirst, frequency of urination, weight loss and, in women, vaginal itching.

Before accepting the diagnosis of diabetes make certain that both you and your doctor are aware of any "water pills" (diuretics) you may be taking, or oral contraceptives, both of which may spuriously elevate the blood sugar. An overactive thyroid gland can do so too, as may, in fact, any severe illness or infection, such as a heart attack or stroke. (That's the reason we don't usually measure blood sugar during such catastrophic events.)

Getting the Sugar to Work

Sugar is the basic fuel that provides the energy required for all body functions—from the beat of the heart to the thought processes of the brain. However, to make that energy available, the sugar molecule must be "broken down" and get out of the bloodstream and into the cells. When that doesn't happen, for one reason or another (usually because the pancreas isn't making enough insulin—a hormone produced by the islet cells in the pancreas), you are left with a lot of sugar just floating in the blood not doing you any good. The body then tries to eliminate it. The best way to do that is via the urine. But since the kidneys can't excrete sugar in lump form, the body must provide enough water to dilute or dissolve the sugar in order to flush it out. The net result of all of this is that you find yourself spending more and more time in the bathroom (voiding the sugar) and at the water tap (drinking the needed extra water). And that's why the cardinal signs of untreated diabetes are frequent urination and great thirst. In women, the urine rich in sugar provides a good medium for fungus to grow in the vagina—hence the vaginal itching.

When Fat Substitutes for Sugar

What alternatives does the body have when there's not enough sugar available for energy? It turns to its fat stores, breaks *them* down and melts them away, accounting for another major symptom of diabetes—weight loss. And when fat reserves are exhausted, protein is the next to go.

Ketones and Fat-Poisoning

The appearance in the urine of the end products of such abnormal fat utilization (ketones) is evidence of trouble. That's why diabetics test their urine not only for the presence of sugar that is being excreted by the kidneys, but also for ketones. Finding them means that the treatment of the diabetes must be adjusted or changed, that insulin is required or that, if already being used, its dosage is inadequate to burn up the circulating sugar. When present in the blood in excessive amounts, ketones are toxic, sometimes literally poisonous, and may eventually render you unconscious. So the major immediate risk of "uncontrolled" diabetes is coma, due to the high concentration of ketones in the blood, when the body has had to resort to the rapid breakdown of fats for energy.

The Different Faces of Diabetes—The Childhood or Insulin-Dependent Variety

For many years, diabetes was thought to be one disease, resulting simply from a deficiency of insulin and hence too much "useless" sugar. We now know that excess sugar occurs in at least two kinds of diabetes. *Insulin-dependent diabetes* usually begins in childhood. As compared to the adult-onset type, it is more serious, difficult to control, is often complicated by premature "hardening of the arteries" in virtually every organ of the body—the eye (blindness), brain (stroke), heart (heart attacks), legs (gangrene, ulcers), kidneys (kidney failure)—leads to infections, and is frequently associated with high blood pressure. For all these reasons, "juvenile" diabetes frequently causes disability and/or death at an early age.

Insulin-dependent diabetes is virtually always due to some trouble with the pancreas. We are not sure what goes wrong. Some researchers think that this organ is damaged by a virus or some toxic agent. Others believe that diabetes is one of those mysterious disorders that we call "autoimmune" in origin. The infection, "injury" or "insult," theories all seem quite credible when we realize that only 11 percent of juvenile diabetics have a parent with this disorder. (In 85 percent of the adult-onset cases, one or both parents have the disease.) Regardless of the underlying causes, almost every child with diabetes requires insulin. There's no second opinion needed about that.

Adult-Onset (Non-Insulin-Dependent) Diabetes—Like Becoming Gray

Patients who develop diabetes later in life also have too much inert, unusable sugar and may develop the same symptoms as the juvenile diabetic. There are, however, several important differences between the two. The first is that the insulin deficiency in adults is probably not due to actual disease or destruction of the cells in the pancreas that make it, but rather to their "wearing out," much as one gets gray with age. Interestingly enough, some adult-onset diabetics who are overweight have lots of insulin in their blood—but appear to be resistant to it. Perhaps this is because the necessary interaction between insulin and sugar can take place only in certain designated cells of the body which contain "insulin receptors." But these receptors also attract fat, and they can only accommodate *either* fat or insulin. So, in obese patients, the fat gets to the receptors first, leaving the insulin to float around with nowhere to go, unable to break down the sugar. That is why, even though 10 percent of adult diabetics do require insulin, the remaining 90 percent, especially those who are fat, need only to lose weight, reduce their alcohol intake and avoid concentrated sweets in order to keep their blood sugar normal. In fact, in such persons, insulin is relatively ineffective.

Complications of Diabetes

The other major difference between insulin-dependent and non-insulin-dependent diabetes is the severity and nature of their respective complications. Why these two types, in both of which there is too much unavailable sugar, react so differently is anyone's guess. In the youngster, despite every attempt to normalize the blood-sugar levels with a proper balance between insulin dosage and diet, the ravages of arteriosclerosis seem inexorable and involve the small arteries of the eyes and kidneys especially. Although adult diabetics are not immune to the complications of diabetes (they have a hundred percent greater incidence of arteriosclerosis than do nondiabetics), many do attain a normal life span, especially if preventive measures are practiced. For example, if you are fifty and have just been found to have diabetes, you are less likely to develop a vascular problem (like a heart attack or stroke) if you lose weight, stop smoking, keep your blood pressure normal and get plenty of exercise. I have many diabetic patients in their seventies and eighties who are in excellent health despite their elevated sugar. Even those who need insulin may have no significant symptoms of arteriosclerosis. One man, a doctor, now eighty-one years old, doesn't even need glasses.

Treatment of Diabetes—A Matter of Controversy

The treatment of diabetes remains a subject of great controversy. This is important for you to appreciate, since a second opinion about any problem in diabetes may differ totally from the first, not necessarily on the merits of the case, but because the physicians involved happen to subscribe to opposite schools of thought.

Insulin—When and Why

Before the discovery of insulin, we had nothing to offer the diabetic but dietary advice. This was not enough to protect the juvenile patient from diabetic coma and death—which usually occurred within two years after the onset of the disease. When insulin became available, it was initially given to everybody with a high blood sugar, regardless of symptoms or the presence or absence of ketones. Such therapy prevented coma deaths in the insulin-dependent diabetic, but didn't do very much for many of the adult-onset or non-insulin-dependent diabetics.

The child, in whom there is so little natural insulin available, must receive it by injection in order to minimize the breakdown of fat. On the other hand, the diabetic adult who is not using his fatty tissue for energy, does not usually need insulin; his disease can often be managed by diet and weight loss alone. So, if you are middle-aged, are found to be diabetic, and are given insulin despite the fact that you have no symptoms, ask for a second opinion, from a diabetologist.

Pills Against Diabetes—Good or Bad?

Some years ago, the observation was made that certain oral medications, chemically related to the sulfa drugs, could reduce blood-sugar levels. These agents were not nearly effective enough to substitute for insulin in the young diabetic, but they were initially prescribed for almost everybody else with high blood sugar, the assumption being that such "normalization" was necessary and good for you—no matter how it was achieved. But a group of diabetologists decided to see just how beneficial these sugar-lowering pills really were. To almost everybody's surprise, it turned out that diabetics so treated didn't do all that well. In fact, the oral medication seemed to result in a greater number of deaths from heart disease than did the treatments consisting of insulin or of diet alone. There was no apparent explanation for this adverse affect, but it was thought to be due to some acute disturbance of heart rhythm.

These findings by the University Group Diabetes Program (UGDP) touched off a controversy that has not yet been resolved. There are many who hold that from a statistical viewpoint, the study was poorly designed, that its conclusions are invalid and that the oral antidiabetic medications are very useful. Other doctors and statisticians believe that the oral antidiabetic agents are actually dangerous. The U.S. Food and Drug Administration has taken a position in support of the UGDP study. At least one of these medications has been withdrawn from the market in the United States, and others now carry a label stating that their use may be hazardous to your health.

Where Does Your Doctor Stand?

It is important for you to know your own doctor's position in this controversy. If he accepts the findings of the UGDP study, he is not likely to prescribe oral antidiabetic agents for you except under very special circumstances. For example, if after following a strict diet you are still thirsty, losing weight and have ketones in your urine, he may decide to give these drugs a try before starting insulin. Again, if for some reason you cannot administer your own insulin and have no one to do it for you, he will reluctantly have you try the oral agents. But he will almost always first attempt to reduce your blood sugar by diet alone. (Ninety-five percent of people who develop diabetes in adult life could probably be managed by diet if they had the necessary will power.)

On the other hand, if your doctor believes the oral antidiabetic agents are effective and desirable, that the UGDP study is an exercise in bureaucratic futility and its conclusions run counter to his own experience, he will probably insist that in addition to a diet regimen you take the pills straightaway.

The most dramatic proof of this difference of opinion among doctors in the United States is the fact that in the estimated five million Americans who have high blood sugar, about one million are given a pill to lower it, some 1½ million take insulin, and two to three million are treated by diet alone.

The Pregnant Diabetic

Despite the fundamental disagreement about the antidiabetes pill and our ignorance about what causes the disease(s), there are several points on which most doctors concur. For example, no one will argue about juvenile diabetics' need for insulin, or that their health and survival demand avoidance of wide swings in the sugar levels. Also everyone agrees that rigid sugar control of the pregnant diabetic is also critical. Any sustained elevation in the pregnant patient is transmitted to the fetus. When that happens, the fetal pancreas responds to the elevated sugar level by making more and more insulin. This may result in episodic *low* blood sugar and possible complications in fetal development, including a high rate of infant mortality.

In the past, young diabetics, especially those with any vascular disease, were discouraged from having babies, because the infant mortality rate was high (30 percent) and the mother suffered many complications. Today, however, as a result of more successful control of blood sugar, selected diabetics whose disease can be stabilized are actually encouraged to have children. In such diabetic mothers there does not appear to be any worsening of the diabetic or vascular status as a result of childbearing, and the infant mortality is now only 4 percent. So, if you have diabetes, want a baby, and are discouraged from having one, don't hesitate to ask for another opinion from a diabetologist.

Understanding the Diabetic Diet

Control of diabetes and to some extent the long-term outlook for the disease hinge on adherence to diet. In every case, simple sugars must be avoided completely, and some carbohydrates must be reduced. How much and what you may safely eat depends on your age and weight. For example, in childhood and adolescence, adequate nutrition is very important for proper growth and development. Since diabetic children are usually thin anyway, calories should not be restricted as they are in the adult. Any adverse impact on the blood sugar of a more liberal diet (but a carefully planned one) can be controlled by adjusting insulin dosage. But if you are an adult diabetic and overweight, you should decrease the total number of calories to about 1,200 per day (people engaged in heavy labor will require more), and within that caloric limitation, you may eat virtually anything you wish. If you don't weigh too much, be sure you keep it that way. It's a good idea for all diabetics to add some fiber to the diet, because enough of the right fiber may decrease the amount of sugar absorbed by as much as 25 percent, and insulin requirements by as much as 20 percent. But check with your doctor about the type of fiber you're eating. They're not all equally good (oat bran is the best). Many simply leave you with alot of gas and the same amount of sugar!

What to Eat and When

If you are an adult on a low-calorie diet and not taking insulin, you may take your meals anytime during the day. But if you require insulin, what you eat and *when* you do so are very important. Blood sugar can rise and fall precipitously if meal time and insulin dosage are not coordinated. For example, should you miss a meal, yet take the same amount of insulin at the usual time, the blood sugar may drop enough to cause a severe insulin reaction or even coma. Insulin-dependent diabetics must also be careful about the *kind* of food they eat at specific times of the day in relation to their insulin dosage, because protein, fat and carbohydrates increase the sugar level at different rates. For example, a candy bar (carbohydrate) will raise it much more quickly than will a steak (protein-fat). If your insulin is geared to take care of a rise in blood sugar due to carbohydrates, and you eat protein instead, you may suffer an insulin reaction because the protein has not delivered as much sugar as the insulin was expected to neutralize.

Since vigorous exercise also burns up sugar, a diabetic taking insulin who "works out" should either eat more or reduce his insulin dosage, in order to avoid a low-blood-sugar reaction. This, however, is not true for the diabetic who is not on insulin.

Whatever kind of diabetic you are, if you have been given a diet that makes life almost intolerable, discuss it with your doctor—or get a second opinion from a diabetes specialist. In view of today's new knowledge, it is no longer necessary for you to endure a lifetime of boring, tasteless food. Almost anything is permitted—in moderation—except simple sugar. The inflexible high-protein, low-carbohydrate diet of yesteryear is rarely needed anymore. In fact, today most diabetes specialists will prescribe a very tolerable 60 percent complex carbohydrate (that is, starches), 20 percent protein and 20 percent fat diet—with liberal amounts of fiber.

Complications and Control

Although the most important long-term complications of diabetes, especially in children, are vascular, the nerves too may become involved. That is why diabetics often develop severe pain, numbness and weakness in various parts of the body, especially the legs.

A key question that remains unanswered is whether these nerve and vascular complications result from the high blood sugar, from excessive ketones or from other causes not as yet identified. In other words, if we were able to keep the blood sugar normal at all times, would diabetics still have all these problems?

The Insulin Pump

Most experts now believe that rigid sugar control at or near normal levels would greatly reduce the debilitating, crippling and lethal consequences of this disease. They believe that even when the blood-sugar level is "acceptable" at the time we measure it, there are peaks and valleys throughout the day and night. An "insulin pump" has been developed to avoid such swings. Especially designed for use in young diabetics, it is worn on the belt and at preset intervals, releases insulin into the tissues through a permanently placed needle. This or similar devices are already available, and you should be aware of them. A totally implantable pump will soon be ready too. Neither of these instruments, however, senses and responds to the blood-sugar level. They simply make it possible for the diabetic to release an extra dosage of insulin in response to an added caloric load.

Frontiers of Research in Diabetes

Efforts to transplant a healthy pancreas, the organ containing the cells that make insulin, into diabetics have not as yet been successful. The major problems with this technique are blood clotting within the transplanted organ and its "rejection."

Another area of current research involves injecting the

islet cells of the pancreas that actually make the insulin into the vein of the diabetic. Hopefully, the cells would settle in the liver, where, it is hoped, they would start producing insulin. The problem with all these theories is that no one knows whether simply replacing the insulin by whatever route will provide the basic answer to the complex disease we call diabetes.

. KEY FACTS TO REMEMBER

Diabetes, with its complications, is the third leading cause of death in the United States. High blood sugar probably represents more than one disease. The two forms currently identified are the insulin-dependent type, more serious and usually found in children, and the adult-onset or non-insulin-dependent form, which often can be managed by diet and weight loss.

Major immediate complications of diabetes result from the body's burning of its fat stores in lieu of the normally available sugar. The end products of such metabolism (ketones) are toxic when present in high concentrations in the blood.

The major area of disagreement about the treatment of diabetes relates to the use of the anti-sugar pill. Many doctors believe that it is beneficial, others think it is dangerous. Consult at least one diabetologist whether you are or are not prescribed this medication.

Insulin is almost always needed by diabetic children. It is much less commonly required in adults. The latter should ask for a second opinion when advised to take insulin, especially in the absence of symptoms.

Control of the pregnant diabetic has reduced complications of the disease in the mother and has significantly reduced infant mortality. Diabetic women should not *pro forma* be denied the right of childbearing. If you are, ask for a second opinion from a diabetes specialist.

Diabetic diets need not be severely restricted. If yours is, ask for an opinion from a diabetologist.

6

Hypoglycemia— Our Most Common "Non-Disease"

Diabetics have *hyper*glycemia, that is, too much sugar in the blood; *hypo*glycemia means an abnormally *low* blood sugar. The diagnostic level is said to be less than 40 mg. percent, but this figure is arbitrary. You may in fact experience symptoms of hypoglycemia even when the blood sugar is somewhat higher.

How It Is Diagnosed

True hypoglycemia causes sweating, rapid heartbeat, weakness, headaches, nervousness, a feeling of hunger and visual disturbances—symptoms easily mistaken for those of emotional instability. When your doctor suspects that you have hypoglycemia, he will ask you to come to his office as soon as the "attack" begins. He will have a blood-sugar analysis done to see whether the level is actually low at the height of symptoms. Or he may have you undergo a glucose tolerance test. You will be given a measured amount of sugar to drink, following which blood samples are taken every hour for five or six hours, or longer. If your symptoms are reproduced at any time during the test and can be correlated with either an abnormally low blood sugar, that is, 40 mg. percent or less, or with an abrupt drop in sugar in a relatively short time, then the diagnosis of hypoglycemia is reasonable. If it is made without that kind of confirmation, well—

Why Argue with Success?

Every internist is besieged by patients, almost always women, who are convinced, or have been told, that they are suffering from hypoglycemia. (It is curious, and I'm not sure that I know the reason, but I have never yet seen a man who has hypoglycemia or thinks he does.) I believe that this diagnosis is made much too often. It is usually arrived at in the following circumstances: An anxious, tremulous, nervous, depressed or exhausted woman is not satisfied when told that her symptoms are emotional in origin. So she asks in desperation, "Maybe I have hypoglycemia?" Unable to find any other explanation, some doctors will agree and prescribe a diet to help the "low blood sugar." And it often does—at least for a while—probably because of the psychological impact of having found the "cause" of the trouble.

If you are convinced that you have hypoglycemia, are following a diet and feeling better with it, continue exactly what you are doing. I never argue with success.

When the Blood Sugar Is Really Low

An individual may become hypoglycemic under certain special circumstances, the most common of which is too much insulin when being treated for diabetes. Also, if you've gone without food or drink for many hours, your sugar level will drop a little, leaving you feeling faint. The reason that Jews fasting on Yom Kippur don't usually develop hypoglycemia is that normally as the blood sugar drops, the pancreas gets turned off and makes less insulin. So, sugar levels do not fall too much. But if the pancreatic response is not deactivated quickly enough by the low sugar and continues to secrete an inappropriately large amount of insulin, low blood sugar with its attendant symptoms may develop.

The Liver as a Sugar Regulator

The liver is also important in maintaining normal blood sugar. It acts as a reservoir, storing sugar and releasing it when levels are low. So if you have severe liver disease, and that extra amount is not available to you when you are fasting, you may become hypoglycemic when normal individuals would not. This is especially true in heavy drinkers, since too much alcohol poisons the enzyme system that allows the liver to release its sugar into the system.

If you are pregnant and thus require more sugar to provide additional energy for the fetus, it is conceivable that your blood-sugar level may drop enough to give you symptoms. If you have some illness, are running a low-grade fever, and have lost your appetite, the increased metabolism resulting from the fever and the impaired nutrition may also reduce the sugar levels in the blood. (Remember grandma's advice to "feed a fever"?)

When Too Much Is Too Little

The foregoing is a description of how an inadequate food intake can give you low blood sugar. You can also develop hypoglycemia *after* eating sugar. It happens this way. When you take some sugar, the pancreas is stimulated to produce insulin in order to burn it off. Once the sugar level drops, no more insulin is made. However, when this feedback mechanism is impaired, insulin continues to be produced and you end up with an abnormally low blood sugar. (Patients in whom this phenomenon occurs may develop diabetes later—almost as if this was the first evidence of something wrong with their pancreas.) The management of this particular kind of hypoglycemia is to eliminate sweets from the diet, thus avoiding the insulin "overshoot."

If you have had a portion of your stomach removed, for example, because of an ulcer, the remaining part of that organ allows the sugar to move quickly into the small bowel, where it is more rapidly absorbed. This sudden increase in blood sugar also causes insulin overshoot and results in hypoglycemia.

Alcohol, Medication and Low Blood Sugar

If you think you have symptoms of low blood sugar, make sure to tell your doctor whether you are taking any of the following drugs: sulfas, oral antidiabetic agents, aspirin, Darvon or Thorazine. These are only some of the medications that may cause hypoglycemia, as can alcohol in "large amounts" (tolerance varies from person to person).

There is also a very uncommon condition in which a tumor of the pancreas (called an insulinoma) produces large amounts of insulin even after fasting for as long as three days. During that time, there is no stimulus for the pancreas to produce insulin since you're not eating any sugar. That is real, true, serious hypoglycemia. Its treatment is the surgical removal of the tumor.

Treating Hypoglycemia

The treatment of *documented* low blood sugar (assuming that an insulin-producing tumor of the pancreas has been excluded) is dietary manipulation. You will feel better if you eat smaller meals, more frequently. You must avoid sugar, reduce carbohydrates generally and eat more protein and fat, both of which result in only a gradual elevation of sugar. A high-fiber diet is also useful, since it reduces absorption in the gut of any sugar you do eat.

KEY FACTS TO REMEMBER

Hypoglycemia is probably the most overdiagnosed "non-disease" there is. If you are told that that is what you have, ask for a second opinion from an endocrinologist. But if the low-sugar diet helps, follow it anyway.

True hypoglycemia may occur in liver disease, among alcoholics, after surgical removal of large portions of the stomach, and in diabetics taking insulin. It may also be associated with the use of certain medications and, in rare cases, with insulin-producing tumors.

7

Disorders of the Ears, Nose and Throat— Too Much Treatment Too Soon?

Not Usually a Matter of Life or Death

This chapter does not deal with life-threatening disorders like cancer, stroke or heart attack. But although the subjects discussed in the next few pages—tonsils and adenoids (whether they should be removed) and sinuses (whether they should be drained)—are more banal, you may find some information which may reduce pain, suffering and expense. If you keep having your sinuses perforated or drained at regular intervals, if you can remember when your own tonsils were removed or if your child has just had a tonsillectomy, you know how miserable life can be.

It's My Sinuses Again

Chronic sinusitis, a recurrent condition that can plague you with recurrent cough, headache and nasal discharge, affects about 25 percent of the adult population of the United States. In the course of more than a million days every year, Americans spend their time having their nasal bones cracked, popping expensive antibiotics down their gullet, or sitting at home, bent over a humidifier instead of going to work. So it behooves you to know about some recent changes in the way we treat this disorder.

Well Protected but Hard to Treat

The sinuses—air pockets surrounded by bone—are well designed by nature to resist infections in the nose and mouth. As a matter of fact, considering all the dirt and contaminants we breathe and the many dental infections we have, it is quite remarkable that our sinuses don't develop trouble more often than they do. But the same anatomic structure that renders them resistant to infection also makes the sinuses difficult to reach and treat, once infection sets in.

The maxillary sinuses (situated in the general area of the cheekbones), are the largest and the ones most likely to give you problems, either because they are irrigated too frequently and too enthusiastically or not often enough. The frontal sinuses (above the eyes), and the ethmoid sinuses (very small, multiple air pockets in the skull) can also become infected and require treatment.

Blame the Woes on Your Nose

Sinus trouble is almost always the result of some problem in the nasal passages. An allergy to pollens may cause the lining of the nose to become boggy, swollen, and, therefore, more vulnerable to infection. Many viruses and bacteria can penetrate the lining of the nose even when it is healthy, but do so more easily when it is irritated by an allergy. If you have a deviated nasal septum that interferes with proper drainage and breathing, or if you have polyps in your nose as a result of chronic infection and allergy, you are a natural target for sinus trouble too. An infected tooth with abscess formation, contaminated bathing water and head injury can all cause sinusitis as well.

Which Antibiotic to Use and When

If the symptoms of sinusitis have not responded to steam and decongestants, and you have begun to blow greenish-yellow mucus out of your nose, you should now take an antibiotic. The best one, at least theoretically, is selected after the mucus is tested to determine which antibiotic will be most effective. Many doctors, however, will empirically give you doxycycline (Vibramycin), penicillin, erythromycin, or ampicillin without actually making such an analysis.

When Is Sinus Irrigation Justified?

Most cases of acute sinusitis do well with antibiotics alone. But if after treatment of the acute attack, you continue to have facial pain, headache, postnasal drip and chronic nasal discharge, *occasional* washing of the sinuses is helpful.

When X rays of the sinuses reveal clouding and the radiologist is not sure whether it is due to an old, burned-out infection or the presence of fresh pus, the doctor may irrigate them in order to find out.

Repeated washing out of sinuses with all its pain, cost and inconvenience is a thing of the past—or should be. If it is done more than three times, you should discuss with the doctor the advantages of an "antral window," in which a permanent opening in the (maxillary) sinus is created. This permits its natural drainage without the need to crack the bones each time.

A Stuffy Nose and Full Bladder

So many people suffer from a chronically stuffy nose. This is usually the result of an allergy, a reaction to changes in the environment (vasomotor rhinitis), a deviated septum, local infection, certain medications, glandular or hormonal problems, or injury or tumor. Whatever the cause, one is tempted to use a nasal decongestant right away. Unfortunately, some of these agents may give you a rebound effect if taken frequently and for prolonged periods of time. They do shrink the mucous membranes of the nose, but as their effect wears off, the congestion may return with a vengeance. Remember, too, that the active ingredient in many of these decongestants is related to ephedrine or adrenaline and may increase heart rate, raise blood pressure and cause disturbances of cardiac rhythm. Most healthy persons can tolerate these effects without danger, but these drugs should be avoided if you have any heart problem or hypertension. Also, older men, or those with any prostate trouble, should be careful about taking these substances, since they can interfere with the ability to empty the bladder. I have seen more than one man in agony due to sudden urinary retention after taking a "harmless" decongestant. For all these reasons, it is a good idea to try simple steam inhalation first. If that doesn't help, then you may use one of the many nasal sprays, drops or oral decongestants available over the counter. Most decongestant preparations also contain antihistamines for their drying and antiallergic actions, in which case they may make you very drowsy. So, take them just before retiring, when you can get a good night's sleep, not in the morning when you are about to drive your car.

You may also find that after a while an antihistamine prescribed for you no longer seems effective. It's almost as if you had become "immune" to it. Changing to another brand doesn't seem to make any difference. Before you and your doctor abandon this group of drugs, and go onto some other, more powerful agent (like steroids), you should both be aware that there are six different groups of antihistamines from among which you can choose. Tolerance to one group does not necessarily mean tolerance to the other five. It's probably a good idea, if you have chronic allergy and take antihistamines fairly regularly, to switch brands, say every two months. That will reduce the likelihood of your becoming "immune" to this medication.

Some allergic patients suddenly develop a flare-up of their symptoms. This may be due to increased exposure to a pollen or other offending substances. Under these circumstances, one may need something "stronger" than an antihistamine-decongestant combination. The usual medication you will be prescribed is a corticosteroid (e.g. prednisone). You can take it in tablet form for a few days, via a slowly absorbed injection, or by aerosol. If steroids are prescribed, be sure to tell or remind your doctor if you're pregnant, have high blood pressure, an ulcer history, diabetes or some psychiatric history.

Remember, too, that not all stuffy noses are due to allergy. You may be taking some drug which may be responsible for the symptoms. Before medicating yourself with over-the-counter remedies, check to see whether you are on anything to lower high blood pressure. Common offenders include the following: Reserpine, hydralazine (Apresoline), guanethidine (Ismelin), methyldopa (Aldomet), prazosin

(Minipres), propranolol (Inderal), nadolol (Corgard) or metro-prolol (Lopressor). Certain tranquilizers will also cause nasal stuffiness, so it's a good idea to check out *any* drug you happen to be taking if you have this symptom.

Tonsillectomy—As American as Thanksgiving Turkey

Tonsillectomy has for decades been a ritual most American children are required to undergo—like kindergarten. At the very first complaint of a sore throat, parents are on the phone making plans to have the tonsils out. Seduced and distracted by promises of ice cream and ginger ale after their operation, our youngsters are led by the hundreds of thousands to this barbaric rite in which the lymph glands in the throat are extirpated. It turns out that the lucky ones are not the kids who get all the goodies, but those whose parents either can't afford to have the operation done or reject it for other reasons.

Although more than a million such procedures (the adenoids are also removed for good measure) are still performed every year in the United States, there is now a very real difference of opinion among doctors concerning the need for this operation.

Doctors have an innate reluctance to excise any organ, especially one whose function is not completely understood, unless there is some compelling reason to do so (when, for example, some part of the body is severely diseased, gangrenous, obstructed or perforated). We wouldn't think of removing a kidney simply because it is infected; we try to control infection with antibiotics. We do our best to save a tooth; we pull it only as a last resort. Why then, after a sore throat or two, are tonsils immediately condemned to extraction?

Tonsils *do* have a function other than to help send surgeons' children through school. These glands consist of lymph tissue and are the first line of defense against infection. They are filters which trap invading bacteria entering the throat and prevent them from getting into the bloodstream. A tonsil that is infected is one that has been doing its job. Of course, after repeated infection, the tonsillar tissue is finally destroyed and then must come out. But it doesn't seem quite right to me to remove the tonsils simply because they are inflamed, especially when one can now treat them with antibiotics, restore their integrity and retain their protective function.

Does Tonsillectomy Really Make a Difference?

Those doctors still in favor of the routine tonsillectomy for children who have had only a few sore throats argue that after the operation the incidence of these attacks decreases. But this assumption is open to question. Recently a large group of children who had had five or six attacks and whose tonsils were *not* taken out were studied. It was found that the number of sore throats dropped substantially—even when surgery was not performed. So the fact that a child has been suffering from sore throats in his first year of school does not mean that he is going to continue to have them. And the fact that they do not recur after the tonsils are removed is not necessarily the result of the operation. Put another way, recurrent sore throats in childhood are probably a naturally occurring phenomenon that is self-limited and usually does not require surgery.

My Son, the Mouth Breather

Is all this true for the adenoid glands too? Like the tonsils, they are collections of lymph tissue, but they are situated in a different part of the throat area and are routinely removed with the tonsils. (That's why the operation is called "T-and-A"—tonsillectomy and adenoidectomy.) Parents are rarely asked for permission to remove the adenoids when a child goes in for a tonsillectomy. It is part of the package. Your child always has his mouth open and snores, doesn't he? When the results of another large series of T-and-A's were analyzed and the adenoids that were removed were examined, they were rarely found to be infected. What's more, there was little if any correlation between snoring, mouth breathing and the size of the adenoids.

Tonsillectomy—Simply Unnecessary or Harmful Too?

Are these operations merely painful and unnecessary, or can they actually cause some harm in the long run? Nobody is really sure. In one study, persons who had had their tonsils and adenoids out in childhood had a higher incidence of Hodgkin's disease (a form of cancer of the lymph tissue) than a matched group in whom the operation was not done. That is not enough to permit any definite conclusion, but it does raise a question, doesn't it?

All this adds up to the following: If your child has enjoyed good health except for recurring sore throats and plans have been made to remove his tonsils the following spring or fall, even though he has been free of attacks in the interval, get a second opinion. If during the next year or two, attacks don't recur, your child may be free and clear, and may avoid the surgery forever. If, on the other hand, the throat infections persist, he may fall into the small group that actually needs the operation. Even then, ask whether the adenoids must come out too.

How We Hear

Sound is conducted through the external ear canal (that's where people who live dangerously poke things to get the wax out), reaches the eardrum, and makes it vibrate. This moves three little bones attached to the drum, which then send messages to the hearing apparatus in the inner ear. The sound signal is subsequently transmitted by nerves to the brain, where it is interpreted. Deafness can result from trouble anywhere along this route. For example, if you've got a big wad of wax in the ear canal, the sound wave will be dampened and your hearing will be impaired. A hearing aid obviously won't do you any good in this situation, because the sound just can't get through. Or the trouble may be due to an eardrum that is scarred by previous infections and therefore doesn't vibrate normally when the sound waves strike it. Or, the three little bones behind the drum may become fused and so cannot transmit the vibrations of the drum to the hearing apparatus in the inner ear, which may itself be diseased or injured. Finally the nerve (acoustic nerve), which carries the impulses to the brain, may malfunction—occasionally because of a tumor pressing on it.

These various potential mechanisms of deafness permit us to divide hearing loss into two major types. The first is *conductive*—in which the deafness is due to some obstruction to the *transmission* of sound in the external canal, disease of the drum or bones. This embraces the entire route the sound travels until it finally reaches the inner ear and the acoustic nerve. Any trouble beyond that point, involving the inner ear or the acoustic nerve itself, is termed *sensorineural*, or nerve, deafness.

People with nerve deafness don't hear high-pitched sounds. Their biggest acoustic problem is the noisy cocktail party where they have trouble understanding a soft-spoken female. At home, they go about their business unaware that the phone is ringing (I often wonder why the pitch of the bell has not been lowered by the telephone company in order to make it more audible to subscribers with nerve deafness.)

Sensorineural deafness is very difficult to treat. Hearing aids are usually of little help; no medicines that I know of result in measurable improvement either. So, if you are told that you have nerve deafness and are advised to get a hearing aid, make sure that you get a money-back guarantee—and never buy one in the first place, except when prescribed by a hearing specialist.

In contrast to nerve deafness, *conductive deafness* is treatable—by simply removing wax or a foreign body from the ear canal, or by operating on the eardrum or the little bones behind it that have become fused. A hearing aid is usually helpful too.

Deafness due to an acute infection in the middle ear will improve strikingly after treatment with antibiotics. However, if you have chronic middle-ear disease, you may benefit from surgical treatment.

A disorder called Ménière's disease, in which there is buzzing and other noises in the ear, dizziness and a fluctuating hearing loss, will sometimes respond to medications, including antihistamines, tranquilizers, low-salt diets or diuretics.

Deafness Can Occur in Healthy Ears

It is important to remember, however, that deafness can be due to several treatable causes that do not originate in the hearing mechanism. For example, as many as 10 percent of patients with hypothyroidism have a hearing loss that will improve, often dramatically, when the deficient thyroid hormone is replenished. Rheumatoid arthritis may cause a conductive type of deafness that may respond to steroids (cortisone-type drugs). About 10 percent of patients with fluctuating hearing loss are found to have diabetes mellitus. Unfortunately, reducing the sugar doesn't always improve the hearing in these cases. Certain disturbances in fat metabolism, characterized by high triglyceride and cholesterol levels, may result in hearing loss. In such cases, reducing the intake of saturated fats and concentrated sweets and losing weight may improve the hearing. Patients with kidney disease may become deaf. Certain medications (antibiotics) may cause hearing loss which is frequently permanent. I have several patients who became stone deaf after taking the antibiotic Streptomycin or ethacrynic acid, a diuretic. I know of heavy smokers who became deaf and whose hearing was restored when the cigarettes were stopped. (I suppose this best can be explained either by nicotine toxicity or spasm of the blood vessels in the ear.) Aspirin in large amounts has been known to produce a hearing loss, which fortunately clears up when the drug is stopped. Allergic reactions to food or inhalants also can cause deafness that may or may not be permanent. So, it's a good idea, when your vanity finally permits you to accept the fact that you're deaf, to consult your doctor first and then an ear specialist. Don't rush off to buy the least obstrusive hearing aid. You may not need it.

KEY FACTS TO REMEMBER

Chronic sinusitis is a disabling disorder affecting 25 percent of the population of the United States. It usually results from chronic allergy and/or infection in the nose. The acute attack can often be managed by antibiotics, but chronic sinusitis may *occasionally* have to be drained. However, repeated irrigation and washing of the sinuses is rarely necessary, and you should see another ear, nose and throat specialist if you're being treated in this way.

Chronic nasal stuffiness is usually, but not always, due to allergy. Most cases can be managed by antihistamine-decongestant pills, but certain precautions should be taken. Some people become "tolerant" to antihistamines. Switching to another type may be all that is necessary to restore the efficacy of those agents. In more severe cases, short-term use of steroid hormones may become necessary.

Tonsillectomies are probably unnecessary in the majority

of cases in which they are done. Recent evidence suggests that sore throats in children usually clear up without the operation. The suspicion also exists that removing the protective function of the tonsils may cause one to be more susceptible to other disorders, including cancer, later in life. Removal of adenoids probably has little impact on mouth breathing or snoring.

There are many different causes of deafness. Various diseases and drugs may induce hearing loss, which is often temporary but sometimes permanent. Deafness due to disorders of the hearing apparatus are of either the "bone" or the "nerve" type. The former may benefit from surgery and hearing aids, but the latter usually do not. Never buy a hearing aid from a commercial establishment without first checking with your ear doctor—and always ask for a money-back guarantee.

8

Asthma—
Preventing and Controlling Your
Wheeze

Musical, but Not a Comedy

Some three million Americans—twice as many men as women—suffer from some form of asthma. That's a lot of wheezing (although asthma can manifest itself as shortness of breath and cough without wheezing). Most asthmatics, perhaps 60 or 65 percent, develop this disorder before the age of five; some outgrow it, others don't. Surprisingly, despite all the new drugs we have for its treatment, five thousand people in the United States still die from asthma every year. Many of these deaths are unnecessary, and that's the reason for this chapter.

Acute, Chronic or Both

Any process that narrows the air passages (bronchial tubes), be it spasm, infection, allergy or mucus, results in wheezing. This constriction may occur only now and then, so that there are long symptom-free intervals punctuated by only an occasional acute attack. When the condition is chronic, the asthmatic patient may become accustomed to his perpetual wheezes, and doesn't really feel sick—until an acute attack supervenes. Then the low-grade wheezing becomes louder, the patient usually develops a hacking cough, and breathing becomes difficult. In many cases, sudden, severe asthma appears "out of the blue," without any previous history.

Spasm and narrowing of the air passages result in obstruction to air flow *out* of the lungs, leaving you with more than the normal amount of air in the chest. In time, in order to accommodate this extra volume, the lungs become distended, and the chest may assume a barrel shape.

Room for Improvement

The first goal in managing the asthmatic patient is to prevent acute attacks. When one does occur, it must be treated quickly and effectively. Once asthma has become chronic, we try to improve the flow of air in and out of the affected lungs and prevent infection. Remember that in *every* case of asthma there is the possibility of *some* reversal. No matter how sick you are, today's newer drugs, alone or in combination, can make you feel a lot better.

It's Either "Intrinsic" or "Extrinsic"

You will find it convenient to think of asthma as occurring in two distinct forms. The first is called *extrinsic*, because it is induced by an environmental substance to which your body is "allergic." This happens mostly in infants and children who inhale something their system doesn't like—a pollen, certain dusts or other irritants. Occasionally, a food will also cause an asthmatic attack. Presented with this "insult" or "challenge," the body responds by throwing the airways to the lungs into spasm and having them make more mucus to entrap any invading organism. The end result is an attack of wheezing (because of the airways' constriction) and coughing (because of the mucus secretions). In time and with experience, vulnerable patients begin to dread certain places or seasons of the year (where and when offending agents are found); they try to avoid friends who wear perfumes that trigger asthmatic crises or who invite them to dinner in a home filled with dander from furry pets.

The other kind of asthma is called *intrinsic*, in which there is no apparent external provocation. The usual picture is one of chronic infections, "colds," or sinusitis, with repeated attacks of asthmatic wheezing. It seems to have nothing to do with where you are, what you eat, or the air you breathe. But the end result is the same as in the extrinsic form— spasm of the airways with wheezing, mucus and cough.

The distinction between extrinsic and intrinsic asthma is an oversimplification of a complex, biological process, but it is a useful guide. I know of no real proof that asthma is strictly an emotional disorder, although many people, including doctors, still cling to this point of view.

Exercise, Aspirin and Asthma

In many asthmatics sudden attacks can also for some reason result from acute emotional stress—fear, anger or sorrow—vigorous exercise, especially in cold weather, and abrupt exposure to cold. You may also become asthmatic because of the kind of work you do (exposure to fumes, dusts, and other "allergens"—occupational asthma) and even from medication. Some twenty-five years ago I reported in the medical literature near-fatal asthmatic attacks in two patients with chronic asthma who had taken aspirin for some minor pain. (Other doctors have described similar reactions to this agent in persons without any previous medical problem.) So, if you have chronic asthma or are prone to acute attacks of wheezing, be careful about *any* drug you use, including "benign" ones like aspirin.

The Causes Are Not Always Obvious

If you have asthma, either intrinsic or extrinsic, you must try to eliminate from your life those factors that bring on the acute attack. They are usually obvious, like cats, dogs, grasses or other pollens. When they are not, however, your doctor can help to identify them. For example, you can be tested for allergy to house dust, pollens, ragweed or animal dander, to mention a few of the common offending inhalants; or to nuts, seafood, tomatoes, a dye called tartrazine, widely used in such products as hot dogs and margarine, and other foods. (Most patients have more than one allergy.)

Anyone Want a Cute Six-Year-Old?

I have found that patients often actually do know what makes them sick, but hide that information from the doctor

and so kid themselves. I used to be one of those "deniers."
Years ago, when my own children were very young, I bought
a German shepherd puppy for them. He turned out to be an
extremely protective, fun dog. He was extremely intelligent
too, preferring me to anyone else in the family. But Christopher
was huge, and he shed all over the place. One child, who had
heretofore enjoyed excellent health, suddenly began to suffer
frequent "colds"—coughing, wheezing and shortness of breath.
These symptoms seemed to come on whenever he played
with his favorite pet. It never "occurred" to any of us, least of
all to me, the doctor, that the boy's trouble could be due to
the dog. That would have been unthinkable—almost like
being told that you are allergic to your wife, husband or
child. My son was also unaware of any association between
the dog and his new illness, not only because he loved the
animal, but probably too because he subconsciously feared
the animosity of the rest of the family should the dog have to
go on his account. As the asthmatic attacks became more
frequent, serious and prolonged, I asked several of my colleagues what they thought the cause of the boy's respiratory
distress could be. Each one pointed to the big dog—hair and
dander. I couldn't imagine how so many experts could all be
so completely wrong. Seven allergists later, all of whom were
in agreement on the diagnosis and recommendation ("Get rid
of the dog"), I still resisted. I was sure there *must* be some
other way, especially since Christopher was now protecting
me on my house calls at night. I conferred with a host of
veterinaries and visited dozens of pet shops, looking in vain
for something to spray on the dog's coat. There is, of course,
nothing that can neutralize the dander from a 100-pound dog
in a five-room apartment, or prevent it from affecting the
lungs of a susceptible six-year-old. After I had tried all the
sticky, smelly, useless sprays I could get my hands on, and as
the child became sicker, I made the inevitable, overdue
decision and gave the dog away.

It is easy to become emotionally trapped by a pet, no
matter who you are and how much you know, or how bad it
can be for your health. (An interesting sidelight to my own
story is that having been deprived of his dog and all other
furry pets, my son developed a great interest in reptiles. He
is now a knowledgeable herpetologist. He and I "enjoy," in

our home, a 35-foot python, an equally large boa, several iguanas, turtles, frogs and lizards—none of which give him asthma. My own reaction is described somewhere in the section on high blood pressure. But whenever I complain about his menagerie, my son reminds me about Christopher and how long it took me to make up my mind.)

An Environment That Defies Control

The first objective, then, in managing extrinsic asthma is to identify the offending allergen and get rid of it. *Promptly.* Of course, except for pets, that is not always possible. There are too many aspects of our environment beyond the control of any individual. You can, indeed, *must* stop smoking, and you can choose the no-smoking section of an airplane, but there are no "no-perfume" areas where you can seek refuge. Nor is there anything one can do about certain noxious industrial fumes, pollens and dust—or is there?

How Effective is Desensitization?

In the typical asthmatic attack, the body is challenged by a substance called an *allergen,* which provokes an immunological or "defense" response. This consists of the release of certain chemicals, one of which is histamine, that constrict the bronchial tubes and cause asthma. Desensitization, or hyposensitization, involves injecting under the skin tiny amounts of whatever it is that you are allergic to. We don't give you so much of the material as to make you sick, but just enough to provide the body with the opportunity gradually to build up resistance to it. Theoretically, when that is achieved, the adverse reaction to the allergen will either be entirely prevented or rendered less severe.

Desensitization usually takes years, is expensive and occasionally is uncomfortable. Does it work? It is said to have an 80 percent success rate in hay fever caused by pollens, ragweed, dander and dust. The reduction in asthmatic attacks is probably much less. And don't expect much in the way of results for at least two years after starting the shots. As far as foods are concerned, desensitization is probably of no value. You simply have to avoid eating anything that makes you sick.

Blue Cross Won't Pay

In cases of *intrinsic* asthma, the kind that develops from allergy to unknown causes (but clearly related to chronic lung or sinus infections), attempts to desensitize patients to their own bacteria led to the administration of vaccines made from these bacteria. This technique is still popular, sounds logical and, theoretically, should work. In actual fact, there is no evidence that it does. As a result, Blue Cross will no longer reimburse you for it. Should this regimen be offered to you, consult with another lung specialist or allergist, unless you're willing to pay for the treatment out of your own pocket.

The Anti-Asthma Armamentarium

So you've done everything *you* can to manage your asthma. You've tried to live in an allergy-free environment, you've stopped smoking, you've identified and now avoid foods that might induce an attack (more important in children than adults); you're careful about exercise and aspirin and you take antibiotics at the first sign of a respiratory infection. You even try to spare yourself unnecessary emotional crises, (but you now know that your asthma does not reflect a disturbed personality). But despite all this, you're still getting attacks of wheezing, for which you are going to need medication. Drugs available to asthmatics fall into three main categories: those that *prevent* the attack, those that are used from day to day to control chronic symptoms, and finally, agents needed to abort an acute flare-up.

Preventing the Attack in the First Place

One medication, cromolyn, blocks the formation or release of the adverse chemicals ("mediator substances") when the provoking agent strikes the lungs. Cromolyn, when it works, is particularly effective in allergic children or young people and those patients at any age whose asthma is induced by exercise. Remember, however, never use it for the treatment of an acute attack—only for prophylaxis. It comes in a powder-filled capsule, which is put in an *inhalator* that pierces the container and propels the powder into the air passages. Children may consider this route of administration inconvenient, while their parents find it relatively expensive. And youngsters generally don't like to take medication prophylactically. But you're lucky if it works, so be sure to ask your doctor about cromolyn.

Many asthmatics can go for long periods without taking any anti-wheezing drugs. Others need something almost continuously to keep their airways open. In this latter circumstance, the xanthine group of drugs are most useful. They are marketed in tablet form as Slo-Phyllin, Theo-Dur, or Quibron (to name those that I happen to use most in my own practice), as a liquid (Elixophylline) to be taken by mouth, or via the enema route, or as a suppository. (For emergency situations the drug can be given intravenously, but there is no aerosol form).

Although the xanthines are the mainstay of chronic anti-asthmatic treatment, they can cause several problems. Some of them are gastric irritants, and give you stomach pain, nausea and vomiting; the rate of absorption may also vary from person to person so that you may require much more (or much less) of the drug than you are taking. There are other toxic side effects like rapid heart rate, nervousness and even convulsions which may preclude their use in any given patient, but these are usually dose-related.

The *adrenaline* family of drugs are time honored agents in the treatment of asthma. Adrenaline itself, injected in tiny amounts, will almost always end a severe asthmatic attack. It is used primarily in emergency situations when the spasm is severe and the patient is in acute trouble. Its major drawbacks, and important ones for cardiacs, are that it speeds the heart, raises the blood pressure and may induce irregularities of heart rhythm. Heart patients with asthma should also avoid most of the beta-blocker drugs like Inderal, for the treatment of their cardiac condition, because those agents can induce spasm of the airways.

Then there is oral *ephedrine*, an adrenaline derivative, which is more slowly acting and less potent than the parent substance, but nonetheless effective. The Chinese had been using it in herb form to relieve asthma for thousands of years. (Bronchitis and asthma are among the leading causes of death and disability in China to this day.) But it wasn't until 1920 that Western scientists discovered its active principle— ephedrine. You can count on it to relieve an attack of wheezing.

Patients with chronic asthma take it three or four times a day to open up a "tight chest." But be careful if you have heart trouble, because, like adrenaline, ephedrine increases heart rate and raises the blood pressure.

Newer Medications

There are several newer compounds (beta agonists) that have the same mode of action as ephedrine and adrenaline, but are often better tolerated. These include Alupent, Brethine and Ventolin. All three effectively relieve bronchial spasm with much less effect on heart rate or blood pressure than either ephedrine or adrenaline. They can be used indefinitely three or four times a day—by mouth or inhalation—for prevention after they have relieved the acute episode. I prefer them to any of the other agents for maintenance therapy.

Steroids Can be Safe

A third group of drugs used in the treatment of asthma are the *steroid* hormones. They are very potent dilators of the bronchial tree, and therefore very effective in the treatment of asthmatic spasm. Throughout this book, you will find notes of caution, and dire warnings about taking the cortisone-type drugs capriciously. Their long-term use is fraught with potential danger. But in some asthmatics, the situation can become so bad that the doctor has no choice. When these steroids are necessary, they should be taken for seven to ten days, no more, and prescribed in declining doses. In other words, you start off with a large amount the first two days. This has an almost immediate effect on symptoms (in association with other bronchial dilating drugs), and you can begin to taper the dosage on the third day. The schedule is so planned that by the tenth day at the latest, you're off the medication completely. And that's usually all you need. If steroids are prescribed for a longer time than that, get a second opinion.

A major advance of which you should be aware is the cortisone now available in an aerosol mist. It acts directly on the walls of the bronchial tubes, and is *not absorbed* into the bloodstream. This drug, beclamethasone, is marketed in the United States as Vanceril. It is effective for the acute attack and can also be taken in small doses as a preventive during a vulnerable phase, for example, the hay-fever season. The combination of beta agonists mentioned above and Vanceril is excellent for most chronic asthmatics and has sharply reduced the need for emergency adrenaline.

Drugs Are Not Enough

You must live by two cardinal rules if you are asthmatic. First, you have got to stop smoking. Tobacco smoke is irritating to the lining of the air passages. Second, any respiratory infection, no matter how minor, should be treated promptly with antibiotics and eradicated. If you fail to do so, the "cold" ends up with your spitting yellowish or greenish sputum. Then you begin to wheeze and are sick for weeks, coughing, spitting and wheezing. Doctors used to refuse to prescribe antibiotics for patients who had only a "simple cold." If you are asthmatic, that conservatism doesn't apply to you.

KEY FACTS TO REMEMBER

Asthmatic wheezing often results when the bronchial tubes become narrowed—by spasm, mucus, infection or allergy. Asthma may be acute and paroxysmal, or chronic. Its causes, external or internal, must be identified and eliminated from your environment. Determination of the responsible factors may require the aid of an allergist.

A number of drugs, some very old, others quite new, are available for the prevention and treatment of asthma. They must be carefully selected and combined for optimal effect—something that may require a second opinion from an allergist or a chest specialist.

9

The Skin—Common Problems Affecting the Largest Organ in the Body

This chapter contains a discussion of some of the more common and difficult skin problems. Since so many are chronic and a few are even life-threatening, you should be alerted about when to get a second opinion and why.

The Easy Life

When I was a medical student, my friends and I used to sit around and muse about our future as practitioners. We speculated with some animation about what each of us might be doing twenty-five years "down the pike." Most of my classmates expected to end up as family practitioners. Others hoped to be specialists in one field or another—endocrinology, cardiology, gastroenterology or surgery. Many, especially those who thought they lacked the necessary technical or mathematical talents, opted for psychiatry. Interestingly enough, anyone who expressed the intention of becoming a dermatologist was accused of taking the easy road, of avoiding a career with either physical or intellectual challenges. After all, whoever heard of a skin doctor getting an emergency call in the middle of the night? And where was the glamour or challenge in treating an itch or a rash?

The Largest Organ in the Body

How times have changed! Cosmetics now constitutes a multibillion-dollar industry and the "dull" specialty of dermatology has become one of the more exciting fields in medicine. We appreciate more and more that the skin is as vital as any other body tissue, and as big. One of my dermatologist friends reminds his patients that he treats the largest organ in the body. What appears on its surface often mirrors important disease processes taking place internally. Do you have a "simple" allergic rash? There is probably a lot more going on inside, possibly involving the heart, lungs, liver or kidneys. If you have an unexplained sore, it may be due to syphilis—a disease that can spread throughout your body. A peculiar tightness of the skin may reflect a disease that also "scars" such internal organs as the heart. Almost any serious malady sends clues to the exterior—to the skin—tumors, arthritis, heart trouble, kidney disease, liver malfunction and glandular diseases, to name but a few. So the dermatologist is no longer perceived as the chap who wanted the easy life. A good "skin man" is an astute biological detective, tracking down the clues that lead to proper diagnosis. In addition to that, however, he is also confronted with the problem of treating some of the most troublesome symptoms known to man. If you have ever been plagued by a serious, persistent itch, you know exactly what I mean. It can be worse than pain. But happily, today's dermatologist has at his disposal a wide range of treatment options (from sophisticated radiation to ointments that eradicate skin cancer), none of which were available to his predecessors.

Psoriasis—It's More Than Just Dandruff

Psoriasis is a chronic, troublesome skin disease that is newly diagnosed in as many as 250,000 Americans each year. It's a bore, it's embarrassing, it's uncomfortable, it's expensive, and occasionally, it can be serious. You can't always spot psoriasis victims because the silver-red scaly plaques which are its hallmark are often hidden by the clothes. But if it affects the patient's scalp, you'll see more "dandruff" on his or her shoulders than you thought was possible.

Normally, the superficial cells in the skin respond to

everyday wear and tear by shedding and multiplying at equal rates. This process is usually imperceptible. In psoriasis, these "top-layer" cells are formed much more rapidly and prematurely. They are, therefore, not really "healthy," and so the superficial skin is scaly and sheds very easily. No one knows why these cells multiply so enthusiastically. It's obviously due to some breakdown in a regulatory mechanism that determines the pattern of cell division.

Psoriasis is easy to diagnose, but difficult to treat. It not only involves the scalp, where it simulates a bad case of dandruff; the typical scaly, silvery patches can occur anywhere—on the elbows, knees, penis, back, between the buttocks and around the anus (which, like the scalp, is one of the few areas where they are likely to be itchy). Nails are commonly affected too. In some cases, psoriasis not only involves the skin, but is also accompanied by a severe form of arthritis.

Inherited, But Not Found Among Blacks

Some four in every hundred whites living in the United States have psoriasis, but it is rarely found in the dark-skinned races. It is often inherited, and thus appears to run in families; it may develop at any time or at any age. Although patients can occasionally tell me exactly when their skin problem started—triggered by a bad cold, a sunburn or some other illness—generally speaking, any relationship between such an event and the onset of psoriasis is probably coincidental.

Treatment, Yes; Cure, No

Once psoriasis sets in, it becomes chronic and often difficult to treat. For that reason, those who suffer from it will go from doctor to doctor looking for a cure. If you have psoriasis, there are two important facts that you should be aware of. There *is no cure* at this time, but the disease *can* be treated. The regimen selected will depend on the size of the area of skin involved (is it just a small, localized plaque or is it widespread?), how long you have had it and whether it is complicated by arthritis. Even if you do respond to treatment, chances are that you will have a recurrence some time in the future.

The psoriatic patches are most commonly treated topically with creams, ointments, lotions and shampoos containing cortisone, tar, phenol, salicylic acid or even simple salt water. Among these, the most effective, at least in my experience has been hydrocortisone. It's also the most expensive. Unlike the oral form, cortisone creams and ointments are relatively safe. In nonhairy areas like the elbow or knee, cortisone ointments covered overnight with Saran Wrap, Glad Wrap or some similar product, reduces scaling and redness.

There are literally scores of these topical steroid preparations now commercially available without a prescription. These are usually the weaker strengths which are appropriate for use in such areas as the face, arms, groin or the armpits. But in scalp, elbows, and knees, higher concentrations of the drug are necessary. In any event, it should be applied three times a day and rubbed in thoroughly. Indiscriminate application of the more potent ones can cause damage to healthy skin, leaving it very thin and sometimes painful. Avoid the chronic use of any cortisone cream or ointment over large areas of the body, since, in addition to its local effect, there is the additional possibility of its absorption into the bloodstream. And keep it away from your eyes too.

Occasionally, an injection of a diluted cortisone solution into individual plaques of psoriasis does yield very good results, but this should be done carefully and only by a qualified dermatologist. Finally, let me emphasize that almost never should anyone with psoriasis take hydrocortisone by mouth. Massive doses are required to achieve any effect and the risks involved in such a regimen are simply not worth taking.

Coal Tar, Messy But It May Be Worth It

In addition to the steroid creams, there is a form of topical therapy still in use today that dates back some fifty years, and which is also fairly effective (but remember, like every other treatment of psoriasis, is not a cure). It involves the application of crude coal tar, followed by daily exposure to ultraviolet rays (the Goeckerman method). This therapy is usually limited to patients with the severe form of the disease because it's so messy and time-consuming. The ointment is applied every two to four hours to the entire skin surface, except the body folds and head. It is removed twice a day and followed by the ultraviolet ray treatment. Plaques usually clear after two to four weeks in most cases, and you may remain free of disease for many months, or even years, thereafter. So if your disease is severe enough, and not responsive to the hydrocortisone, ask for a second opinion about the Goeckerman method. But be sure the dermatologist doing it is experienced, since the proper dosage of the ultraviolet is very important.

Sunlight, Sunlamp and the IRS

I am sometimes asked to write a letter to the Internal Revenue Service to justify a patient's going to a warm climate for the winter. I do so happily and with a clean conscience, because, as in cases of severe heart disease, where cold weather worsens angina pectoris, psoriatics also benefit from exposure to sun and salt water. One of the best places for getting both is the Dead Sea in Israel, where, in addition to sunlight, you can bathe in water with a very high salt concentration.

If it is not practical for you to go South, West or to the Middle East in the wintertime, and if your psoriasis is extensive and severe, try using a sunlamp; like the sun, a sunlamp also emits high-intensity, long-wave, ultraviolet light. If, at the same time, you take a drug called psoralen, the results are even better. This combined treatment, called "PUVA"—"UVA," refers to type-A ultraviolet light (less penetrating and less harmful to the skin than the B type), and the "P" stands for psoralen.

A course of treatment with PUVA will require about twenty office visits to the doctor over a period of six to eight weeks. And it usually works. But be careful. Too much exposure either to sun or to ultraviolet light not only will give you a painful sunburn, but also will increase your risk of developing skin cancer and eye trouble (cataracts), and perhaps changes in your chromosomes. It may be for these reasons that the Food and Drug Administration has yet to approve PUVA for general use.

We worry particularly about skin cancer after PUVA therapy, especially if you had such cancer in the past or have previously been exposed to significant amounts of ionizing radiation. For example, if you were treated for acne in the days when doctors recommended superficial X rays to the skin, PUVA therapy increases your chances of developing skin cancer or cancer of the thyroid gland. But one has to balance the good with the bad. Whether or not you decide to take PUVA depends on the severity of the psoriasis. In any event, after the treatment is completed, have your skin checked very carefully over the years in order to detect the earliest evidence of cancer. The risk of this happening is about 2½ times normal.

When the Psoriasis Is Very Bad

For patients with severe psoriasis, there is available a strong and potentially toxic drug called methotrexate. This is a chemical used in the treatment of various cancers; it slows the growth of rapidly multiplying cells, and in psoriasis such rapid, nonmalignant growth is the basic problem. But since methotrexate may damage the liver, it should really be used as a last resort, only by highly trained specialists, in the lowest possible doses, and for the shortest time necessary to get results. But it does work, and has been approved by the Food and Drug Administration for cases of severe psoriasis.

What's New—and Far Out

The patient with psoriasis, turning in desperation to "outsiders" for help, may end up with some "far out" recommendations. These include dietary changes, sleep therapy, tonsillectomy or antibiotics, none of which I have ever known to make any difference in the course of the disease.

In 1979, an important research development was announced. A derivative of Vitamin A (retinoic acid) taken orally was found, in initial clinical experiments, to result in dramatic improvement of psoriasis. If the early promise is fulfilled, the drug may soon become available. Make sure to check its status with your doctor.

Finally, I have been reading scattered reports of the use of dialysis in the treatment of psoriasis. Dialysis is the process in which body wastes are washed out of the system via an "artificial kidney." I know of no convincing evidence that it works. If this fairly drastic approach is recommended to you, by all means get a second opinion.

Acne—A Plague at All Ages

Acne is predominantly a disease of teen-agers and young adults, affecting some 15 million of them between the ages of 12 and 17. Although benign in the sense that it is not a threat to life, it may be cosmetically and socially disastrous to youngsters. I have written this chapter to help separate fact from the folklore surrounding the causes and treatment of this disorder.

A Matter of Hormones, Not Infection

Acne *looks* like a skin infection and, indeed, infection does play a role, but it is really a hormonal disorder. Usually beginning in puberty, it is worse in girls, and flares up before their menstrual periods, when they start to take the "pill," or more importantly, when they discontinue it. The condition affects boys too and in both sexes often clears up in adult life. It sometimes reappears in slightly different form at the time of the menopause—again presumably because of the change in hormonal status at that time.

How Acne Develops

The sebaceous glands in the skin which produce the oil that gives it its normal texture are under the influence of hormones. As the production of these hormones varies, so does the amount and quality of the grease made by the glands. Bacteria normally present in the ducts of the hair follicles (which receive the secretions from the sebaceous glands) can alter the chemistry of the waxy stuff. Under certain circumstances, they produce an irritating chemical, which then causes the inflammation and the pimples that we call acne. Blockage of the hair duct is the final and crucial element in the causation of the disease.

Acne most commonly involves the face, back and chest, because this is where the greatest concentration of sebaceous glands is found. In adult men, lesions frequently concentrate on the back, and in women around the mouth or lower part of the face. Cosmetics, especially greasy moisturizing creams, can aggravate or even trigger the disease.

So the three preconditions necessary for acne to develop are first, hormonal changes that increase the secretion of the glands, then action of normal bacteria on these secretions, and finally, obstruction of the hair duct.

Old Myths Die Hard

The subject of acne is still surrounded by old wives' tales, the most important of which concerns diet. There is a commonly held but mistaken view, even among some doctors, that acne is your punishment for eating "junk food." The fact is that diet has almost nothing to do with acne; changing it usually will not make any difference in the course of the disease. The only exceptions to this statement are (1) a high intake of seaweed and kelp (not favorite snacks of American teen-agers) may produce an elevated iodine content that can occasionally worsen the condition; (2) some dermatologists believe that a drastic reduction in the amount of fat consumed will improve acne. I don't have any personal experience with kelp eaters, and I'm not sure that the claims about fat reduction are valid.

Here are a few more misconceptions and half-truths. Acne is the result of masturbation or lack of cleanliness. Totally false. Squeezing the pimples will spread the infection. Partly true. "Don't do anything for the acne; you'll outgrow it." Not only wrong but dangerous. Although superficial blackheads or whiteheads sometimes do clear up spontaneously (presumably because of a change in the patient's hormonal status), failure to treat acne can lead to permanent scarring due to the rupture of pus-filled cysts deep in the skin.

The Best Treatment

So, treatment of acne has very little to do with your diet, sex habits or personal hygiene. What you need for the severe inflammatory form is antibiotics to control the bacteria that act on the grease and cause inflammation, infection and blockage of the ducts. Oral tetracycline is the most widely prescribed. It is relatively inexpensive and safe, and that's important because you may have to take it for years to control the condition until your hormonal balance "straightens itself out." Doing so, however, can result in intestinal upset and fungal infections. When tetracycline is not well tolerated, erythromycin (taken with meals) is effective too. In my experience, however, it causes intestinal symptoms more often than tetracycline. The modern therapy of acne that is *not inflamed* involves the topical application of antibiotics and other substances directly to the skin. Solutions of erythromycin, tetracycline or clindamycin can in many cases eliminate the need to take oral antibiotics. One of the objections that teen-agers have to the use of topical tetracycline is that it causes the skin to "glow" under the black light used in discotheques! Another very effective topical antibacterial (but not antibiotic) is benzoyl peroxide, applied to the skin in a gel form. You may also need to apply certain chemicals to help peel and dry the skin. These come in the form of soaps and lotions and include salicylic acid, resorcin and sulfur products. It is also very important that the doctor release any pus accumulated behind the blocked ducts. Occasionally, he may have to inject a weak solution of cortisone directly into the inflamed areas to prevent scarring.

Tretoin (retinoic acid—a derivative of Vitamin A) in cream form opens up the plugged glandular ducts and thus improves acne. It is probably the most effective of the topically applied agents. Since it renders the skin more sensitive to sunburn, always apply sunscreen with it if you're going to be exposed to strong sunlight. If you can, use tretoin every other day. That will give you substantially less irritation than daily application.

Pocks on You

When pockmarks do develop, you may benefit from *dermabrasion*, a kind of sandpapering of the skin, to smooth out the crevices. This treatment is somewhat involved, and the results are not always good. If you are black, think twice about dermabrasion because the resulting keloid (scar tissue) formation can be worse than the scarring from the acne. Also, if you are dark-complexioned and are exposed to the sun after dermabrasion, you may end up with areas of too much pigment, or too little.

There are other types of treatment sometimes recommended for the treatment of acne. Women can take "the pill"—especially types that contain high doses of estrogen. This will reduce the amount of wax produced in the hair glands. You won't see any results for at least three months.

Some doctors are also enthusiastic about giving zinc tablets for acne, others have found it ineffective. You're probably better off without it, especially if you have ulcer problems, since it can cause gastrointestinal bleeding.

Finally, the newest treatment for acne is an oral form of retinoic acid (13-cis-retinoic acid). It's supposed to cut down the wax production of the glands, but there is not yet enough information about its effectiveness or safety.

Just Lying in the Sun

Years ago acne was treated by radiation. Although that did occasionally result in improvement, we're now seeing the late consequences of such therapy—cancer of the thyroid and skin.

Acne does improve in the summertime, a benefit some doctors attribute to sunlight, but that has never been proved. It may be that the irritation of the solar ultraviolet radiation results in increased blood flow to the skin, or perhaps it's simply the tranquilizing effect of just lying in the sun.

Skin Cancers—You Can Rarely Be Sure

Not a day goes by that the general practitioner, internist or dermatologist is asked whether a certain mole, or wart or area of skin discoloration is "suspicious" for cancer. To be perfectly honest, there are many times when I look at the lesion in question and just don't know. My dermatologist friends admit that even they are not always sure whether a growth on the skin is actually malignant or even potentially so. To be sure, they generally biopsy it. I agree wholeheartedly with that approach. Never balk at the suggestion of a biopsy to exclude the possibility of cancer.

The wisdom of that position was driven home to me very dramatically not long ago. One of my patients complained of an itch in the middle of his back. He couldn't see the involved area because of its location, but his wife told him she saw a "pimple" there. He consulted a dermatologist, who wasn't sure either. He doubted that it was anything serious, but suggested that they wait a month and then let him have another look. About six weeks later, my patient returned to the doctor, who happened to be very busy that day. After waiting about an hour, and being an irascible type anyway, he left in a huff to "teach that guy" a lesson. A month later he complained to me that the itch was worse than ever. When I looked at his back this time, I saw what was obviously a melanoma, one of the most malignant cancers there is. Two precious months had been lost—because the dermatologist was conservative and the patient impatient. The cancer was finally removed. In the first edition of this book, I estimated the man's chances of survival at 50 percent. As we go to press with this paperback edition (over one year later), he's still alive and well.

Fact and Folklore About Skin Cancer

There are several popular misconceptions about skin growths that one hears from time to time. "A growth that's painless can't be serious." Not true. Pain has absolutely nothing to do with the diagnosis. "Removal or biopsy of a tumor causes others to appear." Obvious nonsense. Finally, despite the lack of any real evidence, some people still fear that removal or biopsy of a growth causes it to spread.

Most skin tumors are, in fact, benign. They include the common freckle, mole, and what we call 'keratoses.' The latter, which develop as we get older, are small areas of heaped-up skin with a brownish discoloration. They are only of cosmetic importance. Skin tags, especially frequent around the neck and armpits, are completely innocuous.

We used to think that the hairy elevated mole remains benign except in the rarest of circumstances, but the flat, brown variety is a potential troublemaker. I even said so in the first edition, but it's no longer believed to be true. The fact is any skin cell with pigment in it has malignant potential. If in the slightest doubt, check it out with a skin doctor.

Here is a good general rule to follow. *Any bleeding or ulceration on the skin, any growth that itches or changes in color or size, is suspicious.* Show it to a dermatologist without delay.

The Spectrum (and Specter) of Skin Cancer

Skin cancers can be divided into three major types. The first and most common, the basal cell cancers, or *epitheliomas*, originate in the lowermost cells of the epidermis (the superficial layer of the skin). They usually occur in areas of the body chronically exposed to sun, like the face. They grow very slowly, often bleed spontaneously or with slight irritation, and don't really constitute a later threat to your life after their complete removal.

Another kind of skin cancer is the *prickle-cell* epithelioma. It originates a little more superficially in the epidermis than does the basal cell cancer, and it is much less common. Unlike the basal cell cancer, which rarely is found too late to treat, the prickle-cell cancer, when diagnosed, must be attended to immediately before it metastasizes. Generally speaking, however, those that arise in areas of sun-damaged skin rarely spread early, if at all.

The treatment of these first two major types of skin cancer is varied, but burning and scraping them out, as well as cutting them away, are time-honored and reliable approaches.

Finally, we come to that small group of cancers called *melanomas*—among the deadliest of all human cancers. It is only recently that we have recognized several different melanomas, some of which are less threatening than others. The worst kind, the one that spreads earliest and fastest, nodular melanoma, may be black or brown in color, frequently ulcerates or bleeds and may be tinged with red, white or blue. It is usually more elevated than the less deadly varieties. Another type, the superficial spreading melanoma, is curable when treated early enough. Redheads and blondes are more susceptible to the above two forms of melanomas. The black, mottled and large pigmented lesion constitutes the third variety of melanoma. Usually appearing on the face of the elderly, it also is curable if removed early. *Excision is the sole preferred therapy for all melanomas.*

There are some malignant skin lesions (other than melanomas) that can be removed without surgery. Such alternative methods are especially useful for growths on the face, where surgery may cause scarring or disfiguration. Radiation is one nonsurgical technique. Another is a topical anticancer ointment such as 5 Fluorouracil (5FU). Cryotherapy, using liquid nitrogen is also effective. Other malignant tumors can be removed by a technique called chemosurgery (no surgery is actually involved), in which, again, potent topical anticancer drugs are used. So if you are told that you have a skin cancer that has to be cut away, and you want some other option, ask for a second opinion from an experienced dermatologist.

Herpes—Most Everyone Has (or Had) It

I must have been in a great hurry to finish the first edition of this book. What other reason could there possibly have been for omitting at least some discussion about herpes infections generally, and shingles specifically? The herpes viruses are extremely important and common infecting agents. It is estimated that they are present in anywhere from 30 to 90 percent of young American adults and are responsible for the second most common venereal disease in this country. The symptoms they can cause are troublesome, recur unpredictably and are very difficult to prevent and treat. That makes them ideal situations for "far out" remedies, some of which make a second opinion desirable.

The Belly-Button Landmark

There are at least four types of herpes viruses now identified, one of which is the herpes simplex virus (HSV). There are two HSV viruses—Type I and Type II. They differ mainly in respect to when and where they strike, and the seriousness of the illness they cause. Type I almost always infects *above* the belly-button, and occurs mostly in children. It is responsible for those painful sores in the mouth, eyes, and the lining of the upper airways and food pipe. The Type II herpes virus infection hits *below* the belly-button, and is related to sexual contact at any age. I'm going to leave this particular infection for the moment, and will discuss it in the next chapter dealing with sexually transmitted diseases.

Let's get back to the HSV Type I, which affects the young. The painful sores they cause are not effectively treatable at this time. We simply have you keep the viral blisters dry and clean. If your case of herpes virus is severe and recurrent, you may need more than the conventional treatment. Ask for another opinion because there is an explosion of new anti-viral agents becoming available. Most of these, ranging from Interferon to Vidarabine (marketed as Vira-A) are either still in research or unproven. But that can change at any time. Also, have your doctor check on the current status of *lysine*. This is a safe food substance, an amino acid, which has been used by dermatologists here and abroad in the treatment of both Types I and II herpes infections. I have seen it work in a few patients. It is taken by mouth for a period of several months. The only caution is that while on lysine, you must avoid cola drinks, chocolate, and nuts, because these contain another amino acid on which the virus you're trying to get rid of actually thrives.

Shingles—Not For Doctors Only

Herpes zoster or shingles, as it is commonly referred to, is a painful skin eruption caused by a virus related to the simplex oral (Type I) and genital (Type II) strains discussed above. It is, to my knowledge, probably the only infectious agent which can cause two different diseases. In childhood, it usually results in chickenpox; in older patients, or those at any age whose resistance is lowered, it produces shingles. Although shingles is rarely a cause of death, it is a common cause of pain and suffering. People with cancer, or individuals taking what we call "immuno-suppressive drugs" (used in the treatment of certain malignancies and also to prevent rejection of transplanted organs) or those who have received a lot of radiation are all particularly prone to this infection.

The shingles or herpes varicella (V2) virus is usually acquired in childhood, at which time it causes chickenpox. In some cases, the infection may not even be apparent. The virus then travels up the nerve fiber, and settles down in the nerve cells near the spinal cord, where it remains for years and years. Happy in its new home, it doesn't give you any trouble. But, each year, in about three to five unlucky persons per thousand, the virus becomes reactivated for some reason. It then leaves the cell, travels back down the course of the nerve, right to its endings in the skin, and causes the

very painful blisters called shingles. For a few days before the
sores appear, the involved skin is very painful. Symptoms
may be mild, but are occasionally severe, especially if they
involve the eye, or occur during pregnancy. A characteristic
feature of the disease is that it hardly ever crosses over the
mid-line of the body. So if you develop blisters on both sides
of your chest, or back, or face, chances are it's not shingles.
The most troublesome aspect of this infection is that in some
people, after the blisters disappear, the pain persists for
weeks, months, or even years.

There is no cure for shingles at the present time, but you
should be aware of the variety of treatment options available
for severe cases. You should also know about those that are
not effective. Unfortunately, many patients are still being
given therapy which is in most cases useless—like B_{12} shots,
gamma globulin injections or antibiotics. The promising new
agents which may help include Vidarabine (marketed as Vira-
A); high doses of steroids given in gradually decreasing
doses over a three-week period; if the disease is diagnosed
early enough, Interferon, which will no doubt be available in
increasing amounts in the next year or two, may also modify
its course. Other measures which may be effective in some
cases are a form of electrical stimulation called transcutaneous
nerve stimulation, a drug marketed as Tegretol, (normally
used as a pain-killer and anti-convulsant), and certain antidepressants like Elavil and Sinequan.

The point in my going into such detail is if you are suffering from the pain of shingles, don't just sit back and endure it. Ask for a second opinion from a dermatologist experienced in the management of this disorder.

KEY FACTS TO REMEMBER

Diseases of the skin often mirror serious internal disorders ranging from infection to cancer. Their correct diagnosis
and management is, therefore, more than only a matter of
appearances and comfort.

Psoriasis, a very common skin disorder, may affect the
joints in its more serious form. There is no cure for this
disease at the present time, but several kinds of therapy may
result in relief and remission. These include topical ointments, ultraviolet light and a variety of drugs, some of which

are also used in the treatment of cancer. Too much exposure to ultraviolet rays increases the risk of cancer of the skin in later years. Anticancer agents have potential toxicity.

Acne is basically a hormonal disorder, not an infection. It has very little to do with life style, what you eat, masturbation or personal hygiene. Fundamentals of treatment consist of oral or topical antibiotics and measures to prevent scarring.

The great majority of *skin cancers* are easily recognized, removed and cured. A few, especially the malignant melanomas, are among the most virulent cancers known to man. It may take an expert and skin biopsies to differentiate the relatively benign from the malignant kind. The management of malignant melanoma demands early and aggressive surgical removal.

The *herpes virus* family can produce a variety of painful skin conditions ranging from recurrent "cold sores" to "shingles." These are difficult to prevent and treat, but there are new treatment options of which patients with severe symptoms should be aware.

10

Sexually Transmitted Diseases (What we used to call V.D.)

Venereal, Not Venerable

An infection transmitted from one person to another during any kind of sexual act is technically a venereal disease. For most people, the term "venereal" brings to mind only syphilis and gonorrhea. In terms of today's disease patterns, however, it should also include several other common infections, which affect many more people than do the classical two. There are, first, trichomonas, a "benign" organism that is found in as many as one quarter of all normal women and that gives them vaginal discharge, itch and sometimes pain. Chlamydia is also an infectious agent we used to think was a virus, but now know is a bacterium. It may affect the eyes, the lungs or the genitourinary tract. In the latter event, the presence of a discharge raises fears of gonorrhea even though it is watery and not purulent like the typical "dose." Finally, there are viral infections (the most important of which is herpes) and venereal warts.

From the point of view of numbers, and even consequences, the herpes virus is probably the most important. It is very contagious, resists treatment, keeps recurring, harms the infant born of an infected mother, and may even contribute to the incidence of cancer of the cervix.

In the last edition of this book, I said "at this time,

there is no compelling reason to ask for a second opinion if you have a genital herpes infection, except to confirm the diagnosis. There is no effective treatment." That being the case, I completely ignored this important disease even though it is among the most common of the sexually transmitted infections. Since then, however, things have changed somewhat. Although the disease is still "incurable" in the sense that the recurrent herpes sores cannot predictably be prevented, there are several treatments to reduce the severity of symptoms. And you should be aware of them. So let's take at least a brief look at genital herpes.

In the preceding chapter, I discussed some of the characteristics of herpes virus infections generally. Remember, there are two types, I and II. The former usually infects above the waistline; the latter, herpes genital virus, below.

However, both types I and II will "take" at the site of their inoculation, wherever and at whatever level it may occur. For example, if someone with a herpes simplex (Type I) infection of the lip or mouth engages in oro-genital sex, the result may well be a herpes genital infection. Presumably because of the greater frequency of that kind of sexual activity, some 30 percent of genital herpes cases are actually of the Type I variety, the kind that has no business below the belly-button!

No one knows how many Americans have herpes genital virus, since it is not a reportable disease. But the numbers are increasing annually. The Center for Disease Control estimates there are 300,000 *new* cases each year. The statisticians further suspect that as many as 35 percent of the general population has at some time or other been exposed to this infection. Now, since it is clear that one person in three doesn't have the *symptoms* of the disease, there must be a tremendous number of carriers, that is, individuals who harbor and can spread the virus, but who themselves don't suffer from it.

How You Get Herpes and Why It Recurs

After sexual activity of one kind or another with someone who is infected, the virus lands in the area of contact, the mouth, vagina, penis or anus. Then, some 3 to 7 days later, you're apt to develop a burning pain at that site, followed by the appearance of the herpes blisters. These usually persist anywhere from two to six weeks. They then heal completely, without scarring. But that's by no means the end of the story. It's only the first chapter. Because, as in shingles, after the blister clears, the virus travels along the course of the nerves in the area to settle in the nerve cells near the spinal cord. And there it sits until it's ready to come out. That will take place within one year in most patients. What suddenly causes the virus to leave the body of the nerve and to re-trace its step down the nerve fiber to produce the painful sores once more (reactivation) is not clear. Fever due to any cause, heat, sunlight, menstrual periods, sexual intercourse, emotional stress or a "run-down" condition generally may do it. That's a pretty wide spectrum of provoking circumstances, many of which are unavoidable. The natural history of genital herpes infections then is a primary lesion followed by recurrences at varying intervals. You are most contagious to others when sores are visible, because they are teeming with viruses. The frustrating fact is that some persons, especially women, remain infectious even in the absence of any evidence of disease.

Aside from the pain, and psychological problems associated with any sexually transmitted disease, genital herpes is not a life-threatening or dangerous disease—with two exceptions. First, there is mounting evidence that herpes genital virus is associated with an increased incidence of cancer of the cervix. Second, a newborn contracting herpes at birth as he or she emerges through the mother's genital tract, can become very sick, and often die. As a result, many physicians now recommend a Cesarean delivery when the mother is known to be harboring this disease. So if you are pregnant and have had recurrent herpes, make sure you are under the care of an expert in the identification and treatment of this infection. He should work closely with your obstetrician. If the virus is demonstrated to be present in your genital tract near the time of delivery, ask your obstetrician about a Cesarean delivery. Unless he gives you a reasonable explanation as to why it shouldn't be done, ask for a second opinion.

Dealing with the Herpes Virus—Prevention and Treatment

In order to minimize the risk of infecting a partner, anyone with recurrent herpes should abstain from sex while sores or blisters are present. *That's* obvious. Even *between* recurrences, men should use a condom, and women a contraceptive foam. The latter kills many of the viruses present.

Once the sores appear, the purpose of treatment is to get rid of them as fast as possible, and to control pain. But remember that, as of now, despite the fact that experimentally the virus in the sores can be reduced in number with some drugs, *there is no satisfactory, safe medication, either topically applied or taken internally, that will either cure the infection of the skin or eliminate its recurrence*. The best advice I can give you is to use drying agents only in the early wet or blistery stage. Otherwise, I prefer my patients to compress the blisters with salt water, or if not too uncomfortable, to dab them with rubbing alcohol a few times a day. I avoid prescribing calamine lotion because it is a drying agent, and almost always causes crusting, that makes the sores more vulnerable to infection.

When the lesion has begun to dry of its own accord, I prefer a hydrocortisone ointment or cream. In general, it is a good idea to use such ointments (well-rubbed in) on herpes when it affects the penis or vulva. But I must tell you that other doctors think these ointments actually prolong the duration of the infection. So if they are prescribed for you, and don't seem to be working, get another opinion from a dermatologist expert in this field.

As far as treating the symptoms of herpes, keep away from potent pain-killers. This is a chronic disease, and you don't want to end up addicted. Your best bet is plain aspirin. Two will not only give you relief, they are believed also to prevent the spread of the virus.

So much for the treatment of symptoms. What can we actually do to modify the course of the disease, especially the recurrences? You can see the problem we doctors have. No matter how many of the viruses we kill on the surface of the skin by various methods (mostly topically applied agents), their brethren sitting within the nerve cells just waiting to come down go scot free! But there is a great deal of research activity which has generated some exciting claims. You should inquire about them if you are troubled by recurrent herpes infections. Following is a list of some of the newer approaches to treatment:

1. Acyclovir, when applied directly to herpes viruses the first time they appear (as opposed to recurrent sores), results in very early healing. It apparently does not affect recurrence.
2. Lysine, an amino acid, (described in the preceding chapter for herpes Type I), is claimed by some to prevent recurrence. It's worth a try if your doctor finds no reason why you shouldn't take it.
3. Aspirin and other anti-inflammatory drugs like indomethacin (Indocin) may prevent recurrences. If you can tolerate them, small daily doses, after consultation with your doctor, are worthwhile.
4. Laser beam treatment of the herpes as soon as they appear has apparently delayed recurrence in 65 percent of cases, according to some investigators. It also reduces the number of viruses in the sores.

The above four methods may hold promise. There are others, however, which although they have been shown to be ineffective, are still being prescribed. If you're advised to take any one of the following, ask for a second opinion.

1) Smallpox vaccine
2) Levamisole
3) Photo-inactivators
4) Local application of ether
5) BCG vaccine
6) B_{12} shots

What is clearly needed, but *not yet available*, is a vaccine to protect us all from herpes genital virus.

Traditional VD

Gonorrhea and syphilis are two infections that have plagued mankind for centuries. If you think that antibiotics have rendered them obsolete, you are wrong. They continue to infect many thousands each year, but there have been some important changes in their treatment, of which you should be aware.

How Do I Love Thee? Let Me Count the Ways

Gonorrhea is much more common than syphilis, although the consequences of the latter are apt to be more serious. You are not likely to get gonorrhea from using someone else's towel or from a public toilet. (I'll have more to say about that later.) The bacterium that causes gonorrhea (the gonococcus) is spread via the vagina, penis, anus or throat—but not the mouth. If you use your imagination, you can postulate any number of ways in which it can be transmitted between homosexuals, "innovative" heterosexuals, or plain old-fashioned lovers. However you go about it, in the words of Hippocrates, gonorrhea is usually contracted by "excessive" (or unlucky) "indulgences in the pleasures of Venus."

Gonorrhea, My Knee!

Although the portals through which the gonococcus invades are the penis, vagina, throat (gonococcal pharyngitis from fellatio but rarely cunnilingus) and anus (gonococcal proctitis), the infection does not always remain at the site of contact. For if the gonococcus enters the bloodstream, it can end up almost anywhere in the body—for example, the heart (especially if you have a diseased valve there from old rheumatic fever) or the liver. Not infrequently, it even causes arthritis, which usually affects a large joint, like the knee. So if you have had typical gonorrhea, with discharge from the penis or vagina, and days later develop a hot, painful, swollen joint, think in terms of gonorrhea.

Thank Goodness for Antibiotics

The consequences of gonorrhea ("dose," "clap" and other colorful synonyms) have, of course, been modified by the availability of treatment. Before the era of antibiotics, it was a miserable business. Women frequently were left sterile from scarring of the pelvic organs. (Many, untreated, still are.) In men, the penile urethra would become obstructed, requiring repeated, uncomfortable stretching, or dilatation, in order for them to be able to urinate or copulate. In the acute stage, with pus coming out of the penis, the only treatment was painful irrigation. Then, in the middle 1930s, sulfa drugs were discovered, and initially they cured the disease. But the gonorrhea bug soon became resistant to them, and within a few years less than 25 percent of gonorrhea cases responded to those agents.

The Resistant Bug

The phenomenon of *resistance* to antibiotics is an interesting one. It is not the patient who becomes resistant to an antibiotic, but the infecting organism. It happens this way. When the antibiotic you take works, it eradicates *most* but not all of the offending bacteria. A few resistant ones remain, but they are too few to cause symptoms. As they multiply, their subsequent "generations" are also resistant. Should they be transmitted to someone else or multiply in sufficient numbers in your body, they are not sensitive to the original antibiotic. In order to cure this new infection, we now have to use a different antibiotic.

The genes that confer resistance on an organism are not only passed on to the next generation, they also spread, by a process called "transduction," to other bacteria with which they are in intimate physical contact. It is a kind of good-neighbor policy among bacteria, and it is effected and enhanced by bacterial viruses that go from bug to bug, passing along this "resistance factor." The degree of resistance and the length of time it takes to develop depend on the organism and the antibiotics involved. For example, consider two very common bacteria originally sensitive to penicillin, the streptococcus and the staphylococcus. The former are still sensitive to this antibiotic, even though it has been used for almost forty years, while only half of the staphylococcus infections today now respond to it. Generally speaking, however, the longer an organism has been around and the more people it has infected (gonorrhea falls into both these categories), the greater the problem of resistance.

When penicillin was discovered in 1943, it was found to be extremely effective against the gonococcus. All one needed for a complete cure in virtually every case of gonorrhea was one shot of 160,000 units of penicillin-G. Gradually, relatively resistant strains began to emerge, so that more and more penicillin was required. To make matters worse, in the late 1970s we began to observe another phenomenon, which complicated treatment. Some of the gonorrhea organisms were making an enzyme called *penicillinase* which inactivated and rendered ineffective any penicillin with which it came in contact. (The ending *-ase* identifies an *enzyme*—a protein that breaks complex chemicals into simpler compounds. For example, lactase works on lactose, lipase splits fat [lipids], and so on.)

So now there were two obstacles to treating gonorrhea. As a consequence of the widespread use of penicillin over the years, the development of relatively resistant strains made it necessary to increase the dose of penicillin from the original 160,000 to 4,800,000 units today to cure the infection. And now there were penicillinase-producing gonoccoci totally untouched by penicillin. (Such penicillinase-producing gonococci are fortunately rare in the United States.)

It Should Be Reported, but Often Isn't

The combination of changing sexual mores and penicillin resistance has resulted in a worldwide gonorrhea epidemic. In the United States alone, it is estimated that one of every 108 persons is infected. (No one can be sure of the exact number, since gonorrhea is not usually reported, even though the law requires doctors to do so.) There are between three and four million new cases every year, but happily, the incidence has begun to level off.

No Longer a Disease of Men

In the "old days," gonorrhea was basically a disease of men, and the reservoir was the prostitute. That is no longer so. In the British Isles and Scandinavia, for example, the ratio of males to females with gonorrhea is now somewhat less than two to one. Modern contraceptive techniques are probably responsible for this change of incidence in that their use has increased the frequency of sexual activity in women. In addition, the "pill" contains hormones that alter the chemical environment of the vagina, making it, in fact, more hospitable to any gonococcus that is introduced. The result is a 50 percent greater vulnerability to infection in exposed women taking the pill. Also, when a woman with an intrauterine device (IUD) contracts gonorrhea, the risk of it spreading within the pelvis is also greater. We are not sure why this is so, but we suspect that it is due to the changes induced in the lining of the uterus by the IUD—changes which may also be responsible for its contraceptive effect.

The above discussion can be translated into practical terms in the following way. You have just had a sexual encounter with a new "friend" (male or female), and a few days later you come down with gonorrhea. The doctor gives you a shot of penicillin and sends you on your way—ostensibly cured. But neither of you reckoned with so many resistant strains of gonorrhea around. The yellowish discharge and burning during urination doesn't clear up as you expected. A few days later, you return to the doctor to find out why you continue to have symptoms despite treatment. A look at the pus under the microscope shows that you are still infected. Chances are that you will now be given tetracycline capsules, four times a day for five days, for a total of ten grams of that drug. (Remember always to take tetracycline either one hour before or two hours after eating, since food—especially dairy products—in the stomach interferes with its absorption. Also try to avoid this antibiotic if you are pregnant, because it may have adverse effects on the fetus.)

Some doctors now prefer to use oral tetracycline in the first instance when treating gonorrhea, because of the resistance problems with penicillin, the pain of the injection and the ever present possibility of a sensitivity reaction to that antibiotic. (Remember, however, that 30 to 40 percent of the penicillinase-producing gonococci are also resistant to tetracycline.)

There are physicians who prescribe ampicillin or amoxicillin (related antibiotics) in one big dose by mouth for the treatment of gonorrhea. These are also very effective, but not quite as dependable as penicillin or tetracycline.

If none of these four drugs does the job, you will have to be treated with spectinomycin. This antibiotic is administered in a single, intramuscular injection and is effective against penicillinase-producing as well as resistant gonococci. This drug costs four times as much as penicillin and doesn't work very well in cases of gonorrhea in the throat. Neither has it yet been proven to be safe in pregnant women. Also, if by any chance, you just happen to be incubating a syphilis infection contracted at the time you got your gonorrhea, spectinomycin will have no effect on that infection. (Penicillin, tetracycline, ampicillin and amoxicillin, on the other hand, will probably cure it.)

Here are a few additional tips about gonorrhea and its treatment. Before you opt for tetracycline rather than the penicillin (because you don't like shots) bear the following in mind: (a) tetracycline has a 25 percent failure rate when the infection involves the anus, which it frequently does in homosexuals; and (b) if you are pregnant, the drug may adversely affect the fetus. Also, if you are someone who doesn't always remember to take all the pills prescribed for you, a single shot of penicillin is much more reliable than five days of "maybe" treatment with a capsule.

When you are given a shot of 4,800,000 units of penicillin-G for the treatment of gonorrhea, you should also take a pill called probenecid. This drug blocks the excretion of penicillin by the kidney and, so, ensures adequate blood levels for longer periods of time.

If penicillin and probenecid fail to cure your gonorrhea, and days or weeks later you develop the same kind of discharge all over again, before blaming it all on a penicillin-resistant organism, you should think of two other possibilites. First, if you are sexually active with the same sexual partner, and didn't think to have him or her treated as well, you may have simply gotten yourself reinfected. That happens in a surprising number of cases. Then again, maybe you didn't have gonorrhea in the first place. I mentioned earlier that chlamydia, transmitted the same way as gonorrhea, also gives a urethral discharge (although it is watery and not mucus). In fact, in the United States, 80 percent of white males and 30 percent of black males who visit the doctor because of a discharge from the penis after sexual contact have chlamydia, not gonorrhea. Tetracycline will cure both diseases (one of the reasons some doctors prefer to start with this drug rather than penicillin). So if your doctor prescribes penicillin for your discharge *without examining it under the microscope to make sure it's gonorrhea,* ask him about chlamydia, especially if the discharge is watery.

Your Alibi—The Public Toilet Seat

Let's get back to the matter of the toilet seat. Earlier in this chapter, I said that you don't get gonorrhea from using somebody else's towel or from a public toilet. Recently, some scientists who were curious to know whether the gonococcus could survive on a toilet seat long enough to infect anyone, reported the results of their studies. They commandeered several different men's and ladies' rooms, and put live gonorrhea organisms on the toilet seats. (I presume the facilities were closed to the public for the duration of the experiment.) To their surprise, they found they survived for periods of up to two hours—long enough for the next several users to contract the disease. Even so, how the bug, alive or dead, could get from the seat into the penis or vagina is not clear to me. I suppose a theoretical case could be made for its entering the anus. The organisms continued to live even longer when placed on toilet paper.

Did that "scientific study" really prove anything? Not necessarily, because in its next phase, a random examination of several toilet seats was made for any gonorrhea that had not been put there by the researchers. You will be relieved to know that none was found. So even though this represents an inconclusive experiment, if you ever develop gonorrhea and need an alibi about how you got it, you might refer to this work.

Gonorrhea Vaccine?

There is talk about the possible development of a gonorrhea vaccine in the foreseeable future. If successful, that might well eradicate this disease. But don't hold your breath. Those who anticipate it are probably overly optimistic.

Syphilis—Every Little Breeze Seems to Whisper "Lues"

Syphilis (lues) is a much more serious, but far less common, venereal disease than gonorrhea. It disseminates more vigorously from the point of contact than does gonorrhea. Untreated, years after you contract the infection, syphilis can affect almost any part of the body—the brain, heart, liver; you name it.

Penicillin remains the most effective antibiotic agent against syphilis. However, since the causative organism (*Treponema pallidum*) divides very slowly and penicillin is active only against the dividing forms and not the fully developed ones, a single shot of the regular penicillin such as is given for gonorrhea is not enough. To cure the syphilis, you will either need several such shots over a period of time, or one injection of a slowly absorbed, long-lasting preparation in order to obtain a prolonged level of the antibiotic in the blood. If you are known to be allergic to penicillin, you can be treated with oral tetracycline for fifteen days or erythromycin for thirty days.

Remember, that when you get gonorrhea, there always is the chance that you contracted syphilis at the same time. The amount of penicillin needed to cure gonorrhea will usually, but not always, eradicate syphilis. But if it doesn't, syphilis will continue its insidious spread and become apparent much later. So, if you have been treated for gonorrhea, even successfully, always have your blood checked for syphilis a month or two later—just to be sure.

How reliable are the blood tests for syphilis (VDRL, Wasserman)? If you think you were infected and noticed on your mouth or genitals a suspicious "sore" that cleared without treatment, take care, because the blood test for syphilis may be negative for a few weeks after exposure. Also, if you are completely "innocent" and, in the course of a routine blood test, are told that you have syphilis, don't panic. A widely used test (VDRL) sometimes gives "false positive" results. Hold your ground with the doctor. He will then send the blood for a very specific test which does not lie. Imagine him accusing *you* of having syphilis! (The interesting thing about the false positive test for syphilis is that the disease such a result reflects is usually much more serious than *treated* syphilis.)

KEY FACTS TO REMEMBER

The term "venereal disease" usually conjures up images of gonorrhea and syphilis among the promiscuous. In our society, however, there are many other infections that are of equal or greater importance which can be transmitted sexually. These include genital herpes and chlamydia.

Syphilis and gonorrhea are both curable, if recognized and treated adequately—and in time. Penicillin is the drug of choice for both, but penicillin-resistant gonorrhea organisms are emerging and may present a problem. In such cases there are effective alternative antibiotics.

Only a small percentage of vaginal and penile "discharges" are actually gonorrheal in origin, the majority being due to organisms that mimic this disease.

Syphilis, if unrecognized in its acute form, may then go "underground" for many years, surfacing later in a lethal form. Expert consultation is desirable in those late cases because of the complexities of treatment.

Herpes genital virus is the most common of the sexually transmitted diseases. While not usually serious, it can be life-threatening to the newborn and may also increase the risk of cervical cancer. Pregnant women with this infection should consider Cesarean section. If this is not suggested, a second opinion should be obtained.

Most treatment of herpes genital infection is an attempt to control symptoms. There is no cure or vaccine as yet. Several new treatments hold promise; other older ones have been shown to be ineffective. Whatever treatment is recommended to you, a second opinion is advised.

11

The Heart—Still Our Number 1 Killer

Why This Is the Longest Chapter in the Book

This chapter was written to inform you about the major types of heart disease and your many options both for their prevention and treatment. It is entirely proper for it to be the longest in this book—for two reasons: heart trouble is the number-one killer in our country, and I am a cardiologist.

It's Likely to Kill You

Chances are that when "your number is up" (in many instances, long before it should be) you will die from some disease or disorder related to your heart or arteries. The condition that, statistically speaking, is most likely to do you in is called *arteriosclerosis,* or "hardening of the arteries." There are, of course, other heart nemeses—birth defects, rheumatic fever, infections, spasm of the coronary arteries, and some injury or other, but these are statistically of relatively minor importance as compared to arteriosclerosis.

Your Friends, the Experts

As a result of our great and justifiable preoccupation with vascular disorders, we are swamped by a variety of self-styled experts—the news media, friends, doctors, government, the

119

meat and dairy industries and voluntary agencies—all of whom are full of suggestions, dicta and warnings about what we must do (and avoid) to "prevent" disability and death from heart disease. Their advice focuses currently on control of the "risk factors"—high blood pressure, cigarette smoking, obesity, cholesterol and other dietary constituents, personality characteristics, elevated blood sugar, and the sedentary life. This plethora of theories, some valid, others conjectural, stems from the fact that we have not as yet identified the real, fundamental cause(s) of arteriosclerosis. In this chapter, I will review the status and validity of the more important concepts presently in vogue, and to what extent understanding and acting on them may affect your health and longevity.

The Kind of Heart Disease You're Born With

Infants and children are vulnerable to a special kind of heart trouble resulting from some error in development while still in the womb. Mother may have provoked nature's aberrations if she contracted German measles while pregnant. (She should have gotten herself deliberately exposed to this otherwise harmless, viral infection before she became pregnant, or taken the vaccine which is now available to prevent it. And if she wasn't sure whether she ever had German measles, there is a blood test that could have told her.) If she smoked excessively, drank too much or took some "harmless" medication, her chances of giving birth to a child with such congenital heart disease were increased. The classic example was thalidomide, a very effective sleeping pill widely used in Europe for several years. Children of women taking it were born not only with incompletely formed limbs (the most dramatic and obvious consequence) but also with serious heart deformities.

Some 25,000 children are born each year in the United States with one or more of thirty-five different cardiac defects. Treatment when feasible or necessary, is almost always surgical. If done in time, as many as 15,000 of those lives could be saved. But it is a good idea to get a second opinion from a pediatric cardiologist when an operation is recommended to make sure that it is needed and that the timing is right.

When to Operate, and When to Wait—Alternatives to Surgery

Some malformations of the heart are so severe that unless the infant is operated on immediately, he or she will soon die. (Surgery either corrects the problem, or is only palliative—that is, improves but doesn't cure it.) But some abnormalities are not immediately life-threatening, and it may be better for the repair to be done when the child is older, stronger and better able to withstand major heart surgery. Also, in some types of congenital heart disease, for example, those with a "hole" in the wall between the two ventricles (*ventricular septal defect*), the defect may close spontaneously later on. Even when closure of the "hole" is advised, it can sometimes be done without surgery. In a new technique, a small umbrella-like device, in the closed position, is slipped into the heart by a catheter. When in place at the site of the defect, the "umbrella" is opened, sealing off the hole.

Another congenital heart condition, called *patent ductus arteriosus*, can be cured by medication without surgery. In such cases, the baby is born with a large artery that should have closed off at birth but remains open. The role of this blood vessel during development was to carry blood rich in oxygen from the mother's placenta to the fetus, since the fetus' lungs do not function while it is still in the uterus and so cannot provide oxygen. At birth, when the infant starts breathing the ductus arteriosus begins to close, a process that takes several weeks. If it fails to do so and remains open, the result is a "blue baby." For years, we treated such infants by tying off or cutting this "extra" artery at surgery. One day, someone observed that taking Indocin (a drug used in the treatment of arthritis) actually caused this vessel to contract and close of its own accord. But this therapy works only when started early, a good reason for every newborn baby to be examined carefully at birth. If any suspicious murmur is heard, a pediatric cardiologist should be called in for consultation.

The "Floppy Valve"

There is one very common abnormality of the heart that only fairly recently has been recognized, although it is responsible for a host of symptoms. We think it is present in at least 10 percent of "healthy" women, and probably 6 percent of "normal" men. It is usually suspected when the doctor hears a little click when he listens to the heart with the stethoscope. There may or may not be an accompanying murmur (a sound produced under many different circumstances when blood flows in a turbulent manner through the heart). We used to think that this click and murmur were just a variation of the normal heart sounds and of no significance. But the introduction of cardiac sonography (in which sound waves bounced off heart structures are carefully analyzed) has enabled us to "view" the interior of the heart without actually penetrating it. As a result, we now realize that the click and murmur are the result of one of the heart valves, the mitral valve, closing somewhat abnormally. We are still not sure what causes this condition. It sometimes is present at birth, or it may first be heard only later on. It goes by a variety of names—Barlow's Syndrome, mitral valve prolapse—but the most popular designation is "floppy valve." In the vast majority of cases, such a valve neither interferes with normal heart function, nor reduces life expectancy. In a certain number, however, it is associated with symptoms we used to consider "neurotic" —as, for example, unexplained "atypical" chest pain, palpitations, migraine headaches and fainting for no apparent reason.

The "floppy valve" does not usually require surgery, except in those cases where the distortion is severe and the valve leaks. When it is detected in young women (whom we used to consider "nervous" or "maladjusted," before we identified the disorder), it may cause anxiety about whether or not the "heart condition" will interfere with childbearing. It almost never does. There is, in fact, no reason for you to change your life style in any way, except that you should probably take antibiotics when you are having any dental work or gynecological or urological intervention—there is said to be a risk of the valve becoming infected by bacteria that get into your bloodstream when any of those procedures are performed. In my own practice, I prescribe such antibiotics only when the click is accompanied by a murmur and not usually when the click alone is present.

You might wonder how this mild, mechanical derangement of the heart valve sometimes causes these bizarre symptoms. We are not quite sure, but according to one of the theories, persons so affected may secrete too much of an adrenaline-like substance; this may account for the palpitations, nervousness and chest pain. There may also be an association between the "floppy valve" and body build, migraine headaches later in life, and other congenital heart lesions. Unless your doctor listens very carefully to your heart he may miss the diagnosis and you may go through life unfairly branded a neurotic. (But remember, there are many more real neurotics than there are "floppy valves.")

Hearts Not Easily Broken

A final thought before leaving this brief review of congenital heart disease. The heart has a very special place in our culture and folklore. Even though it is probably the toughest organ in the body, working constantly every moment of our lives, day and night, we still regard it as fragile. And any heart "problem," no matter how trivial, generates great fear and anxiety. Society stigmatizes the "cardiac" as someone not quite like the rest of us. This attitude can be devastating to a child who may have a perfectly innocent heart murmur, but is physically and emotionally overprotected by anxious parents. The result is often severe psychological crippling that dwarfs the consequences of any real physical impairment. I know of many children, now adults, who because of some harmless heart murmur grew up to be emotionally inadequate—cardiac neurotics—due to unwarranted parental anxiety. So, if you have a child with some congenital heart condition, remember that, with today's sophisticated surgical procedures, chances are that he will be able to resume virtually normal activities. And when surgery is not required, follow the medical advice that you are given, and allow your child to live without fear.

Rheumatic Fever—"It Licks the Joints and Bites the Heart"

Hearts normal at birth may become diseased as we go through life—sometimes early on. In adolescents and young adults, the coronary arteries in the heart have not yet significantly narrowed. Therefore, heart attacks are not common in this age group. However, the valves that control the flow of blood in, through and out of the heart are frequently distorted by disease, usually rheumatic fever. The real trouble actually starts much earlier than do the symptoms. It begins in childhood with an acute attack of rheumatic fever, which usually appears as painful joints, "growing pains," or "arthritis," following a history of sore throats. The heart itself may seem not to be affected, but it frequently is. The joints clear up, and the patient is left without any apparent trace of disease. Years later, usually during a routine physical exam, a heart murmur is heard. The first question asked is "Did you ever have rheumatic fever?" You either may not remember that you did or were unaware at the time that it was, in fact, rheumatic fever.

How does rheumatic fever cause the murmur? During the acute attack, the lining of the heart valves becomes inflamed, and as a result gradually develops scar tissue. Instead of moving freely to direct blood flow within the heart, the scarred valves are now rigid and stuck. When they fail to open properly so that blood is prevented from *leaving* a given heart chamber, the condition is called *valvular stenosis*. On the other hand, when the valve leaflets open normally, but do not shut tightly upon closing, blood *leaks back* into a chamber from which it has been squeezed out, a condition called *valvular regurgitation* or *insufficiency*.

Stenosis and insufficiency often occur together in the same valve, or one set of valves may be stenotic and another insufficient. Valve distortion if severe enough strains the heart muscle, which now has to pump harder to get blood across a narrowed opening, or dilate in order to accommodate the extra volume of blood that has leaked back. After years of such malfunction, surgery usually becomes necessary and almost always means replacing the diseased valves with artificial ones. The decision about what kind of operation is needed and when it should be done depends on your symptoms, the results of special diagnostic tests and the response to medical treatment. Such a decision should never be made without consulting at least one experienced cardiologist.

Your doctor decides that you need valve surgery when he sees evidence that the heart is laboring, and that further stress to it may be dangerous and irreversible. That evidence is accumulated in many ways and includes your description of the symptoms, the physical examination, and an array of tests. What you tell the doctor and how he interprets the story are most important. Some of the special procedures done are easy, painless and inexpensive, like the ECG or chest X ray. Others are more costly, uncomfortable and, on occasion, risky. You should know what tests are available to you, the information they yield, and in what sequence they should be done. It is obviously foolish to start with the most complicated, painful, dangerous, and expensive ones before simpler ones have been exhausted.

Diagnostic Cardiac Tests

First there is the *ECG*. You never need to balk at that. It tells the doctor a great deal about how you are doing—whether your heart rhythm is normal, whether it is damaged or getting any bigger as a result of whatever cardiac problem you have, and whether it is under strain.

The *chest X ray* is also informative, because it indicates heart size and shape, as well as evidence of congestion (fluid) in the lungs—proof of heart failure.

You should also know about *echocardiography*, done as easily and painlessly as an ECG. This sonar technique is now highly developed and tells a great deal about how well (or poorly) the valves are functioning, and how the heart muscle is withstanding any stress. An echocardiogram can be done in your cardiologist's office, if he happens to have that piece of equipment, or, more usually, in a hospital laboratory. It does not require your being admitted to the hospital. Unlike cardiac catheterization, it is noninvasive, that is, nothing is introduced or injected into the heart.

The newest method of evaluating heart, and more specifically, valve function, is the radionuclide cineangiogram (RNCA). Like echocardiography, this test does not involve "breaking and entering,' as far as your body is concerned. Nor does it require your checking into a hospital. You simply go to a laboratory for about an hour. You are given a tiny tracer dose intravenously of a short-lived radioactive substance (usually technetium) which goes to the heart. A computerized gamma camera, in effect a big Geiger counter, is swung over your chest, and the activity of the radioactive particles in the heart is monitored at rest and after exercise. This provides additional useful information about valve function, and to what extent its distortion is hurting your heart.

Cardiac Catheterization

The initial non-invasive evaluation may now indicate the need to proceed with *cardiac catheterization*. That often but not necessarily means that "it looks like go" as far as surgery is concerned, and that the doctors, especially the surgeons, require more detailed information about the interior of the heart and its functioning. Cardiac catheterization is done in the hospital. Usually, you come in the night before, and leave the day after the test. The procedure involves the passage of a thin tube (catheter) into one of your veins or arteries (depending on which side of the heart is being studied—veins go to the right side, the arteries to the left), and threading it up into the heart. Its progress is followed by a fluoroscope. None of this requires general anesthesia. The only discomfort you have is when the skin is broken to introduce the catheter and that is well taken care of by just freezing the area with novocaine. Once in the heart, the catheter records the pressures on either side of the diseased valve, and measures oxygen content and blood flow, thus gauging the severity of the disorder. When these data are obtained, iodinated dye is then injected through a catheter into the heart. We follow the passage of the opaque material and identify the size and thickness of the various cardiac chambers. If this study is done on a patient over fifty years of age, and there is the possibility of subsequent valve surgery, we will also, for good measure, take a look at your coronary arteries to see whether they are narrowed. If they are, they must be fixed first in order to minimize the risk of the more difficult valve operation, which is done at the same sitting.

The Risk Is Minimal—In Good Hands

Many thousands of cardiac catheterizations are done every year, and are rarely associated with complications. But occasionally an accident does occur, usually clot formation, or *embolus*. In addition to that, the procedure is expensive, time-consuming (about one to one and a half hours on the table, plus two hospital days) and can be uncomfortable. So it is better to get as much information from the noninvasive techniques first. When cardiac catheterization is advised, asking for a second opinion to see whether the other tests have provided enough data is not unreasonable.

When to Operate and When to Wait

Suppose that after the "workup," the diagnosis of valve disease is confirmed and you are told you need an operation. Your options now depend to a great extent on your symptoms. You can tell, however, that an operation should be done if you are becoming increasingly short of breath after less and less exertion. That is an indication that your heart muscle is weakening and cannot expel all the blood returning to it. The extra volume of blood that cannot be squeezed out by the failing heart then backs up into the lungs, leaving you breathless. When that happens, surgery is in the cards sooner than later. But you can buy some time with medications that decongest the lungs (water pills), strengthen the contraction of the heart (digitalis), or reduce its work load (Apresoline, nitroglycerin derivatives). I have had many patients who continued for several years this way, delaying operation, during which time their condition remained stable, and surgical technology and operative statistics improved considerably. In any event, don't rush into surgery before consulting another cardiologist.

Why Prosthetic Valves Need Careful Watching

My personal philosophy about almost any heart surgery is that the longer you can delay it *safely,* the better-off you are—provided that a reasonable quality of life can be maintained. You might well ask, "Why not replace the valve at the earliest sign of trouble?" First, there are the risks inherent in any operation—risks that are constantly decreasing as newer techniques in anesthesia and better artificial valves are developed. For example, patients undergoing valve replacement in the 1980s are being given prostheses with fewer long-term complications than those operated in the 1960s. Also, the artificial valve, although it corrects the abnormality of flow within the heart, requires lifelong care and supervision and is itself vulnerable to disruption or infection.

Most such devices demand indefinite anticoagulation ("thinning") in order to prevent little clots from forming on their surfaces. These can break off and travel to different parts of the body—the brain, for example, where they cause strokes. When your blood is being thinned, you must have it tested at least once or twice a month for the rest of your life, because the correct dosage of anticoagulant varies virtually from day to day. It can be affected by other medications you happen to be taking. The amount that was just right last week may now leave your blood too "thin," putting you at risk for an internal hemorrhage somewhere. Or it may not be thin enough, so that you may develop an embolism.

The prosthetic valve like the diseased rheumatic valve it replaced can also become infected. That is something else that you will have to be extremely careful about for the rest of your life. A minor dental procedure, manipulation of the prostate, indeed, any infection that releases bacteria into the bloodstream can result in their settling down on the valve. These infected clumps may then be seeded throughout the body. This condition, called *endocarditis,* is often difficult to control once it sets in and may require a second operation to replace the artificial valve. (A diseased valve that has not been surgically treated is also vulnerable to such infection.) Although this is most likely to happen within the first few months after surgery, late infection occurs in about 1 percent of patients per year.

A word here about preventing infection, not only on prosthetic valves, but in "floppy" valves and those diseased by rheumatic fever. I have found a great deal of confusion among patients (and doctors) as to which antibiotic should be given, in what circumstances, in what dosage, and how soon before and after the "event" that is being covered.

Generally speaking, if your valve is vulnerable, you should have antibiotic prophylaxis when you undergo *any* operation. No fever should go undiagnosed and untreated for more than a day or two. Antibiotics should be prescribed for sore throats associated with temperature elevation. If you need catheterization of your urinary bladder for whatever reason, you should be covered with the appropriate antibiotic. As far as dental work is concerned, no matter what problem brings you to the dentist, the moment you open your mouth, there should be an antibiotic aboard. But I find some patients dosing themselves with drugs several days before and after the cleaning and extraction. That's unnecessary and undesirable. All you need is two grams of an oral penicillin preparation like Penicillin V (it comes in ½ gram tablets) thirty minutes to two hours before the procedure, followed by 500 mg. every six hours for about six or eight doses. That's all. If you're allergic to penicillin, use erythromyin— take 500 mg. (the usual tablet is 250 or 500 mg.) ½ to two hours before the dental work, and 500 mg. every six hours for six doses. If you have a prosthetic valve, the antibiotic should preferably be given by injection.

Endocarditis can also disrupt the suture lines that hold the artificial valve in place so that it no longer opens and closes normally. Even in the absence of infection, some artificial valves, especially earlier models, sometimes degenerate or break down. They may soak up fats in the blood, swell and crack. Or, as the blood rushes across the artificial surfaces, the red blood cells disintegrate, releasing their pigment and causing jaundice and anemia.

In short, valve replacement means lifelong vigilance and monitoring. It is not like having your appendix or your gallbladder taken out, after which you are through with it. But despite these potential problems, when you really need to have it done, there is no alternative to a spanking new heart valve. The dire consequences mentioned above happen in only a small number of patients. But the procedure should not be performed before it is necessary. The matter of timing is a delicate and critical one. You must not wait too long, because then the heart may become irreparably strained or damaged. The final judgment is one that must be made by you and your doctor, and you may both want to share that responsibility by asking for another opinion from an experienced cardiologist.

Picking the Surgical Team

Suppose that everyone agrees that you need valve replacement now. There are still some very important options to be exercised. The first is the decision about where the surgery should be done. One of the problems in American medicine today is that so many hospitals vie for prestige. They feel the need to impress boards of trustees, donors and government agencies with their ability to do virtually every sophisticated procedure. Many smaller institutions often have the most modern surgical equipment and an excellent cardiac surgeon or two. But it takes more than one surgeon and a pile of machinery to perform successful heart surgery. It needs an experienced team that consists not only of good surgeons, but also trained nurses, respiration therapists, lab technicians—a team that operates several times a day or week. The expertise of the senior surgeon must be supplemented with experience enhanced by a large volume of cases and a group effort. Some hospitals have better surgical results than others for those very reasons. But you can't go on statistics alone. A hospital with a superb cardiac surgical team may have higher mortality figures than one less good because it is tackling more difficult, high-risk cases that have been turned down elsewhere. So, once the decision about surgery has been made, ask around before you decide where to have it done.

An Alternative to Valve Replacement

There are other options of which you should be aware, and one relates to the kind of surgery that will be done. For example, consider repair of the mitral valve. If you are young and the valve is not yet hardened and rigid due to deposition of calcium, it may not have to be replaced at all. Instead, the surgeon cuts into the valve, freeing the leaflets and enlarging the opening. This is called a *commissurotomy*. It takes less time, is less hazardous than replacing the valve and (except in special circumstances) does not require subsequent anticoagulation—three very important advantages. Several of my patients have had this procedure done, some as long as fifteen years ago, and are still fine. In others, the valve cusps became stuck again and needed replacement, usually some five to ten years later.

Of Homografts and Heterografts

If the diseased valve cannot be repaired as described above, it is cut away and replaced, usually with an artificial device. Such prosthetic man-made valves work very well in most cases, but usually require anticoagulation for reasons discussed earlier. In recent years, we have been using heterograft valves made from pig (porcine) or cow (bovine) tissue as well as homografts from other parts of your own body. Although these have the advantage of not requiring permanent anticoagulation, we are not entirely sure about their long-term durability. But, if you are about to undergo valve replacement and for some reason cannot take anticoagulants, ask about these newer techniques.

Diseased Heart Valves and Pregnant Women

An important question often raised by young women with rheumatic valvular disease is whether it's safe for them to have a baby. The gynecologist may be either too conservative or not cautious enough in his advice. This decision should always be made in consultation with a cardiologist, regardless of how the gynecologist rules. We have come a long way in the medical (and surgical) management of rheumatic heart disease, so that today many women so affected may safely give birth.

Hardening of the Arteries—Anywhere in the Body

We now come to the major problem of vascular disease—*arteriosclerosis* (or "hardening" of the arteries)—which, though declining in incidence in the last few years, still causes almost a million deaths every year in the United States alone. Before middle age, it is mainly an affliction of men, but when women reach the menopause, the two sexes are affected in approximately equal measure. Wherever this disorder occurs, the affected artery is narrowed by plaques along its lining. These are rich in cholesterol, calcium and other fats. They become progressively larger until complete occlusion of the vessel takes place. In a smaller number of cases, blockage follows spasm of the artery or bleeding into one of the plaques.

When the coronary arteries are involved, the result is a heart attack; when it takes place in the blood vessels of the brain, it produces a stroke; it causes kidney disease when it strikes the renal arteries; aneurysms of the aorta and vascular disease of the extremities result from involvement of those blood vessels; and blindness is often the consequence of hemorrhage from the arteries in the eyes.

The two major theories about arteriosclerosis are (a) hardening of the arteries, like fever, is a manifestation of many disorders. This accounts for its affecting different arteries with varying rates of progression and severity, so that some patients live with it for years while others die quickly; and (b) it is, in fact, only one disease due to several contributing causes. Whichever of these two theories is correct, your vulnerability, as you will see, depends on several factors.

Suppose that you were to consult me because one or both of your parents had died young (before the age of sixty) from heart attacks. So did various aunts and uncles, and perhaps one or two grandparents. You have been reading all about the prevention of heart attacks. You feel perfectly well, but want to know how you can avoid the premature heart disease that runs in your family. The following pages contain my advice based on current knowledge and opinion.

Where There's Smoke, There's Heart Disease

I will first ask whether or not you smoke cigarettes, how many and for how long you have been doing so. If you use more than ten cigarettes per day you are at a major disadvantage right off the bat. As a practicing cardiologist, I see so many patients who suffer heart attacks in the prime of life. Many of them have a "good" family history, their cholesterol level is normal, they are not overweight, they exercise, and their blood pressure is "perfect". But, alas, they smoke cigarettes rather heavily. So let's consider that risk factor first.

I could write a short monograph about all the excuses people make in order to continue smoking. "But, Doctor, I don't really inhale." (Nonsense, everyone inhales.) "Cigarettes are not bad for *me*. I only smoke them halfway down." (That's still bad because a half is worse than none.) "What you're telling me doesn't apply to my brand of cigarettes, because they are very low in tar and resin, and have a marvelous filter." (A cigarette is a cigarette is a cigarette.) "If I stop smoking, I'll get as big as a house. Wouldn't that be worse for me than cigarettes?" (If one has to choose between two hazards, overweight, in my opinion, is preferable to and less dangerous than cigarette smoking.) "But a cigarette relaxes me so much. Isn't nervous tension more dangerous than tobacco?" (Decidedly not.) "Okay, I'll stop using cigarettes, but I'd like to smoke a pipe or cigars because I hear they're pretty safe." (Less dangerous, but not "safe," and it would depend on how many you smoked anyway.)

How Cigarettes Nail the Coffin

After we dispose of all these excuses, the reluctant patient petulantly demands to know exactly why and how cigarette smoking is dangerous. Regardless of the mechanism(s) (which we don't fully understand), cigarette smokers have been shown to be at fifteen times greater risk of developing heart attacks than nonsmokers, especially when this habit is associated with high blood pressure and an elevated cholesterol level. (And, by the way, it will probably give you an early menopause as well.)

There are several theories about how tobacco does you in. Experiments in humans and animals have shown that when cigarette smoke is inhaled, blood vessels in various parts of the body constrict, presumably because of the nicotine. When such spasm affects the coronary arteries, the blood supply to the heart muscle is reduced. If these vessels have already been somewhat narrowed by arteriosclerosis, this additional constriction can be critical. Or, perhaps, cigarette smoke releases a substance that promotes clotting of the blood within the arteries. Also, smokers generally have higher cholesterol levels than do nonsmokers. Persons who have an irregular heartbeat often tell me that their palpitations are worse when they smoke. (Remember that sudden death may occur when the rhythm of the heart becomes abruptly disordered, even if the coronary arteries are not completely blocked.) As you puff away, the increased concentration of carbon monoxide inhaled makes less oxygen available to the heart. This too may play a role over a period of time in the causation of angina and arteriosclerosis. Finally, a fascinating piece of work was recently reported from Denmark. One scientist there postulated that women who continue to smoke heavily during pregnancy may predispose their children to arteriosclerosis at an early age. He analyzed the umbilical arteries in infants of such mothers after birth, and found evidence of severe damage to the vessel walls. It may be that this kind of injury also occurs in other blood vessels in the fetal heart or brain and lays the groundwork for premature arteriosclerosis in adult life.

Whatever the underlying mechanism, most doctors are convinced that cigarette smoking does increase your vulnerability to heart attack, and significantly so. When your doctor insists that you stop (even if he can't kick the habit himself), don't bother looking for another opinion.

If you need any further inducement to stop smoking, let me remind you that cigarettes are also believed to be an important cause of lung cancer and the aggravation of stomach ulcers. They may also have an adverse effect on the unborn child when used during pregnancy.

Why You Don't Stop

They may play dumb, but most people know very well that smoking is hazardous. It is written right there on every package, where the Surgeon General reminds them about it every time they light up. So why don't they stop? Why, indeed, doesn't the very same doctor who pleads with you to break the habit always follow his own advice? Why do even some patients who have had heart attacks or lung disease continue to smoke?

The Cigarette Addict

The answer to all these questions is that cigarette smoking is more than a bad habit—it is an addiction. I believe people who tell me that they can't sleep, feel nervous, are depressed, suffer from headaches and eat compulsively, when they try to quit smoking. These classic symptoms of nicotine withdrawal are much milder in light smokers than in heavy users.

Is Any Cigarette "Safe"?

Smokers are always searching for the "safe cigarette", one they can smoke with impunity. The ads emphasizing less tar and nicotine are meant to assuage the fear guilt and anxiety of the tobacco addict. But serious doubts have been raised whether these cigarettes are in fact less harmful. It had long been suspected that given a weed with less nicotine, the addict will puff it more frequently, smoke it down to a shorter butt, and light up more often than he would the high-nicotine brand. In other words, he needs a certain daily "fix," or quota, of nicotine, and if the cigarette he smokes contains less, he simply puffs more and smokes more in order to meet that requirement. Furthermore, he also inhales more deeply and retains the smoke in his lungs for a longer time. (Nicotine in the smoke is transferred from the lungs into the bloodstream to be delivered to the heart, brain, and other blood vessels.) In order to determine whether or not this was so, the Medical Research Council in Britain undertook a scientific study of cigarette smokers and their habits. The results, reported in November 1981 reaffirmed the suspicion that the "weaker" the cigarette, the more it was smoked, and the more you smoke, the more carbon monoxide you inhale.

Some scientists believe the carbon monoxide to be the most harmful substance in cigarettes; not tar, resin or nicotine.

Cardiac patients driving cars on congested freeways, or guards working in heavily trafficked tunnels, have decreased exercise tolerance, presumably because of the increased carbon monoxide to which they are exposed. So, in the long run, you may be doing yourself more harm with these "safer" cigarettes.

Pipe tobacco and cigars do contain less tar and nicotine, but they actually give you more carbon monoxide, because of the manner in which the smoke is delivered to your lungs from the bowl of the pipe or the leaf of the cigar. Also, when a cigarette smoker switches to pipes and cigars (whose main "benefit" is that he inhales them somewhat less), the smoking technique to which he became accustomed when he used cigarettes leads him to inhale the pipe and cigar smoke very much as he did the cigarette smoke.

The sum and substance of this focus on the dangers of carbon monoxide is the suggestion that perhaps heavy smokers should substitute nicotine tablets or chewing tobacco for cigarettes, thus eliminating consumption of carbon monoxide. But there is little consolation even in this alternative. Areas of the country where tobacco is chewed have a dramatically higher incidence of cancer of the mouth, throat and pharynx.

Cold Turkey Is Best

If you have decided to quit cigarettes, it is probably better to do so abruptly—cold turkey—than to taper (although SmokeEnders reports considerable success with gradual withdrawal). Sudden cessation may leave you temporarily with more intense symptoms of nicotine deprivation, but then in a matter of days, if you can hold out, you are through with it. You may continue to yearn for a weed now and then, especially after a heavy meal, but you can handle that. On the other hand, when you "cut down," rather than quit, and reduce your nicotine intake but don't eliminate it, the result is chronic withdrawal, and ultimate return to the habit. I know very few heavy smokers who have cut down their cigarettes to just a few a day for any length of time.

The Risk of Hypertension

Tobacco, then, is a key risk factor for arteriosclerosis. High blood pressure, which is also the most important cause of strokes is another. We could probably reduce heart attacks by at least 30 percent if everyone in America stopped smoking and had a normal blood pressure. *In my opinion, hypertension of any degree, from mild to severe, should always be treated and normalized.* Weight reduction, regular exercise, and decreased salt intake are all important in managing elevated pressure, but quite frankly, what it almost always boils down to in the end is medication. Since this involves a lifelong commitment, it should never be made casually. Make certain that the diagnosis is based on several recordings taken over a three- or four-week period. And after you have started the medication, if you find that it gives you unpleasant side effects, don't just stop taking it. Your doctor has enough alternative agents at his disposal with which to normalize your blood pressure in a tolerable manner. If he doesn't seem to be able to do so, get a second opinion from someone specializing in the treatment of hypertension.

The Great Preoccupation

Let's get back to the hypothetical subject with a strong family history of premature arteriosclerosis. He will listen politely to the cigarette and hypertension data, but for some reason, what really moves him is his cholesterol level. The Western world, particularly Americans, is totally preoccupied with blood fats and diet. The other day, I sent a man to the hospital with an acute heart attack. Hovering between life and death, he was concerned about two things only: when he would move his bowels, and his cholesterol level.

The world is full of cholesterol "authorities," each with his own theory about its role in the causation of arteriosclerosis. Every doctor has his own opinion and offers his own brand of advice on whether to avoid eggs like the plague, eat them at will, or simply be "prudent" and consume them in moderation. So do I, but instead of telling you what I think, let me first present the available data to you objectively and let you decide whether or not cholesterol is a precipitating or a causative factor.

Pasta, People and Populations

It is a fact that many people with high cholesterol attain old age without significant arteriosclerosis. The converse is also true. Individuals with normal or even low levels may suffer from this condition. Among the patients with heart disease I see every day, cholesterol levels seem to bear little if any relation to their *individual* dietary habits. For example, a person who eats lots of pasta, cheese, butter, eggs and other such foods (anathema to the cholesterol purist) may not have any more cholesterol in his blood than someone who follows a more "prudent" diet. This may reflect the fact that two thirds of our cholesterol is manufactured in the body regardless of diet, and only one third is derived from what we eat. As proof of this observation, a study was recently reported in which 116 healthy men with normal cholesterol levels were fed either one or two eggs every day for three months. At the end of that time, there was no significant change in the cholesterol levels of those who either had one egg daily or two. Yet, among *populations,* as opposed to individuals, cholesterol levels *do* appear to reflect eating habits. What's more, the higher that level, the greater the statistical association between arteriosclerosis and heart disease.

Cholesterol—The Other Viewpoint

There are some very distinguished scientists (not all of whom are representatives of the dairy, egg and cattle industries) who believe that the alleged hazards of cholesterol and the benefits of lowering it are pure eyewash. Their reasoning goes something like this. The high cholesterol in the blood of those who have heart disease is but a *symptom* of some underlying disorder. The real cause of arteriosclerosis is not known. When the plaques begin to form in the arteries early in life, they do *not* contain cholesterol. Even later, when hardened, fully formed and already narrowing the arterial wall, only 50 percent of these plaques have cholesterol in them. Also, there are two noncardiac conditions—one in the kidney and the other in the thyroid—that are associated with very high cholesterol levels. Yet patients with these disorders do not have more coronary-artery disease than does the "normal" population. (But, of course, under those particular circumstances the elevated cholesterol has not been there for forty or fifty years.) They also point out that in all the trials in which cholesterol has been lowered either by diet or by drugs, there has been no significant impact on the number of heart attacks or the incidence of death. In some cultures, where very little fat is eaten, there is no less heart disease than where fat consumption is high. How do these critics explain the fact that experimental animals that are fed massive amounts of butter develop "lesions" in their arteries? Simple, they say. Such "unnatural" changes in the arterial wall are different from the plaques of arteriosclerosis that cause all the trouble.

The "anti-anticholesterol" buffs conclude by warning against tampering with cholesterol levels especially with drugs. They point out, for example, that clofibrate, a drug that lowers the amount of cholesterol in your body, may give you cholesterol gallstones. Changing the composition of the bile in any way, they believe, may also account for the higher incidence of cancer deaths in some studies where cholesterol was lowered by drugs. They even attack the excessive use of polyunsaturated fats, the basis of all good cholesterol-lowering regimens. In their opinion, these substances may damage the lining of the arterial wall and have an effect quite the opposite from what was intended. In fact, Israel, which has a very high ratio of unsaturated to saturated fats in its diet, nevertheless has an impressive incidence of coronary disease.

Another argument they use is the as yet preliminary report by an international team of researchers from the National Cancer Institute, Massachusetts Institute of Technology, other American and Canadian facilities and the Chinese Academy of Medical Sciences in which these "protective" polyunsaturated fats increased the risk of breast and bowel cancer in animals. Given the choice, most people would prefer a nice mild heart attack to even a "touch" of cancer. As I look at the data, it seems to me that suspicion falls on *all* fat, not only the polyunsaturates.

There is current interest in the possible relationship between *too low* a cholesterol level and cancer. So much so that the National Heart, Lung and Blood Institute, an arm of the U. S. Government, has cautioned Americans against reducing those levels below 185 mg.%. So many of my patients returning from the Pritikin and similar clinics are delighted with values of 140 or 150. I just wonder, in view of all the doubts, how wise or beneficial so great a drop really is.

If Not Cholesterol, What Is the Culprit?

What then do the "nonbelievers" of the cholesterol theory think *is* the cause of arteriosclerosis? They feel that the plaques form in the arterial wall, at the site of some prior injury caused by any one of a number of possible factors, including increased blood pressure, infection (perhaps some virus early in life), an abnormal immune response, or abnormal architecture or angulation of the particular artery involved.

So Whom Should You Believe—and What Should You Do?

How should one react to this controversy in practical terms? I suggest, pending the accumulation of more data, that you follow the middle road between compulsive avoidance of *any* food containing cholesterol and complete reckless abandon. If you are healthy, have a normal cholesterol level (220 mg. percent or less), and do not have a bad family history, there is no need to change your eating habits. With a cholesterol that low, you (or your body) must be doing something right.

But if you are *under* sixty-five, with a cholesterol level above 220 mg. percent, and there has been a lot of heart disease in the family, you should follow a "prudent" diet. That means cutting down on your consumption of butter, cheese and other dairy products, and limiting your intake of eggs to four a week, or less. In addition beef should be replaced by chicken, veal and fish, and all visible fat should be avoided.

Above sixty-five years, regardless of whether you have heart disease, paying homage to the cholesterol hypothesis is, in my opinion, futile—too little and too late to have any significant impact on the disease or its prevention. And so, I permit such patients to eat whatever they like, as long as they maintain a good weight.

I am not sure how important any of this dietary advice really is, but it does have some psychological impact. Together with weight reduction and exercise, it helps to allay patients' anxieties, makes them feel that they are at least doing *something* to reduce their vulnerability to heart attack— and maybe they are.

Should You Bother Measuring Your Triglyceride Level?

I do not believe that triglycerides, another blood fat, constitute an independent risk factor for arteriosclerosis. When they are elevated, it is often in conjunction with some other abnormal finding like a high blood sugar. If your triglyceride level is being checked, make sure that the blood sample is taken only after you have been fasting (had nothing to eat or drink except black coffee, tea without milk or sugar, or water) for at least fourteen hours. So many patients come to me worried about a high triglyceride detected in a screening survey. When repeated after appropriate fasting, it is often found to be normal.

Triglyceride levels may be useful in determining the *kind* of blood-fat abnormality you have. For example, when the cholesterol is high, its dietary management depends to some extent on whether the triglycerides are normal or elevated. If the cholesterol and triglycerides are both up, it is more important to restrict carbohydrate intake than to limit cholesterol and fats. But when the triglycerides are normal, and the cholesterol high, we do limit cholesterol and fat intake.

Good Guys (HDL) and Bad Guys (LDL)

More recently, we've been measuring the *lipoproteins* in the blood, as well as the cholesterol level. Since fat and water don't mix, in order for the fatty cholesterol to circulate in solution or dissolve in the watery bloodstream, it must be "transported." The "vehicle" which attaches itself to the cholesterol molecule and does the "carrying" is a lipoprotein (*lipo* means "fat") made in the liver and intestine.

Lipoproteins vary. We divide them into three kinds—high-density lipoproteins (HDL), low-density lipoproteins (LDL) and very-low-density lipoproteins (VLDL)—according to their chemical weights and composition. Now try to visualize the many cholesterol molecules in the bloodstream, each being dragged around by its own lipoprotein. It seems that the *kind* of lipoproteins you have, and their amounts, may be more important than the cholesterol level itself. The more HDL you have, the better off you are. But LDL and VLDL are bad news. The reason for the difference is related to how the wall of the artery responds to the lipoprotein. When HDL, carrying its cholesterol load, approaches the arterial wall, it is turned away. Cholesterol circulating in the bloodstream doesn't do you any harm—only when it is absorbed into the wall of the artery may it eventually cause arteriosclerosis. Since HDL-attached cholesterol is not sucked in by the artery wall but remains in solution, it presumably is less of a threat. In addition to being rejected by the lining of the artery, the HDL is also thought to attract cholesterol already in the wall, sucking it out—a sort of chemical Roto-rooter.

The same cholesterol molecules, however, when transported by the LDL or VLDL proteins get deposited into the blood-vessel wall. As more and more of them settle there, the artery becomes progressively narrower and may finally close.

Several epidemiological studies, including the famous one at Framingham, Massachusetts, seem to support the theory that the most important thing about lipids is the manner in which they are transported, and that persons with a high HDL content are at reduced risk for developing premature coronary disease. That is why HDL blood levels are now done routinely by many doctors.

Research is currently directed toward finding some medication that will increase the HDL concentration, thereby keeping the cholesterol out of the arterial wall and removing that already in it. Oversimplified, but that basically is where it's at.

How to Get the HDL Up

Although we don't, as yet, have a drug that elevates the HDL, there are other ways to increase your HDL level. For example, stop smoking; cigarettes lower HDL. Exercising and losing excess weight raise the HDL. So do fish, garlic, brewer's yeast and lecithin. (It is interesting in how many "primitive" cultures garlic is intuitively thought to be beneficial.) Absolute teetotalers have a somewhat higher incidence of heart disease than the social drinker who takes one or two drinks a day. It seems that alcohol, in moderation—a couple of drinks a day—raises the HDL. (But if you are a reformed alcoholic and have had a lot of trouble getting and staying on the wagon, don't throw it all away just to elevate your HDL. That is still only a hypothesis. Alcoholism is a fact.)

And so it turns out, at least in terms of HDL, that all the things we knew were bad for us over the years, like emotional stress, physical inactivity, obesity, cigarette smoking and the like, all lower the HDL. Good clean living, with lots of exercise, lean weight and drinking in moderation help get the HDL up.

The Cholesterol–HDL Ratio

Despite the fact that HDL concentration may be more important than cholesterol level, analyzing both values together is probably more revealing than either alone. When we calculate the cholesterol–HDL ratio, the lower the value, the smaller the statistical risk. Below 4½–1, you are in good shape; between 7– and 9–1, you are at twice the risk of having a heart attack; a ratio greater than 13–1 triples the chances.

Pritikin's Program

A few years ago there appeared in the lay press glowing reports of "miracles" being wrought by the "Pritikin Regimen" —a diet tough to follow for any length of time coupled with a substantial daily walk. This program is now being administered in "live-in" centers throughout the country, and, in addition, thousands of patients with heart disease (or a vulnerability to it) are following the regimen on their own. If you choose to go to a Pritikin Center (there are now several operating throughout the country), you'll sign up for a three to four week program (at a cost of about $5,000). You will be put on a stringent low-fat (5 percent to 10 percent of daily intake), low-cholesterol diet (no more than 100 *milligrams* per day), consisting basically of complex carbohydrates. These are, for the most part, whole grains, fruits and vegetables. Processed or refined foods are taboo. Within the permissible categories, you can eat as much as you want. Tobacco, alcohol (haven't they heard about HDL?) coffee and tea are forbidden.

You will use no sugar and only tiny amounts of salt. When packing your bags for the trip, you might just as well leave all your vitamin and mineral supplements at home. They are considered "no-nos" by Mr. Pritikin.

You will also walk at least 30 to 60 minutes twice a day.

Soon after Pritikin began getting publicity, a few of my patients enlisted in his program. They returned reporting much less angina, normalization of previously high blood pressure without the use of drugs, significant lowering of cholesterol and triglyceride levels, weight loss (usually 12 to 15 pounds) and, among the diabetics, reduction of their blood sugar levels to the point when insulin was sometimes no longer required. Patients who hadn't been able to get "from here to the door" without chest pain were now able to walk five and more miles a day. And age was apparently no barrier. People in their eighties, some of them "too far gone" to have heart surgery, were coming back "rejuvenated."

I asked among my colleagues whether they too had heard such reports, and what they thought of them. Very few knew anything about Pritikin and most of those who did said it was just "ballyhoo." Formal comment from the medical "establishment" was also negative.

At this point I decided to visit Mr. Nathan Pritikin myself, accompanied by an experienced nutritionist. I found him to be personally engaging. He is not a physician, but he obviously knows a lot about nutrition. He can very effectively motivate his audience. I interviewed several patients, examined their records, which were made available to me, and I left impressed with what was being done. Most of the "guests" with whom I spoke assured me that they did, in fact, feel better since starting the program. The majority had lost weight; high sugar levels did come down; elevated blood pressures were frequently reduced if not normalized, without medication. It was clear to me that many of Pritikin's claims, even if not statistically documented, were apparently justified at least over the short term. Stress tests done after the regimen was completed did reveal improved conditioning, so that patients were able to perform an increased work load before attaining a given heart rate. I could not, however, substantiate any objective electrocardiographic evidence of improved coronary blood flow. Despite that, patients were able to walk further, and with less pain. When the main problem lay in narrowed arteries in the legs, discomfort in the calf muscles induced by exertion seemed also to be lessened.

So, while there is no hard evidence yet that the Pritikin regimen does prolong life or cause regression of arteriosclerotic plaques, most of the patients who follow it feel better for a while, at least.

I have now had several years in which to make some kind of assessment of Pritikin's technique among my own patients. Several conclusions seem justified. First, his method does not harm. What can be bad about cutting out cigarettes, losing weight, going for long walks, avoiding salt and sugar, eating lots of fresh vegetables together with some chicken and fish? But here's the other side of the coin. Not many people, at least in my experience, will adhere to this regimen indefinitely. The spirit is willing but the flesh is weak. Usually after a few months, most patients begin to "cheat" a little, then a little more, and soon are back to their old eating habits. But some do not, and the majority, I have found, end up in the middle-road, and that boils down to the "prudent" diet that most doctors and the American Heart Association advised in the first place. And here's an interesting follow-up on that. In a recent Canadian study, evaluating the long-term benefits of the Pritikin program as compared to that recommended by the American Heart Association, there was no significant difference! In all fairness to him, Pritikin rejects these findings on the grounds that the investigators never consulted him as to how his program should *really* be carried out.

So, I encourage any patient to follow this program only if he or she can make a lifelong commitment to it. Three or four weeks of it or any fitness and diet program are not going to make any real impact.

What Makes Sammy Jog?

Whether modifying risk factors other than hypertension, tobacco and abnormal blood fats will have an impact on arteriosclerosis, is more controversial. Consider exercise.

Hundreds of thousands of people are into jogging, running and exercising in other ways. What is particularly good about it is that many have also stopped smoking, have lost weight and have had their blood pressures checked. Believe me, jogging with a cigarette hanging out of your mouth isn't going to help you much. In fact, one study showed that in men who smoke heavily and exercise vigorously, there is a substantial risk of developing a heart attack during the workout; even among those under 35 years of age.

I believe exercise is the best tranquilizer there is, even though its impact on the prevention of arteriosclerosis and heart attacks remains to be shown. Young people who enjoy jogging should certainly do so, if they have no orthopedic problems (muggings and traffic accidents en route are another matter).

Young women, classically immune from the ravages of arteriosclerosis, may, however, find that the athletic life can result in menstrual irregularities and even failure to menstruate. This is particularly true in those who become lean and "hard," with loss of body fat due to their excellent physical condition. Nature seems to think that potential mothers need a certain amount of fat to nourish the fetus and to make lactation possible. When the female athlete loses this store of energy, she may also lose the ability to conceive—sort of a protective act on behalf of the unborn child. So if you're exercising vigorously, feeling great, but can't conceive, before submitting to a complicated hormonal work-up, remind your doctor about your physical activity program.

There's nothing to match the feeling of a good workout, regardless of whether it will prevent heart attacks some time in the distant future. Mind you, there are some data indicating that the physically fit withstand a heart attack or major surgery better than those who are not. Also when hundreds of Harvard graduates were asked about their exercise habits years after graduation, those who were dedicated to ongoing, *very* rigorous, regular workouts, without lapse or respite, year after year, did show definite protection against heart attacks. But the level of exercise required was so strenuous that it precluded its performance on a sustained basis by more than a small fraction of the population, at least in my opinion.

A Normal ECG Is No Guarantee

So, exercise is great for the young. What about "healthy" middle-aged people? Again, I think that, if it makes you feel better, you should do it. However, never start on such a program without seeing your doctor and getting clearance, based not on a superficial examination and a normal ECG, but on a thorough history, physical evaluation, and a treadmill (or other equivalent) stress test. As many as 75 percent of people with *underlying heart trouble* have normal electrocardiograms taken at rest. (That is why insurance companies require a stress test when you apply for a particularly large policy.) Only when the tracing is taken *during* and *after* exercise can the presence of coronary-artery disease be excluded, and even then it is not foolproof.

After you obtain such clearance, you may begin to exercise, but always follow these cardinal rules. Start at a low level and increase it gradually to whatever goal you have in mind. You must commit yourself to doing it routinely at least forty minutes a day three times a week. Should your program be interrupted for any reason for longer than two weeks, you must start again at a lower level.

From time to time, joggers drop dead on the run. Sometimes they are young, more often they are middle-aged. Most had previously been given a clean bill of health. When their hearts are examined at autopsy, the majority are found to have some form of heart disease, occasionally congenital, that was undetected during life. Rarely, the victims' hearts appear normal, the precise cause of death is never really established and is assumed to have been caused by sudden coronary artery spasm or electrical instability of the cardiac muscle. Now and then we find that the muscle fibers that sometimes normally surround a coronary artery have become thickened, thereby constricting and occluding it. Although about one in four of us have these muscle bridges, it is believed that in about one of two hundred the bridge can constrict dangerously (that's 0.5 percent of the total population). The danger of sudden death in this group, however, may be reduced if you keep your heart rate below 150 beats per minute while exercising.

Can Fat Be Healthy?

Obesity is considered a minor risk factor for arteriosclerosis. Your "optimal" weight can be found in the life-insurance tables, but a rule of thumb that I find handy is that a man should weigh approximately 115 pounds, plus five pounds for every additional inch over five feet. This formula is not quite applicable to women, partly because of differences in bone size and structure, and partly for cosmetic and cultural reasons. For example, my wife who is 5'8" tall weighs a "perfect" 122 pounds. Can you imagine her reaction if I were to tell her her optimal weight by my table?

Can You Ever Resign from Type-A Membership?

Your *personality type* may also be important in determining vulnerability to coronary disease. Persons who are tense, aggressive, time conscious, always working on a tight schedule—in short, those who make the world go round (or think they do)—the so-called Type A's, are said to have more arteriosclerotic heart disease than do the easygoing, more placid and contented Type B's. I'm not sure that psychiatric intervention can change one's basic personality, although after suffering a heart attack some people do make substantial adjustments in their life style (at least overtly).

Welcome to the Coronary Club

Let's assume that you have done what you could to prevent or delay heart disease and were unsuccessful. You have become a "cardiac." Usually it happens like this. You are perfectly well until one day, while rushing home in the evening, running to get the bus some cold morning, or in the setting of a severe emotional reaction, you experience a sense of oppression, tightness or pressure in the center of the chest. It lasts only a moment or two. Most people ignore it at first, and the symptom may not bother you again for days, weeks or months. But then it recurs, again and again, until you finally come to realize that there is something seriously wrong.

Sooner or later, depending on how willing (or unwilling) you are to face reality, you consult your doctor. Chances are that, on the clinical exam, he will find nothing amiss, and more often than not, your electrocardiogram will also be entirely normal. But if *you* know, deep down, in your "heart of hearts" that all is not well despite reassurance that your complaints are "nothing" because you have a good electrocardiogram, ask for a stress test. Most doctors these days will do it anyway, but some still do not, and so may miss the early diagnosis of heart disease. Persons with angina usually have a diagnostically abnormal electrocardiographic stress test, confirming your intuition and your doctor's suspicion that you have important heart trouble in need of treatment.

You May Die Before You Know It

Although angina is usually due to narrowing of one or more coronary arteries (either by plaques or by spasm), and a heart attack results from their complete obstruction (by the same mechanisms), the time between your first chest pain and your heart attack is entirely unpredictable. My father, who had his first symptoms of coronary artery disease at the age of forty-seven, did not develop a heart attack until he was eighty, and he lived three years after that. Also, even though angina is sometimes the first indication of coronary disease, many patients have a sudden heart attack without any warning, and in many cases, sudden, instantaneous death is the first (and last) objective evidence of trouble.

Now That You Have Angina

Once the diagnosis of angina has been made, your doctor will carefully review any contributing risk factors and try to eliminate them. He will bug you about your smoking; if your blood pressure is high, he will reduce it with medications; if you are overweight, he will prescribe an appropriate diet; if your sugar is borderline and your triglycerides and cholesterol are high, he will emphasize weight reduction and a decrease in sugar intake rather than any major restriction of cholesterol; if your cholesterol is high (above 300), and your triglycerides are normal, you will be told how to limit your cholesterol intake.

Should You Be Taking Cholesterol-Lowering Drugs?

There is recent evidence that cholesterol-lowering agents, when combined with a vigorous low-cholesterol diet, may reduce the size of arteriosclerotic plaques in humans and in animals. If this turns out to be really so, it may revolutionize our concept of the prevention and management of this disorder. For that and other reasons, some doctors, in addition to offering dietary advice, still prescribe drugs to "normalize" your blood fats. For many years there was great enthusiasm about clofibrate (marketed as Atromid-S), but I understand that, as a result of several large studies, both in the United States and in Europe, fewer doctors (including me) are now recommending it except in very special circumstances. These studies showed that in patients with heart disease, lowering the cholesterol with Atromid-S seemed not to have any appreciable effect on survival. Neither did the drug protect healthy persons with elevated cholesterols from subsequently developing heart disease. I have already referred to the increased incidence of gallstones in persons taking Atromid-S. Some specialists in the United States still give it to patients with very high cholesterol and triglyceride levels, who are at high risk for heart disease by virtue of other reasons as well, and who have not responded to dietary management. If your doctor prescribes Atromid-S for you, you should discuss with him his reasons for doing so, and ask why he thinks you would benefit from it.

In addition to an increased risk of developing gallstones, here are some other side effects you may expect from Atromid-S: (a) impotence and/or loss of interest in sex; (b) aches and pains in your muscles and joints; (c) skin rash; and (d) occasionally hepatitis. In exchange for that, you will enjoy some decrease in LDL and VLDL, which, as you have seen, are thought to increase the risk of heart disease. Worth it? In most circumstances, my personal view is that it is not.

Should you consider any of the other cholesterol-lowering

drugs? Any second opinion you get on that subject will depend on the philosophy of the doctor you consult. In my own practice, I rarely use any of them except where the cholesterol levels are sky high and the family history of premature heart disease is especially bad. The drugs available for this purpose are Questran and Colestid, nicotinic acid, probucol (marketed as Lorelco), Cytellin, Choloxin and ne-omycin. They all work differently, but have the common goal of rendering your blood fats less abnormal. The first two, *Questran* and *Colestid*, cause increased excretion of choles-terol in the stool. They produce annoying intestinal side effects—notably gas, constipation—so much so that many patients just won't take them as prescribed!

Nicotinic acid lowers cholesterol and triglycerides, and offers the additional bonus of raising the HDL. It's also very inexpensive. Unfortunately, in doses large enough to be effective, it causes profound flushing and itching (which be-come less intense with time) and can raise the blood sugar and uric acid levels (so avoid them if you're diabetic or have gout).

Probucol, the newest addition to the group, has very few side effects, but it lowers the HDL, as well as the cholesterol, and how desirable that is over the long run, I'm not sure. *Cytellin* has been around a long, long time. It goes back to the days when I was a medical student! It simply sits in the stomach and prevents the absorption of any cholesterol you eat. Because it has a mild laxative effect, some doctors prescribe it together with Questran and Colestid, which have a tendency to constipate you. *Choloxin*, a thyroid derivative, is one drug I wouldn't use for lowering cholesterol if I were you. In the large Coronary Drug Project run a few years ago in this country to determine the impact of reducing choles-terol levels in patients who had had heart attacks, this agent was withdrawn from the study because it was associated with an *increased* number of cardiac deaths and heart attacks. Finally, *neomycin* is an antibiotic which, because it is poorly absorbed, sits around in the gut interfering with cholesterol absorption by acting on the bacterial composition of the intestine. It's all right to use if necessary, but not unless your kidneys are working normally.

If you have reservations about taking any of the above, you might simply eat foods, for example, cookies, made with bean gum from the locust tree. Enough of this appetizing snack consumed regularly (and they're going to have to put it in something other than cookies) has been known to drop cholesterol levels by about 20 percent. That's as good and better than most of the pills made for that purpose.

A Life Style for Angina Patients

If you have been told you have angina, try to lead a normal life, especially psychologically. If you are a workaholic, if you get up at the crack of dawn and don't come home until late at night, or if you frequently find yourself in situations of chronic stress, tension and anxiety, try to modify those aspects of your life style. That definitely does not mean retirement, which in my opinion will bring on a heart attack sooner.

Angina and Exercise—A Safe Combination?

Earlier we discussed the role exercise might play in the *prevention* of heart disease. How important is it in someone who already has a "condition"? Remember that heart muscle is supplied by a network of blood vessels which course through it very much like the branches of a tree, and which become narrowed by arteriosclerosis. In *The Complete Medical Exam* I described what we call "collateral circulation," in which new channels open up to take over the job of the diseased ones. When we inject dye into the coronary circulation and take X rays to visualize the blood flow within the heart (angiogram), we can actually see these collaterals.

Many cardiologists recommend exercise to patients with angina in the hope that it will provide a further stimulus to the development of an effective collateral circulation, improve exercise tolerance and, so, create a sense of well-being in patients worried about their future. Indeed, I am more enthusiastic about exercise as a therapeutic than as a preventive measure. Suitable supervised programs are widely available in "cardiopulmonary rehabilitation centers" throughout the country. If your doctor tells you that you have to take it easy because you now have angina and must not engage in any physical exercise, or shouldn't "strain yourself" (whatever that means), he either knows something about your condition that you don't, or he is of the old school. Find out which it is.

The Exercise Prescription

The *kind* of exercise you do, its amount, and whether or not it is supervised by doctors or trained paramedical personnel are all very important considerations if you have heart disease. A workout must be prescribed as carefully as if it were a potent drug. No doctor would ever give you a bottle of "heart pills" (or any medication, for that matter) and tell you to take as many as often as you like. The same should be true of exercise. It must always be done, at least initially, under medical supervision in cardiac patients. The work load and pace selected should be based at least in part on the results of a treadmill or other stress test that indicates the heart rate at which your ECG becomes abnormal, and whether or not any life-threatening disorders of heart rhythm are provoked. Given this information, a safe level of exercise *for you* can be determined. What is good for your friends and neighbors may be too much or too little for you.

Do It in the Right Amount at the Right Place

Make sure that the exercise facility where you work out has the personnel trained to handle any complication or emergency, as well as the necessary equipment to do so (defibrillators, intravenous sets and cardiac drugs). Accidents can and do occur, although fortunately, they are uncommon. (Such treatment and resuscitation capabilities should be available not only in rehabilitation centers, but wherever stress tests are done—including your doctor's office. If you are scheduled for a stress test, don't be shy about asking whether emergency facilities are at hand, with trained personnel.)

Exercise should be enjoyable if you are to remain motivated to continue it for any length of time. Some forms are safer than others. In my own experience, isometric exercises, in which pressure is exerted against an immovable object, raise blood pressure and are not usually well tolerated by patients with angina. I prefer dynamic exercises, such as walking, biking, running or swimming. Remember that such a program, once started, must be continued on a regular basis. *Always begin your exercise with a warm-up period and taper it off as you finish*. Never just get right into it and then stop abruptly. Neither should you take a hot shower afterwards—

a tepid one is safer. There have been deaths reported among persons taking hot showers after vigorous exercise, the deaths presumably caused by a drop in blood pressure.

Jogging in the Park with Your Tailor

I have found that cardiac patients who perform their exercise regularly and conscientiously and become physically fit can increase the level of the work load before any chest pain or electrocardiographic abnormalities are apparent. For example, if at the start of your program, it took a certain amount of effort to raise your heart rate to 110 beats per minute, at which point you experienced chest pain or pressure, after several months of training you may be able to perform far more work before you reach that critical rate.

I am somewhat ambivalent about having my patients with heart disease go jogging. I prefer them to exercise under the supervision of medical personnel, rather than running around the park with their stockbroker, lawyer or tailor. I know there are some doctors and many jogging enthusiasts who will take exception to this attitude, so you decide what is right for you, physically and emotionally.

Even as their risk factors are controlled or eliminated, most patients with angina pectoris will still require medication to minimize their symptoms. Let me tell you what drugs are available, so that, when they are prescribed, you will understand how they work and what side effects if any you may expect.

The Little White Pill Under the Tongue

The hallmark of the patient with angina is nitroglycerin— the little tablet you slip under the tongue either when you expect chest pain or after you have developed it.

There are several noncardiac causes of chest discomfort, which neither you nor your doctor may be able, at least initially, to distinguish from true angina. These include hiatus hernia, chest-wall pain, muscle strain, arthritis in the neck and various neuralgias, ulcers and gallbladder disease, to name but a few. Since nitroglycerin has a specific action against angina, relieving it almost immediately, it is useful in the differentiation of cardiac from noncardiac pain. But you must appreciate that when this drug is, in fact, abolishing your symptoms, it does so within thirty seconds to three minutes. Patients so often tell me that their "nitro" worked, and eliminated all pain in about twenty minutes! Under those circumstances, the credit definitely should not go to the nitroglycerin; the pain likely would have disappeared by itself and was probably not angina to begin with.

Another important factor to remember about nitroglycerin is that it works by dilating the blood vessels—not only within the heart, but elsewhere as well. Thus, when it acts on the cranial arteries, it causes headaches. This is a sign not of drug toxicity but of effect. A couple of aspirin tablets usually afford relief, and, if you can stay with it for a while, the headaches will gradually become less frequent and disappear. If, however, you cannot tolerate the nitroglycerin, ask your doctor for a weaker strength.

Fainting After Nitroglycerin

Since nitroglycerin also dilates the larger arteries, your blood pressure may drop after taking one. If you happen to be standing at the time and the fall in pressure is substantial, you may faint. So, if possible, always sit down before using it.

The life span of most preparations of nitroglycerin is fairly short—between six and twelve months, after which they lose their potency. So, be sure to ask your pharmacist how long he has had the bottle he sells you on his shelf and always check its expiration date. Remember, too, to protect the bottle from light and to keep the reserves not in your pocket, but in your refrigerator.

Nitroglycerine also comes in a paste or ointment which is applied anywhere on the body you find it convenient to do so. Instinctively, however, and for psychological reasons, many patients will apply it on the chest. Nitroglycerin applied there, though messy, has a rapid onset of action and its effect is substantially longer than when taken under the tongue.

The "Nitro" Complex

Finally, and perhaps most important, don't develop a complex about taking nitroglycerin. So many patients think that to take one is to "give in"—an admission of weakness, a stigma of some kind. That is nonsense. Nitroglycerin is good for you when you need it. It is not habit-forming; it does not worsen your disease; you do not become "used" to it or dependent on it. It can, in fact, save your life. Take it as freely as necessary. However, if your chest pain persists after taking three within fifteen minutes, call your doctor. You may be having a heart attack. Also, if your angina begins to come on at rest or during the night, if nitroglycerin is less effective than it used to be, and you are taking many more than formerly, let your doctor know. These symptoms may indicate that one or more coronary arteries are closing off faster than your collaterals are opening up.

When Longer Action Is Needed

Unfortunately, the effects of a nitroglycerin tablet persist for only twenty or thirty minutes. When pain recurs chronically during the day, other longer-acting drugs are required. Some are related to nitroglycerin; others are not.

The mainstays among the antianginal preparations in the nitroglycerin family are the nitrates, derived from nitroglycerin. They are marketed under a variety of names in the United States, the most well known of which are Isordil, Sorbitrate, Peritrate, Cardilate, Nitroglyn, and Nitrobid. They can be swallowed, chewed, or dissolved under the tongue. The oral preparations are of several strengths, with different rates of absorption from the stomach and varying duration of effect. Like nitroglycerin, they usually cause headaches at first, and for the same reasons. But as you continue to use them, this side effect gradually disappears.

Revolution in Treatment—The Beta-Blockers

The beta-blocking drugs are extremely important in the treatment of angina. Five are now available in the United States (Inderal, Lopressor, Corgard, Tenorim, and timolol), but an influx is expected in the next year or two. The oldest and still the most popular one in this country is Inderal (propranolol).

This group of drugs benefits the angina patient by reducing the heart rate and the oxygen requirements of the heart. The net result is an increase in the amount of exercise that you can do before the onset of pain. It also lowers blood pressure, so it is especially useful in patients who have both angina and hypertension—a common association. These medications have made life more comfortable for the patient with angina and much easier for his or her cardiologist.

Another important effect of the beta-blockers is their beneficial action on disturbances of heart rhythm which frequently complicate arteriosclerotic heart disease.

The symptomatic improvement resulting from the use of the beta-blockers is not due to a "pain-killing" property. These agents don't merely mask angina. You feel better taking them because they really help the heart.

Yet I still see people with angina who have not been prescribed one of these most important drugs. If you are among them, get another opinion—fast—especially if you have severe angina, or bypass surgery is recommended, and you either have not been given any beta-blockers, or not enough.

They Also Prevent Heart Attacks

The beneficial effects of a beta-blocker drug will soon become apparent to you if you have angina. But, in addition to controlling symptoms, does this medication also prolong life by delaying heart attacks or preventing sudden death? In 1964 it was first suggested that Inderal did just that. Later, British researchers studied another beta-blocker called practolol, widely used in Europe at that time to answer this crucial question. The results were dramatic. There was a reduction of nearly 50 percent in the incidence of sudden death and fatal heart attacks in patients given this medication. Just as we were making plans to start using practolol in the United States, other, dangerous side effects of this medication became apparent, and it was withdrawn from the market worldwide. So the critical question remained. Aside from the toxicity of this particular product, were its observed benefits common to other beta-blockers which did not have adverse side effects?

In order to find an answer, several studies were launched at approximately the same time in various Western countries, using different beta-blockers. The first to be reported came from Norway, in 1981. There it was found that timolol (Blocadren) had the same protective effect as practolol. Then from the United States came the results of a beautifully designed study using propranolol (Inderal), which has been available here for many years. Again, great success, as with the other two beta-blockers. Similar results were reported for atenolol (Tenormin) and metoprolol (Lopressor). So it appears that all the available beta-blockers not only control your symptoms, but prolong your life as well. And that's a very important fact for those patients who are contemplating coronary artery bypass surgery to know. At the time of writing, although these beta-blockers are all available in the U.S., only timolol is specifically designated as preventing death. I'm sure the others will soon be too.

Beta-Blockers Are Not for Everyone

There are certain situations when beta-blockers may have to be avoided. For example, they can worsen heart failure. So, if you have swollen legs and difficulty in breathing, beta-blockers are probably not for you. In diabetics, they may mask the symptoms of an insulin reaction. You may still use beta-blockers if you need them, but be doubly alert about the symptoms of too low a blood sugar. Finally, the beta-blockers can provoke spasm of the bronchial tubes in asthmatics. Newer members of this family of drugs are referred to as "cardio-selective," that is, their main action is on the heart and they have much less effect on the airways, so if you are asthmatic you may take them if you have to, but with caution and in the smallest dosage necessary. The cardio-selective beta-blockers now available in the United States are Tenormin (atenolol) and Lopressor (metoprolol). Corgard (nadolol), Inderal (propranolol) and timolol (Blocadren) are not.

There is an important characteristic about the beta-blockers for you to remember. Never stop taking them abruptly if you have severe angina. Doing so may result in a "rebound phenomenon," so that in about 3 or 4 percent of cases, their sudden discontinuation and the consequent acceleration of heart rate may result in worsening of the angina or even a heart attack. Most patients who stop taking them abruptly do so because their prescription has run out. They hesitate to bother the doctor about refilling it, since they will be seeing him in a few weeks anyway, and they are not sure that he will prescribe the same medication again. Never do this with a beta-blocker. Get a refill to keep you going until your next visit.

Beta-Blockers and Impotence—Real or Imagined?

Some questions have been raised about beta-blockers causing impotence. They do in some men. That effect, however, is a difficult one to assess. After all, the specter of angina in a previously healthy man is very emotionally stressful. The ability, desire, self-confidence and abandon necessary to perform the sex act adequately are very much dependent on one's state of mind. The anxiety generated by the diagnosis of serious heart disease can in itself result in impotence, yet so often this symptom is attributed to the disease or whatever medication is prescribed to control it.

However, although psychological factors may contribute toward impotence in some individuals, this group of drugs does indeed have this effect in a significant number of patients. When only Inderal was available in this country, someone so affected had a difficult decision to make. But now, with five beta-blockers from among which to choose (and more on the way), if one renders you impotent, try another. There are enough differences among them so that one may give you a particular side effect, while another does not.

While on the subject of side effects of beta-blockers, there is another I have observed, and which is not often discussed. That's the feeling of coldness in the hands and feet. If that's happening to you, again, switch brands. It may help.

Newer Antianginal Agents on the American Horizon

Nitroglycerin, the nitrates, and the beta-blockers constitute the basis for the medical management of uncomplicated angina at the present time. There are several exciting newer drugs just appearing on the American scene, but which have been available in Europe for some time. These are the calcium antagonists, represented by nifedipine (now marketed as Procardia) in 1965, verapamil and diltiazem. Interestingly, I was given a supply of verapamil to evaluate in 1965, and I found it good for the treatment of angina at that time. What has held up the release of this agent for so many years in this country was the finding of cataracts, which disappeared when the drug was discontinued—in beagles! This is a reflection of the caution with which the pharmaceutical industry and government regulatory agencies move.

The calcium antagonists appear to have very little toxicity and are reported to reduce dramatically the severity of angina, especially the kind that is due to spasm of the coronary arteries. They also correct several important disturbances of heart rhythm. They are currently available for patients who need them under special research protocols.

The "Hasty" Angiogram

When your doctor makes the diagnosis of angina, he will almost always prescribe the drug regimen described above. But every now and then, the first "anginal" encounter with the doctor may be frightening. The following scenario is not uncommon:

You visit the doctor, not at all sure that you have heart disease. But by the time you are ready to leave, not only have you been told the diagnosis, which is bad enough, but you are also scared out of your wits because his discussion includes terms like "coronary angiogram" and "bypass surgery" —all this and you haven't even had a heart attack!

Why would the doctor spring this on you at your very first visit, and what should you do about it? Clearly, this is the kind of situation for which second opinions were made. No matter how mild or severe your symptoms are, you owe it to yourself to obtain another opinion from a cardiologist at the first hint that cardiac surgery is being considered.

The Threat of a Main Stem Obstruction

What is it, in your condition, that would generate talk of heart surgery? Your doctor may have been so impressed with the severity of your symptoms and the electrocardiographic abnormalities (either at rest or after exercise) that he felt it necessary to determine with some precision the extent of the disease within the coronary arteries. One can find an analogy in a tree in which the trunk is so severely affected that the nutrients coming up from the roots cannot pass beyond it to reach the branches—and so the whole tree dies. By contrast, if the same disease strikes a peripheral branch, the branch may fall off but the rest of the tree remains intact. And so it is in the heart. If the *main-stem* coronary artery (from which most of the coronary blood supply derives) narrows critically (and this can often be suspected from your symptoms and other tests), you are at great risk if and when that artery finally closes. For at that time, your heart muscle will suddenly lose most of its life-sustaining nutrition. The result is, at best, a serious heart attack and, at worst, death. If your doctor believes that that is what you have, he will urge you to undergo further testing.

The Radionuclide Angiogram

If he plans to go directly to coronary arteriography, ask about doing a *radionuclide cineangiogram* first. This is a relatively new painless, risk-free, noninvasive cardiac diagnostic technique now in fairly widespread use that makes invasive arteriography unnecessary in some cases. It involves the intravenous administration of a small amount of a radioactive tracer element (similar to radio-isotope scanning of any organ of the body—the brain, liver, thyroid, etc.). The radioactive material goes to the heart, where its pattern of distribution is assessed by a special computer camera. We look to see whether the radioactive material is uniformly distributed through the heart. A gap, or "hole," in the cardiac image when you are at rest suggests the presence of dead tissue—evidence of an old heart attack. Then you perform a stress test after which the nuclear scan is repeated. When one or more coronary arteries are narrowed and unable to deliver adequate amounts of blood to the exercising heart, "gaps" appear in the distribution of the radioactivity, gaps that were not present at rest. Also, abnormalities in the way the heart contracts can be detected in this test, which is almost as sensitive as the coronary arteriogram for making the diagnosis of significant disease of the coronary arteries. Of course, if surgery is contemplated, then an arteriogram is necessary, since that's the only method presently available that actually permits us to see the arteries and to pinpoint the exact location of areas of obstruction.

The Coronary Arteriogram

The coronary arteriogram involves the passage of a thin catheter from an artery near the groin or in the arm, to a point very near the heart where the openings to the coronary arteries are situated. The dye is then squirted into them. The procedure is done under local anesthesia.

The procedure may be uncomfortable and does involve an overnight stay in hospital. Unfortunately, angrography is sometimes recommended not because of any imminent threat, but because there are doctors who believe that *all* patients with angina should have surgery, that a bypass procedure protects virtually everyone against heart attack and death, and that the operative risk in properly selected cases (usually somewhat less than 2 percent in good hands) is worth it. Although the data thus far accumulated suggests that successful bypass surgery done by expert teams does reduce the risk of heart attacks and, in fact, does prolong life in properly selected cases, it is not true for every patient. In my judgment, you should not have an arteriogram or consider heart surgery until you have had a fair trial with all the medicines that are now available. But if you continue to have frequent, debilitating chest pain, and if noninvasive tests show ominous changes, then surgery may well be necessary and you should have the coronary arteriogram. But this is a recommendation that should be made at the time of your first visit only if there is a very strong suspicion of left main stem blockage or serious obstruction of all the major coronary arteries. And if it is, ask for a second opinion from an experienced cardiologist.

Coronary Bypass Surgery—Protective or Only Palliative?

The entire question of bypass surgery—when, why and where—is something that every patient with heart disease should fully understand. The decision about having this operation is one that you must share with your doctor, and frequently with a second physician (a cardiologist). Whether or not you should undergo a bypass operation depends on the severity of your angina, to what extent it interferes with your life style and whether you have been treated optimally with medication. The other factors that go into making the final decision—the presence of certain ECG changes, response to exercise testing, results of your radionuclide test and coronary angiogram—are all a matter of professional expertise.

But given the same tests and even interpreting them the same way, doctors will not always agree on the question of bypass surgery.

My Present Position on Bypass Surgery

I used to recommend bypass coronary surgery only when the angina could not be controlled by medical means—or when the left main coronary artery was involved. I now recommend this operation much more frequently than before, because in the last few years I have seen so many people live more comfortably and, I think, longer after it was done. I know this is at variance with the attitude of some other cardiologists. However, most results reported from large centers seem to bear out my own clinical impressions. In one study, reported in late 1981, among 1,760 patients with angina operated on between 1974 and 1979, the operative mortality was only 1.3 percent, and the four year survival rate was 92.5 percent. This compares with a five-year survival of 90.7 percent in the general population matched for age and sex. In other words, the operation conferred a normal life expectancy on patients with angina. So I now recommend for surgery (a) anyone who has angina so severe that it interferes with the quality of his life and in whom medication is not effective; (b) patients with left main-stem obstruction regardless of age or symptoms; (c) patients whose angina is getting worse despite all efforts to control it with medication; and (d) those who have already had one or more heart attacks and have continued to suffer from debilitating angina despite all the drugs we give them. You must make sure that your own doctor is neither too conservative nor too liberal in this regard. Always get a second opinion, whether the first one says yes or says no.

A word here about the operation itself. The very first patient I sent for surgery had it done back in 1970, when the procedure was in its infancy. It was a triple bypass, that is, three of the arteries were severely obstructed and we were unable to relieve the angina with the medication then available. The operation lasted more than twelve hours, and was a tour de force. (Incidentally, the man is still alive and well). Today, with newer surgical techniques, the same bypass can be done in about two hours. The risk is much less too.

Properly selected patients whose surgery is performed by a skilled team face a risk of under 2 percent! The majority can leave the hospital in seven to fourteen days, and can resume normal activities shortly thereafter. More than 80 percent become pain-free, and are able to discontinue most of their antianginal medication. There are, of course, some operative failures, and sometimes surgery is necessary a second or even a third time. But such unfortunate results constitute a very small minority of the more than 100,000 bypass procedures done in the United States each year.

Coronary Spasm—Heart Attack Without Arteriosclerosis?

No discussion of angina is complete these days without a discussion of the phenomenon of *coronary spasm*. For years, doctors have been aware that some patients—usually but not always those with documented heart disease—suddenly develop chest pain that to all intents and purposes is typically anginal. But the pain comes on while the patients are at rest, not after exertion. Also, upon examination of the hearts of some individuals who have died suddenly, the coronary arteries may show little or no evidence of arteriosclerosis. It was assumed that spasm was responsible for these events. Recently, in a large series of elegant studies done by a group of cardiologists in Italy, the spasm was clearly demonstrated by arteriography. In a few cases, the coronary arteries were otherwise normal except for temporary spasm, which narrowed them dramatically. In most, however, the spasm was superimposed on vessels already narrowed by arteriosclerotic plaques.

Why coronary arteries go into spasm is not clear. But we have already made one important observation in this group of patients, namely, that the beta-blockers, so effective in treating angina due to arteriosclerotic disease of the coronary arteries, are not usually helpful in relieving spasm. In fact, they may worsen the symptoms. So if you have angina and are no better with the beta-blockers, there are two possibilities. You either have run of the mill angina and are not taking enough of the drug, or your angina is due to spasm. In the latter circumstance the nitrates and the calcium antagonists are the best agents to take. On occasion, the failure of your angina to respond to the beta-blockers may, therefore, not necessarily mean that your coronary artery disease is so severe that you need surgery, but that the main problem is coronary artery spasm. And in that case, you certainly shouldn't have an operation.

Lofty Goals for the Lowly Aspirin

In the chapter dealing with strokes, you will read about the prophylactic value of aspirin in preventing clotting within the arteries of the brain. It is only logical that the question of a similar protective action in the heart should be raised and investigated. Several studies to check this hypothesis have already been done and more studies are currently in progress. The data to date suggests that aspirin does afford some protection, although the findings are by no means clear cut. Part of the problem in evaluating aspirin's role in preventing heart attacks is that no one really knows the best dose to give. We used to think that two or three tablets per day were optimal. Now, however, it seems that that is too much, and that a half tablet—or at most, one—may be better. If that is true, then the studies that showed no benefit from aspirin were invalid because we were giving too much, not because the aspirin itself failed the test.

Given our present knowledge, it would seem to me to be entirely reasonable for anyone with coronary-artery disease to take small doses of aspirin (unless you are allergic to it or have ulcers) or any of the other drugs that prevent the platelets (formed elements in the blood) from clinging together and forming a clot (Persantine, Anturane).

It may be simpler, however, just to eat more Chinese food, at least the cuisine that uses black tree fungus (called "tree ears" or mo-er). It apparently has the same anti-platelet function as aspirin and the other drugs mentioned above.

As you read these pages, you begin to see why I stated early on that medicine often does not speak with one voice on many issues. The role of anticoagulants (blood thinners) in the treatment and prevention of heart attacks is a case in point. As long as I can remember in my professional career, this question has been the source of great disagreement, often passionate and even bitter. Careers have been made by doctors taking the pro or the con stance—and the patient is caught in the middle. Whom to believe? There is no question that if you develop angina or suffer a myocardial infarction, your own doctor will be on either side of the fence on this issue. A second opinion will probably not help you either, because what you're told will be based on the philosophy of the consultant you happen to ask. My own view is generally against the use of *long-term* anticoagulants like warfarin (Coumadin) in most cases. The complication of internal hemorrhage, though not great, always exists, even when blood tests are performed at regular intervals. On the other hand, if you have a chronic or intermittent disturbance of cardiac rhythm, it may be a good idea. If this treatment is recommended to you, be sure to discuss all its implications with your doctor.

Blowing Up the Plaques—Bye-Bye Bypass?

Recently, there has been reintroduced and popularized a concept and technique first used in 1964 in the United States—*percutaneous transluminal angioplasty.* A very thin catheter is inserted into the diseased artery. Once in place, a smaller catheter with a soft, flexible balloon at its top is threaded into it. This balloon, when inflated, compresses the plaque obstructing the artery, thereby widening the lumen or diameter of the vessel and permitting more blood to flow through it. When it can be done, this technique is preferable to surgery.

Although angioplasty has promise, it is not without its own risks and must still be considered experimental. It can be done only in special cases, where the offending plaque is in a straight line with and can easily be reached by the catheter. (Some are situated too far down in the artery.) It seems that, because of the limitations of the technique, only 10 percent of patients are candidates for it. Among these, it is successful in about 70 percent. I worry about the balloon rupturing the wall of the artery, or a piece of the clot breaking off and completely obstructing the vessel further down and thus causing a heart attack. For these reasons, when coronary angioplasty is done, there is always a surgeon standing by ready to operate on an emergency basis should the need arise.

Coronary angioplasty is becoming more and more sophisticated and more widely used, though it is not likely ever to replace bypass surgery in the great majority of cases.

When You're About to Have a Heart Attack

Let's move along, then, from the patient with chest pains who has not yet had a heart attack to one who has. Although many heart attacks occur suddenly, without any prior symptoms, in others it is preceded by a progressive worsening of angina. The symptoms become more and more severe, are provoked by progressively less effort or begin to occur at rest (especially at night) and the number of nitroglycerin tablets required increases significantly.

Angina that becomes "unstable" in this way is as much an emergency as is a frank heart attack. Patients with such symptoms are in what we call the "premonitory" or "impending" phase of a heart attack. Under these circumstances, your doctor will restrict your physical activity, keep you at home or preferably send you to the hospital for observation. Your medication will be adjusted or changed, and with rest and a bit of luck, you may be able to avert the threatened attack. If you don't, then you have the added protection of being right there in the hospital when the final closure of the diseased coronary artery takes place. The necessary treatment can be administered without delay. So, if you have "unstable angina" and your doctor recommends this regimen, don't argue. It is sound advice, the kind that does not normally require a second opinion.

If, after you are hospitalized and the treatment is adjusted, you still suffer chest pain at rest, you will very likely be advised to have a coronary arteriogram. At this point, that is good advice, but again, that is the time to consult another cardiologist.

The arteriogram will likely show the kind of critical left main-stem location of disease discussed earlier, or severe obstruction in two or three of the larger coronary arteries. Bypass surgery will then probably be recommended. A second opinion is desirable at this point, even if all the pieces as I have related them fall into place. The purpose of a consultation now is to determine that you are in the best hospital in which to have the operation, and that the surgical team is experienced. If there is any question about these two preconditions, have yourself transferred elsewhere if it is still safe to do so.

A bypass operation is "open chest" and not really "open heart" surgery. The heart is exposed, but the coronary arteries, on which the surgeon does his work, are actually on the surface of the heart. The heart is not entered into as it is, for example, in valve surgery. For these reasons, the risk of bypass surgery is considerably less than for valve replacement.

In the Event of a Heart Attack

Suppose that you do not develop a "premonitory," "warning," "impending," or "unstable" phase of your angina, but simply continue to have your usual degree of discomfort on exertion. Then one day, and for no apparent reason, you develop a heart attack.

Here is a typical scenario:

It is the middle of the night. You are awakened by a more severe heaviness, or pressure, in the chest than you have ever had before with exertion. Unlike your usual angina attack, this time it doesn't go away when you take nitroglycerin. You feel faint, nauseated, and you begin to perspire. The symptoms become more severe, your jaw may begin to ache, or there is pain in either arm (more commonly the left one) or through to the back.

Interestingly enough, statistically, all this is most apt to happen on a Monday. Whether that's because there's too much revelry and drinking on the weekend, for which you pay the price when it's all over, or the re-exposure to occupational stress after a period of relaxation is not clear. But in men without a previous history of heart disease, Monday is the day they're most likely to have their heart attack—when it comes.

No Time for Heroics

Whenever it happens, this is no time to be unselfish or a hero. Wake your spouse and get to the hospital the fastest way you can. I encourage my patients to call me immediately, but not to wait for my response in the event I am not near a phone at that precise moment. Nor will I waste precious time by having them wait for me to make a house call. The first thirty to forty-five minutes are critical at this time. Call an ambulance service, preferably with a paramedical team, or the local police emergency squad. If you are not too sick and you think it may be faster, take a cab. The objective is to get to the nearest emergency room as quickly as possible. Pending the arrival there of your doctor, the personnel will institute the necessary treatment. Here, time, not a second opinion, is of the essence, because of the threat of sudden death.

The Denial Mechanism

As I wrote in *The Complete Medical Exam*, a host of different conditions may mimic an acute heart attack. These include a pinched nerve in the neck, a blood clot to the lung, a hiatus hernia, gallbladder disease, ulcer, gastritis, inflammation of the sac surrounding the heart (pericarditis) and arthritis of the chest wall. But whatever *you* think the symptoms may be, don't fall into the trap of the "denial mechanism." So many patients are convinced that if they don't call the doctor, the trouble, whatever it is, will go away. This unwillingness to face reality is responsible for many deaths. Remember, delay during the first critical hour after the onset of symptoms may be fatal.

Should You Go to the Hospital or Stay Home?

There has been some talk recently, prompted no doubt by the high cost of hospitalization, to the effect that patients with acute heart attacks may be treated at home as safely as in hospital. One report from England purported to show that those who suffered "mild heart attacks" did just fine at home. But that study involved a screening process in which a paramedic or doctor first evaluated the case before deciding whether hospitalization was necessary. Although the statistics reported by the English physicians look good on paper, I prefer a coronary-care unit or similarly equipped facility with trained personnel for my patients. I do not believe that it is always possible to distinguish a "mild" attack from a "serious" one early in the game. It is, however, very easy to do so in retrospect. If a patient experienced pain only briefly, then had no further trouble and was sent home after two uneventful weeks in the hospital, I can say to him in confidence, "You have had only a mild heart attack." But when someone starts off with the same nondescript pain, it may very well persist or get worse in a few hours. Blood pressure may drop or there may develop serious disturbances of cardiac rhythm—in short, it turns out to be a "bad" attack. It is all a matter of hindsight and it is virtually impossible to tell, in the first thirty minutes or one hour when the decision must be made, which patient is going to do what.

If you are having an ostensibly mild heart attack and are told that you can be treated safely at home, ask for a second opinion. I fear that in the interests of economy and "cost effectiveness" some of us may get short-changed at one of the most critical times in our lives.

Treating the Heart Attack

Treatment of the acute heart attack depends on your symptoms and what we find when we examine and monitor you in the first few hours and days. First we relieve your pain with a narcotic, usually morphine. At the same time, you will be given oxygen by mask or via little prongs in the nostrils. (We don't use the tent any more, because it is not nearly as efficient.) At one time, we wondered whether oxygen did any good. We reasoned this way: If the affected coronary artery was blocked and not delivering any blood at all, what was the use of increasing the oxygen going to a completely obstructed artery? None of it would get beyond the blockage to the heart muscle anyway. Although that argument is logical, I never argue with success, and oxygen does seem to help patients with heart attacks. There is also speculation that the amount of heart tissue damaged is reduced when oxygen is administered.

You will also be hooked up to a monitor, that is, an electrocardiogram projected on a screen which can be viewed constantly by the nurse or intern in the room, or at a central console in the coronary care unit. It is watched carefully for any heart-rhythm disturbance that may result from injury to the cardiac muscle, and an alarm is triggered should anything go awry.

The Problems of an Irregular Heartbeat

If your heart begins to beat irregularly, you will be given one of a variety of drugs, usually intravenously, to suppress the irritable foci in the damaged area. The most important of these agents are Lidocaine (which, interestingly enough, is a local anesthetic too), procainamide (Pronestyl), quinidine or digitalis.

Occasionally, if the cardiac rate becomes very rapid, it can cause your blood pressure to drop quickly and decrease the blood supply to the brain. In that event, your doctor may decide not to wait for medication to take effect, but will apply direct-current electroshock to the chest. This usually normalizes the disordered rhythm immediately. "Cardioversion," as it is called, is not needed very often, especially these days, when you can be given drugs. Should you learn, however, that it was required, as you sit in the anteroom of the coronary-care unit, anxiously wondering about a loved one inside, don't despair. Such emergency intervention does not necessarily mean that the outlook is bad. It is needed simply to pull the sick heart through what is often an acute, temporary emergency. Availability of such equipment has significantly reduced the early death rate from heart attacks in hospitalized patients.

Blood Pressure During a Heart Attack

Your blood pressure too will be monitored. If the injury to the heart is substantial, pressure drops considerably. In that event, we try to maintain it at an appropriate level—otherwise "shock" sets in. (The heart is so severely damaged that it cannot pump enough blood to keep the circulation going through the body.) Under these circumstances, drastic measures are required. We sometimes have to insert an artificial auxiliary pump in the aorta near the heart to help that ailing organ pump the blood more adequately. We leave the pump there for a few days to help sustain the circulation, buying time for the stricken heart to regain some of its strength.

There are two new and important approaches in dealing with the very severe heart attack of which you should be aware. The first is a growing tendency at least to consider doing emergency bypass surgery very early after symptoms of the acute attack. When all the tests point to the fact that the attack is evolving into a massive, life-threatening one, there is some evidence that operating on the blocked artery may improve the outlook. This decision is such a grave one that it should never be made without adequate consultation.

The second intervention during the very early phase of a heart attack is still experimental, but holds great promise, in my opinion. It involves injecting an enzyme, streptokinase, directly into the obstructed coronary artery in order to dissolve the fresh clot. Several score of patients have been so treated, and the technique frequently works. However, timing appears to be the critical factor. This procedure has not yet been perfected for routine use. If it is suggested to you at this time, ask for a second opinion.

Modest reduction of pressure in response to injury is often a natural protective mechanism that reduces the work of the sick heart. In fact, during a heart attack, we now sometimes deliberately lower the blood pressure with medicines (especially if it is elevated) in order to ease the burden on the heart.

The vast majority of heart attacks turn out well. In most good hospitals, among every hundred patients who are admitted with that diagnosis, about eighty-five survive. Before the introduction of the coronary-care unit, some 30 percent died.

What I have described above—treatment of arrhythmias, maintenance of dropping blood pressures, management of shock, use of intra-aortic balloons (auxiliary pumps)—are not usual in a heart attack. Furthermore, none of these measures, when necessary, usually allows time for a second opinion. They are all emergency steps and must be taken without delay. The more common course of events in a heart attack is not very dramatic. You have pain for a few hours, it responds to medication, and the rest of the time is spent badgering your doctor to send you home. No drama, no resuscitation, no shock. But it is a good idea to ask for a cardiology consultation immediately after your admission to the hospital if your own doctor is not a heart specialist, in the event of any unexpected emergency that requires extra skill and expertise.

How Long in Hospital?

Until fifteen years ago, we used to keep heart-attack patients in the hospital for at least six weeks. Then, we began to be aware that prolonged bed rest itself was hazardous, mostly because of clots forming in the stagnant veins of the immobile individual. Patients discharged much earlier did just as well over the long term. Today, I generally discharge my patients who have had an uncomplicated heart attack in about fourteen days. Many of my colleagues send them home in ten days. Anything less than that is too soon, in my opinion.

Life After Your Heart Attack

What kind of life can you look forward to after a heart attack? Years ago, you would have been "finished"—unemployable and treated like an invalid in every respect. Today, the questions are not *whether* you will go back to work but *when;* not if you will make love again but *when?* We have had this change of heart (no pun intended) because in most cases the damaged cardiac area forms a tough scar that will not likely cause you any harm in the future. Your attention and your doctor's focus must now be to prevent another heart attack, not worrying about the one you have already survived. The world is full of patients who have had "coronaries." The great majority are living normal, active lives. Others have had new careers writing about their cardiac experiences. In about six weeks to two months, most patients in sedentary jobs can return to work. If you don't have chronic chest pain, are not short of breath, and your feet are not swollen, yet your doctor advises you to retire, get a second opinion. There is nothing worse than forced and unnecessary retirement. You may not be able to return to your former job if it involves an inordinate amount of physical or emotional stress, but that does not mean that you have to stay home and do nothing. Your local medical society or heart association can direct you to job-retraining programs in your community.

Cardiac Rehabilitation

After an uncomplicated coronary, every patient should whenever possible enter a cardiac rehabilitation program individually tailored on the basis of the history, physical examination, the treadmill exercise, Holter monitoring and radionuclide scanning. Such a program is conducted under close supervision at least three times a week, for three or four months after you leave the hospital. Once you have finished that, you should continue it at home or at a local gym. There's nothing better for your morale.

The stress test done before entering the program is a

mild one and can safely be performed about three or four weeks after leaving the hospital; some centers even have you do it before going home. The results help determine your vulnerability to trouble in the near future and how much exercise you may safely do.

The Holter monitor involves applying electrodes to your chest in the doctor's office or cardiac clinic. You then go about your business for the next twenty-four hours, during which the ECG is recorded on a small, light-weight portable tape recorder. You return the monitor the next day, and the tape is analyzed. This technique is especially useful for the detection of irregularities of cardiac rhythm that may be occurring at rest, or while eating, sleeping, making love, and so on. Such rhythm irregularities, of which patients are often unaware, may be life-threatening and are often preventable.

Sex After Your Coronary

With respect to intercourse after a heart attack, many doctors are too permissive, too strict, or more commonly, they ignore the matter entirely. Intercourse, regardless of how it is done—up, down or sideways—requires effort; so, I advise my own patients to abstain for about one month after a heart attack. And as some physicians insist, after that time "only at home" for the next six months. There is more truth to this than humor, because the stress and guilt of an illicit sexual relationship, may constitute an intolerable burden for a recently damaged heart. That may explain the fact that 80 percent of all deaths occurring during intercourse do so when the activity is extramarital.

Up the Staircase and into Bed

I also give my patients some practical advice as well. I tell them that they will know they are ready to make love again when they can climb a couple of flights of stairs at their own pace, without chest pain or undue shortness of breath. If after their heart attack they continue to have angina, I insist that they take a nitroglycerin *before* sexual relations. And, even though I am not a Masters or a Johnson, it is clear that the traditional "missionary" position, with the male on top supported by his elbows, involves more work for the man, because, in addition to performing the sex act, he has to support the weight of his own body. It is easier to assume the side-by-side position or have the woman on top. Also, try to avoid intercourse right after eating a meal or drinking alcohol and when it is: too hot, too cold, you're overtired, or you've been having more than the usual number of angina attacks.

Fear of Sex

Although most patients can't wait to resume their sexual activity, others have to be encouraged to do so. They need reassurance, because they fear the consequences of any sexual activity. It is estimated that in 3 out of 4 men there is at least some temporary interference with sexual performance. At least 10 percent become permanently impotent—for psychological, not physical, reasons. And of those who do resume sexual activity, two thirds permanently decrease its frequency to less than 50 percent of what it was before they became sick. There are no figures to document the problem in women, but any experienced cardiologist will tell you that they react in very much the same way as men. The attitude of a man's mate is critical to his sexual enjoyment and performance after a heart attack. Many women are so afraid of literally killing their husbands by loving them physically that their caution becomes counterproductive and renders the husbands impotent. If your husband or lover has had a coronary, discuss his condition frankly with him and the doctor. After being instructed in the *do*'s and *don't*s of your relationship, proceed accordingly.

Unfortunately, most men who have had myocardial infarctions (heart attacks) are not given useful advice about sex. Your doctor's attitude in this regard will largely determine how well, how often and with what abandon you will enjoy making love in the years to come. Ask him to spell out the rules in the kind of detail you need. Do not accept generalizations and vague instructions. Make sure that the advice given you in this regard is tailor-made to your own cardiac status. That can be done only after objective stress testing. The days when "take it easy" was the only advice given patients after a heart attack are over—or should be.

Death in the Saddle (*Morte d' Amour*)

We recently read about a prominent figure who died suddenly allegedly during sexual activity. The actual risk of this happening to you is very small, no matter how active your social life. Take comfort in the fact that fewer than 1 percent of all sudden deaths occur "in the saddle."

Advice about sexual activity after heart attacks is generally focused on the male, a reflection of the fact that this illness strikes men with alarming frequency in their prime of life and is uncommon in women before the menopause. Any woman who has suffered a heart attack should follow the same guidelines about sexual relations as men.

When Symptoms Continue After a Heart Attack

Every now and then a heart attack will leave you with certain symptoms that require ongoing care. If you experience persistent angina, it will be treated very much as it was before your coronary. If the attack left a large amount of heart muscle damaged, the remaining portion may not be able to pump sufficiently to meet the demands of the body. This is called "heart failure," and is treated mainly by prescribing adequate rest, a low-salt diet, diuretics and digitalis. All beta-blocking drugs are stopped. In more severe cases, we now use a combination of agents which act to reduce the work load of the heart by dilating the arteries and veins. These include Apresoline, the nitrates and several others. You will also have to delay or postpone indefinitely any exercise program until your heart has been substantially strengthened.

Another problem with which we sometimes have to deal after a heart attack is some *disturbance of heart rhythm*. But remember that not every "palpitation" or "extra beat" is serious or requires treatment. When it does, the drugs currently available for that purpose are often toxic and potentially dangerous. So, if you have a heart-rhythm disorder needing drug treatment and you are miserable because of the medication's side effects, do not hesitate to ask for a second opinion from a cardiologist experienced in their use. Before you take any agent, however, make sure you have eliminated from your diet those substances that render the heart more irritable—caffeine in coffee, tea, and many cola drinks; liquor in all its forms; and, of course, cigarettes. I remember one woman whose irregular heartbeat was puzzlingly resistant to all the medications we gave her—until I learned that she was taking eight cups of black coffee and smoking two packs of cigarettes every day.

Drugs for the Irregular Heartbeat

Cardiac agents now available for oral use in the United States for restoring or maintaining a regular heartbeat include digitalis (marketed as digoxin, Lanoxin, digitoxin, Crystodigin), quinidine (Quinidex, Cardioquin, Quinaglute), procainamide (Pronestyl), Dilantin (not for epileptics only), the various beta-blockers and disopyramide (Norpace). There are several other very good drugs on the horizon, some of which are less toxic and more effective than those we are now using, but which are not yet available in this country. If you have a rhythm problem that *must* be treated, yet you seem to be unable to tolerate any of the agents that your doctor prescribes, request a second opinion from a cardiologist who has experience with and access to these newer medicines.

I will now briefly discuss the most important anthiar-rhythmic drugs currently available, so that you may know what benefits and adverse side effects to expect and how to recognize them.

First there is *digitalis*, of which there are several forms. They are not all interchangeable, since each has its own rate of absorption, duration of action and route of excretion from the body. The major use of this agent is not so much to regularize a disordered rhythm as it is to slow a speeding heart. Its greatest application is in the control of atrial fibrillation and flutter, cardiac rhythm disturbances whose major threat to you lies more in their tendency to cause a rapid rate than in their irregularity.

When You Have Too Much Digitalis on Board

Digitalis in the proper dosage is safe and usually without side effects. I find, however, that many older persons require less of the drug, and when given "normal" doses, end up getting too much. This is especially likely if they have some impairment of kidney function. The first evidence of that is a distaste for food—especially meat—followed by weight loss. When the digitalis is stopped for a few days, then restarted in lower dosage, these symptoms clear completely. So, if you have been given a digitalis preparation for whatever reason and find that you are gradually losing your appetite, tell your doctor about it. Don't be shy about suggesting to him the possibility of digitalis excess. He will be grateful to you (especially if you are right).

The amount of digitalis in your blood can be measured by a technique called "radioimmune assay." You are more likely to develop such digitalis toxicity if, after you have been taking it for a while, a quinidine preparation is also prescribed. This is a recent and important observation. Whenever quinidine is added this way, the digitalis dose should usually be reduced by half straight away.

The Beta-Blockers as Antiarrhythmics

Beta-blocking drugs like Inderal (used for the treatment of hypertension and angina pectoris) also help to regularize heart rhythm. But if you are being treated for heart failure or asthma, they must be taken under close medical supervision or not at all.

Quinidine—Lots of Side Effects, but the Best Available Today

Quinidine is perhaps the most useful antiarrhythmic drug we have, but difficult for some patients to tolerate. It frequently causes diarrhea or soft stools, skin rashes, hearing problems and blood disorders. But certain commercially available forms are less troublesome than others. So if you are given a quinidine preparation and you experience any of these problems, let your doctor know. There are alternatives to going through life with chronic diarrhea.

Pronestyl—Effective but Potentially Toxic

An alternative drug to quinidine is procainamide (Pronestyl). It is about as effective as quinidine, but also potentially toxic. Unlike quinidine, which just makes you miserable, Pronestyl's side effects are important. This drug can cause persistent, severe arthritis, or a serious disease called lupus, and a host of other symptoms. I try not to prescribe this agent over the long term, but often find I have little choice. If you are taking it, and you develop arthritis or other unexplained symptoms, let your doctor know immediately. If he doesn't take your complaints seriously, get an opinion from another cardiologist.

Norpace, But Watch Your Prostate

A newer antiarrhythmic agent is Norpace (disopyramide). It is used in circumstances similar to those in which quinidine or Pronestyl might be prescribed—for the prevention or treatment of certain kinds of "extra beats" originating in the ventricles. Although it appears to be better tolerated than quinidine and Pronestyl, it can depress heart function. It should also be used with caution in men over sixty years of age because it can cause difficulty in urination.

From time to time we encounter patients with life-threatening arrhythmias who either are not helped by or cannot tolerate any of the drugs now available, either singly or in combination. If this applies to you, get a second opinion from an expert cardiologist. There are several new, better agents in use in other countries and/or in research here. These include: NAPA, a form of Pronestyl. (We don't know much about it yet, except that it may possibly be less toxic than Pronestyl but probably not as effective.) Aprindine, a powerful drug under active research and investigation. (It is very effective but has significant neurological side effects.) Lidocaine, available and widely used in the United States, can now be given only by vein. It is very effective in controlling the life-threatening cardiac-rhythm disturbances that occur during the acute heart attack. Heretofore, an oral form has never worked because of its inactivation in the stomach. But there are two agents, Tocamide and Mexilitene, now in development, that are effective and can be taken by mouth. Two more promising medications are Encainide and Verapamil, now prescribed in Europe and expected to be released here soon. There is also Amiodarone, widely used in Europe and South America. In addition to all the above, there is a whole group of new beta-blocking drugs that will be trickling onto the American market in the near future and which also have anti-arrhythmic properties.

The Cardiac Pacemaker

There are certain rhythm disturbances that require not drugs, but a pacemaker. A tiny piece of tissue in the heart called the sinus node is responsible for regularizing the rate and rhythm of the beat. When it becomes damaged, usually by scar tissue, there may result intervals during which your heart beats either very rapidly or too slowly. Medication to decelerate the rapid rate may slow the heart too much. When the dosage is reduced, the heart speeds up again. This slow-fast situation is called a "sick sinus syndrome." A pacemaker can be programmed to guarantee a minimal heart rate. For example, it can be set so that your heart will never beat slower than, say, fifty beats per minute. With this protection, we can then give you medication to control the rapid heart beat without worrying that it will make the rate too slow. The heart beat may slow down too much, without the rapid component seen in the sick sinus syndrome. This is usually due to a condition called "heart block." (The block is an electrical one, not in an artery.) Symptoms here depend on the heart rate. If it is slow enough, you may suffer attacks of light-headedness, dizziness or loss of consciousness, in which event you may need a cardiac pacemaker.

Once the cardiac impulse is formed in the sinus node, it spreads throughout the heart, finally causing the muscle to contract and pump the blood. In order for this to happen normally, the pathways along which the electrical wave travels must be intact. Sometimes, due to disease or even surgical injury, it is not. As a result, the heart beats too slowly, and this is yet another situation in which a pacemaker may be necessary.

No Big Deal

A pacemaker is no "big deal" anymore. Even though your life may depend on having one, a pacemaker will not prevent you from carrying on normally; there are throughout the world more than three hundred thousand patients who have pacemakers and who lead normal lives. The surgical procedure itself entails little risk, and it is usually done under local anesthesia. The chest is not opened. A small electrode slipped into the heart through a vein (just like a catheter) takes over the job of regularizing the heart beat from your own diseased sinus node. It is triggered only when your own heart fails to beat—in other words, it functions on demand. (That is why it is called a "demand pacemaker."). It can be set to ensure any heart rate considered desirable for you. The electrode that stimulates the heart is powered by a small generator sewn under the skin.

A cardiac pacemaker does nothing for the heart muscle itself. Nor does it prevent heart attacks, or permit you to live forever. It simply ensures the fact that your heart will never again beat too slowly.

While a pacemaker is great if you need one, it shouldn't be inserted without a valid reason. Occasionally, the heart beats too slowly because of some medication you are taking. I have seen patients referred for an opinion about the need for a pacemaker, when their problem was simply that they were getting too much digitalis or Inderal or reserpine or even Lithium—medications that decrease the heart rate. Simply stopping the responsible drug, or reducing its dosage, restored the heart rate to a satisfactory level. The generator powering the pacemaker electrode formerly had to be changed every two or three years. Newer technology has permitted us to extend that interval to at least seven or eight years—and longer.

Selecting Your Pacemaker

The field of pacemaker technology is changing rapidly. Before you have one put in, make sure that the surgeon who will be doing it discusses with you and your cardiologist the kind that he plans to use. Ask for a programmable model, one in which the heart rate can be varied *after* the unit has been inserted. (In conventional devices, it is more difficult to change the heart rate once the pacemaker generator has been sewn in under the skin.) This can be done simply by holding a potentiometer next to the body. So, if the original heart rate at which the device was set is not the best for you, it can be slowed down or accelerated. Also, the pacemaker impulse as it appears on the ECG does not permit interpretation of what is going on in the heart. All we can tell is whether the pacemaker itself is working. If your chest pain has changed in character and we suspect some heart damage, a pacemaker

ECG is of no help. But if you have a programmable one, it can be temporarily slowed so that your own heartbeat shows up on the tracing and can then be interpreted.

You have several other options when selecting a pacemaker. Ask about the *size* of the battery pack. If you are going to be spending time on the beach, or at the health club, and don't want to advertise your pacemaker, get one of the smaller ones.

Then there is the matter of the *power source* itself. The first generation of pacemakers had mercury-zinc batteries, which lasted only two to four years. The most important recent improvement in the energy source is the lithium battery, currently the most widely used. There are five types, all very much alike. They are reliable and will last as long as twenty years. You can even have a pacemaker with rechargeable batteries. You literally plug yourself into the wall for an hour or so every week, instead of replacing the generator every few years. Personally, I think this a nuisance and no longer necessary in light of the availability of the lithium-powered units.

Finally, there are *nuclear pacemakers*, powered by plutonium 238 with a life span of ten to twenty years. The isotope itself is encased in metal, which prevents the emission of its radiation. There are some three thousand of these nuclear pacemakers now in use.

Should you consider a nuclear pacemaker (assuming that you can afford it, because it is more expensive)? Not if you're elderly. Current statistics show that 44 percent of the patients who have pacemakers die within five years. This is due not to pacemaker failure or any rhythm trouble, but to the fact that the disease that caused the heart-rhythm disturbance in the first place is usually progressive. But if you are young and fully grown, or an adult who needed a pacemaker because of injury to the sinus node during heart surgery or cardiac infection, you should consider the nuclear unit.

What about children? Some youngsters have congenital abnormalities that require pacemakers. But as the child grows, the implanted pulse generator has to be changed to compensate for the development of his body structures, and so the nuclear device is not feasible until growth has ended.

Heart Transplants

The four most dramatic scientific events in my lifetime were the detonation of the first atom bomb, the launching of Sputnik, man's first step on the moon and Christiaan Barnard's heart-transplant operation.

The drama of removing someone's heart and replacing it with the beating organ of a "dead" person was to me an event of staggering scientific and emotional proportions. Some cardiac surgeons I know were not so overawed. Technically, this procedure is apparently not difficult to do, given the kind of skill and back-up teams available at most cardiac centers. Christiaan Barnard had both and, in addition, more than the usual share of imagination, vision and courage. After his initial operations, followed by a flurry of "me-too" procedures throughout the world, heart transplants fell into disrepute because survival was so short due to rejection, the cost was so high, and suffering was so great. But despite the fact that the headlines stopped, serious interest has continued in this operation for selected cases in a few university hospitals here and abroad. Without the original hoopla and fanfare, some five hundred transplants have been done throughout the world, about 200 by the team at Stanford University in Palo Alto, California.

I refresh your memory about all this because if you find yourself in a situation in which you or a loved one has "end-stage" heart disease and there is no hope, ask about the feasibility of a heart transplant. Chances are slight that you will be a candidate, but you never know until you ask. The fact is that for very selected patients, transplant does offer the possibility of survival and near normal function. Several recipients are alive today, years after the operation. Some have even outlived their doctors. At least one patient continues to survive after ten years.

Who Gets the Transplant—and Who Doesn't?

Suitable candidates for a heart transplant must meet strict requirements formulated on the basis of the experience of the teams who have been doing this procedure over the years. For example, patients over fifty-five years of age do not do well and are rarely accepted for the surgery. But if you are younger and have no other important medical problems, your chances may be acceptable. You must also have the personality and psychological makeup to endure the great stress associated with a transplant operation. Remember that it usually fails, not for technical reasons, but because the body rejects the implanted organ. Although we have learned a great deal about matching donor and recipient hearts and, thus, about reducing the risk of such rejection, a heart transplant nevertheless means a "life time" of testing and medication, which only the emotionally strong are willing and able to endure. The same medications that decrease the risk of rejection make you vulnerable to infection, so that continued surveillance is mandatory on that account too.

In Stanford, at last count among their patients, 65 percent lived one year and nearly 50 percent are alive five years after the operation. Most of those who have survived enjoy a "satisfying" life, and some have even returned to work. Those are pretty good statistics, all things considered.

KEY FACTS TO REMEMBER

Heart disease is still by far the number-one killer in most Western countries. A better understanding of the factors that contribute to "hardening of the arteries" has resulted in a significant and impressive decline in the cardiac-death rate. There are many far-out theories about how to prevent heart attacks, but the only proven ones are control of high blood pressure and elimination of cigarettes. There is growing evidence, but not yet definite proof, that normalizing your cholesterol level, exercising regularly, watching your weight, modifying your ambitions so that you are less tense and frustrated, may all delay the onset of arteriosclerosis.

There are three major kinds of heart disease—the one you are born with (congenital); forms that result from infections acquired in early (or later) life (rheumatic fever); and arteriosclerosis.

Congenital heart disease often results from some toxic effect in the mother during pregnancy (thalidomide is the classic example) or infection (German measles). Their children may be born with various cardiac malformations—holes in the heart, deformed valves, or other structural abnormalities. Almost all can now be corrected surgically, but the decisions about if and when to operate, and who should do it, are critical. These should be made only after appropriate consultation with a pediatric cardiologist. Some congenital disorders can be corrected nonsurgically.

A recently recognized common cardiac disorder involving the mitral valve (floppy valve), is now believed to account for many of the symptoms we used to attribute to "nerves," especially in young women. Make sure that isn't your problem before you sign up with a psychiatrist.

Acute rheumatic fever, a disease of childhood and young people, follows streptococcal infections. The development and use of penicillin has resulted in a marked decline in its incidence in the last twenty-five years. The major consequences of rheumatic fever may not be apparent during the acute stage of the disease, appearing only years later, when the heart valves become scarred and distorted. Eventually, these damaged valves must be removed. As in congenital heart surgery, timing of the operation is critical. This depends on a careful description of your symptoms to the doctor, together with his use of appropriate diagnostic heart tests. Make sure that the invasive, uncomfortable and costly ones are done last.

With regard to preventing arteriosclerosis, we are currently limited to control of "risk factors." Cigarette smoking is a major hazard. There is no such thing as a "safe" cigarette, since reduction in nicotine may result in increased use of "less toxic" tobacco with increased exposure to the harmful carbon monoxide in the smoke.

There's no such thing as "benign" high blood pressure. *Any* elevation has been shown to be dangerous over the long term, and should be normalized.

The cholesterol controversy still rages. On the one hand, there are those who are fanatics about reducing blood levels as much as possible (e.g., the Pritikin diet). The other school of thought has it that high cholesterol is only one symptom of a complex disorder, that lowering by drugs or manipulating diet is of no benefit and may be harmful.

It is now widely believed that measuring HDL concentration (the kind of protein that transports cholesterol in the bloodstream) may be more revealing and prognostic with respect to heart disease than the actual cholesterol level itself.

Regular exercise is the best "tranquilizer" there is. Evidence is accumulating that it may reduce the risk of heart disease when done in the proper way and right amount. However, no one with any history of, or particular vulnerability to, heart disease should embark on an exercise program without prior medical clearance and ongoing supervision. For cardiac patients, the amount and kind of exercise should be carefully prescribed, as is any potent medication.

Angina pectoris refers to chest symptoms due to too little blood reaching the heart muscle. It is usually the result of narrowing of the coronary arteries by arteriosclerotic "plaques," but may also be caused by coronary spasm—an old theory whose validity has only recently been proved.

The most important drugs for the prevention and control of angina belong to the nitroglycerin family and beta-blockers, but new effective agents, calcium-blockers, have recently been introduced. The proper dosage and selection of the best antianginal agents often require expert consultation. Side effects may be important, but can usually be minimized.

Coronary bypass surgery is an important advance in the treatment of reduced blood flow to the coronary arteries. When done by experienced surgical teams, in properly selected patients, the risk of the operation is under 2 percent. In the great majority of cases, it eliminates or substantially reduces the severity of angina pectoris. There is a growing belief that bypass surgery also reduces the likelihood of heart attacks and prolongs life. Defining the need for such surgery requires a careful history-taking, physical exam, ECG stress tests, radionuclide scans and, ultimately, coronary arteriography (angiogram).

A new technique, not yet widely available, permits relief of coronary-artery obstruction without surgery. Called percutaneous transluminal angioplasty, it has been successful in selected cases.

Most heart attacks are uncomplicated and are followed by excellent recovery. However, some are severe, require expert care, and leave the patient with symptoms that may require treatment later. Both categories can benefit from sound advice about life style, medication and "cardiac rehabilitation."

Cardiac pacemakers are easy to implant, with only minimal risk. They are used in certain situations when the heartbeat becomes too slow. The decisions concerning when to have a pacemaker and what kind it should be may require a second opinion.

Heart transplants are now feasible in selected patients under fifty years of age. Survival is increasing, and the procedure is now being done successfully in several centers throughout the world.

12

Hypertension—The Silent Killer

High blood pressure (hypertension) left untreated is one of mankind's most important afflictions. Over the years, it pounds away silently at key arteries throughout the body, weakening their walls, helping to clog them up and occasionally causing them to burst. In most cases, while all this is going on, the patient has no telltale symptoms until it is too late. Then, after a "free ride" of several years, the ravages become apparent with a stroke, heart attack, ruptured aneurysm, blindness, kidney failure, cardiac weakness, or hardening of the arteries in the legs or elsewhere in the body. The only way you can ever know, before it is too late, whether you are destined to suffer or die in this way is to have your blood pressure measured. If it is high, see that it is treated effectively.

Black and White

The incidence of hypertension is substantially higher, and is likely to be more severe, in blacks than in whites. Our genes determine the diseases to which we are susceptible, and genes do differ among races (for example, sickle-cell anemia, which occurs in about 0.3 percent of blacks in its full-blown form, is never found in whites). Perhaps there are genetic factors, as yet unidentified, which render blacks more sensitive to salt and hence to hypertension.

So Why Not Just Treat It?

Why not indeed? If it is all so straightforward, why am I devoting a chapter to this question in a book dealing with the need for second opinions? For the following three reasons: (1) unfortunately not all physicians are as vigorous as they should be in normalizing elevated pressures; (2) there is still some disagreement as to what levels of blood pressure are "high" and require treatment; (3) problems in drug therapy may, if not resolved, require consultation. I will elaborate on each of these points as we go along.

It is hard to imagine that only a few years ago there were many doctors who did not believe that high blood pressure needed any therapy at all. In their opinion, as long as you had no symptoms, you could safely be left alone. They even called the condition "benign, essential hypertension"—"benign" because so many people, especially women, *seemed* to be none the worse for it; "essential" because that's what we call any disease whose cause(s) we don't fully understand.

In all fairness, I think this attitude was to some extent influenced by the fact that, unlike today, doctors did not have the drugs with which to lower blood pressure safely, effectively, and for long periods of time. The nihilistic point of view was sometimes passionately defended. One of my colleagues actually "flunked" a certifying exam because he told the professor that he would treat anyone with high blood pressure, no matter how well they felt. The distinguished examiner did not agree, and my friend did not pass the test. If you are being treated by someone who has not caught up with the times (and there are still a few around), pats you on the back and says the high pressure is "normal" for you, run, don't walk, for a second opinion.

Dr. Freis and Mrs. Lasker

Although most physicians suspected that normalizing blood pressure would delay or prevent its terrible consequences, it remained for Dr. Edward Freis and his colleagues to prove it in the Veterans' Administration study in 1970—the first large-scale controlled trial of this hypothesis. When their data showed how important it was to find and treat every case of high blood pressure, the Congress was further motivated by Mrs. Mary Lasker (America's own Florence Nightingale). As a result, the National Heart, Lung and Blood Institute embarked on an intensive educational campaign directed at doctors and the public alike.

The Impact of Action

The truth about hypertension has spread like wildfire among health consumers everywhere—in government, industry, and in the private sector. In just a few short years, the number of cases detected and treated has increased substantially. The result has been a dramatic and continuing drop in deaths from strokes and heart attacks in the United States alone during the last decade.

In view of this experience, and given the increasing number of effective new drugs available for the treatment of hypertension, there is no excuse for anyone to be walking around with an elevated pressure, no matter what.

What Is High?

The *definition* of what blood-pressure levels are "abnormal" and require treatment remains a matter of some controversy. In my opinion, there are still too many doctors who accept as "normal" readings that are too high to be left alone. There are probably two main reasons they do so. Even though Dr. Freis and his colleagues showed the benefit of treating hypertension, he did so only in patients with pressures that were quite high. It was not until the end of 1979 that the need to treat even "mild" elevations was also proved. Furthermore, doctors do not, as a rule, like to give potent medications to patients who feel well. As far as hypertension is concerned, such reasoning is both incorrect and dangerous.

Important—But Boring

Suppose that you are in "excellent" health (as far as you know) and have gone to the doctor only for a checkup. He suddenly announces to you that your blood pressure is high. If you both act on that information, things will never be the same for you. From now on, you will be constantly reminded and hounded about subjects that were never important to you before—what you eat and how much you weigh; the hazards of tobacco; the risks of salt; the perils of cholesterol; the need for exercise and the benefits of equanimity. It's all a bloody bore, and most people resent such massive intrusion into their life styles.

Patients react initially to these fiats in several different ways. Those who are intelligent and understand the implications of untreated hypertension will follow the advice conscientiously. Some will "behave" for a few weeks and then revert to their old habits with the subconscious denial of the high blood pressure. ("After all, I feel so *well*.") Others refuse to cooperate at all ("I'll just take my chances. Life is too short for that sort of regimen.")

I Wouldn't Sell You Life Insurance

I wouldn't sell life insurance to anyone in the latter two categories, and I would suggest that you defer trying to buy any until your pressure is down—unless you are prepared to pay a stiff extra premium. You see, the insurance companies know the score. In statistics accumulated over the years from millions of subscribers, they have found that even in "border-line" cases, persons with blood pressures of 138/88 (we still consider 140/90 the cutoff point for the normal range), the chances of death are 36 percent higher in men and 22 percent higher in women. When we look at readings of 158–167, the risk is 110 percent greater in men and 67 percent greater in women.

Unless You Comply

But suppose that you are a complier. You realize that lowering your blood pressure is important, especially since you have read the projection that if all thirty-five million Americans with high blood pressure were adequately treated, the over-all death rate from strokes and heart attacks would probably drop another 20 percent. You were also impressed by the fact that 68 percent of patients who develop a heart attack and 75 percent of those who sustain strokes have a prior history of untreated high blood pressure. So you faithfully follow the advice given you. You adhere to your diet, lose weight, reduce your salt intake and try to "relax" as best you can. You come back a few weeks later hoping and expecting that your blood pressure will now be normal. But you are disappointed to find the levels only slightly reduced. You are told you will need medication, which the doctor now prescribes. (Remember, you have gone to him without serious complaints in the first place, other than perhaps an occasional headache or nosebleed.) As you leave the office, armed with a prescription for pills that you will probably have to take for the rest of your life, you are at least a little resentful—toward yourself, your bad luck and your doctor. The pills cost money, as will the revisits to check their effectiveness.

Getting Angrier and Angrier

In the next few weeks, your anger and frustration increase. You are nervous as hell, because you are not smoking. You long for forbidden foods. And now, to top it all off, you have begun to notice some side effects from the drugs. At this point, some patients throw in the towel. They quit the regimen and stop going to the doctor.

This doesn't exactly leave the doctor happy either. He has failed to make his point and he has lost a patient in the process. This happens so often that many doctors don't prescribe drugs for the control of high blood pressure until they "really have to"; they leave "borderline" values, which are also dangerous to you, untreated. To protect yourself against that possibility, always ask your doctor what your pressure is and write the numbers down. Be prepared to discuss with him whether you should be treated. Pressure readings are not a secret to be shared only by your physician and your insurance company for the purposes of determining premiums. There is the matter of your life—its quality and duration.

The Numbers Game

What are the numbers for which you require treatment? There is still no unanimous agreement, but the criteria are coming down with every new study reported. It seems that the lower the pressure, the better your outlook—regardless. For example, even though 140/80 is "normal," and nobody would give you medication to lower it, if you happen to have a pressure of 110/70, you are less likely, at least statistically, to come down with one of the complications of arteriosclerosis at some future date.

My Personal Technique

I use the following criteria in my own practice. If there are three successive readings, on different days, greater than 140/90 in persons under sixty years of age, I begin treatment. Beyond age sixty, as the arteries become more rigid and less flexible, I accept 160/90 as the upper limit of normal and treat any values above that.

Sometimes, especially in the course of an insurance examination, the "friendly" doctor who finds a "borderline" blood pressure, will turn the light out and have you lie down, and rest so that your pressure will drop to an "acceptable" level. Such "tranquil" pressures are good for purposes of reducing the insurance premium. They should not, however, constitute the basis for any decision about treatment. You and I should know your pressure response in "the real world" —not in a darkened room, where you are relaxing on a couch.

I have even had patients, when told that their blood pressure is high, plead for another chance. They go home, load up on tranquilizers and come back a few days later looking like zombies. They are surprised when I tell them their readings are unchanged. Although stress and anxiety do raise the pressure, true hypertension is not really a consequence of emotional disturbance. It is a complex biological disease involving many factors—nervous and hormonal. Tranquilizers and other sedatives may help you deal with some crisis in your life, but these are not antihypertensive drugs and should not be used as such over the long term.

How Much Testing Before Treatment?

At this point, you may be confronted with another problem that requires a second opinion, the matter of how thoroughly the *cause*(s) of your hypertension should be medically evaluated. Although we know what happens in association with high blood pressure—the arterial walls are in spasm, hardening of the arteries is accelerated over the years, the level of certain hormones, like renin, circulating in the bloodstream is sometimes increased—the basic, underlying mechanisms responsible for all of this are not understood in the great majority of cases. But in about 5 percent of patients with hypertension, specific, curable causes *can* be identified and eliminated, after which the blood pressure usually remains normal without need for any medication. These forms of hypertension include certain tumors of the adrenal gland and particular types of kidney disease. In order to diagnose such unusual situations, a fairly extensive and expensive workup is required—chemical, hormonal and radiographic.

Now, the question you may face at some point is whether you should submit to such a complex diagnostic evaluation. Years ago, most physicians, especially the "purists" among us, insisted that *everybody* with hypertension (and that included the 95 percent of cases where no cause is ever found) be thoroughly screened in order to identify the meager 5 percent of patients who have the curable form. That approach soon became impractical, especially after the nationwide campaign for the detection and treatment of hypertension was launched. There just isn't enough money in the public treasury, nor are most people willing or able to spend the amounts necessary to undergo tests that are so unlikely to yield any positive results. However, since the tiny number of these curable cases occur, for the most part, in younger individuals, the compromise to which most doctors have agreed is that when significant hypertension is found in persons under forty years of age, a thorough workup is recommended. If you are in your fifties or sixties, are found to have high blood pressure with nothing to suggest that you fall into any of the unusual categories, and it is recommended that you undergo CT scans, kidney X rays and sophisticated biochemical testing, ask for another opinion from a hypertension specialist.

How to Cope with Side Effects of Medication

Now let us get back to the hypothetical situation in which you find that doing your best to lower the blood pressure by changing your life style and eating habits is not enough. Chances are, mind you, that if you are overweight, and succeed in losing a substantial amount of weight, you might not need any medication whatsoever. But suppose you can't—or won't. You are then given medication that seems to have some side effects. In almost every instance, these are either temporary or tolerable—or the blood pressure can be controlled by some other drug that you will be able to handle more easily. (But remember, there are no side effects as disastrous as a stroke, kidney failure, blindness, heart attack or death.)

If you are still unhappy with the medication that you have been given and your doctor tells you that it is the unavoidable price you must pay for normalizing your blood pressure, that "every blood pressure medication has side effects," get another opinion. It is almost always possible to adjust your regimen so that you are virtually symptom-free.

How Antihypertension Drugs Work

In order to understand how and why we use certain agents to lower your pressure, you must first appreciate what happens to the circulation when the pressure is high. The level of the pressure depends, to a great extent, on the caliber of the arteries within which the blood flows. If you fish or canoe or swim, you know that the wider the river, the more languid the water; the narrower the stream, the more quickly it seems to flow and the greater is the apparent pressure of that flow. In the disease that we call high blood pressure, the arterial walls are taut, and it is this tension that is largely responsible for the elevated pressure within the vessel.

The volume of blood within the artery also contributes to its pressure. Blood volume is increased by salt. So, treatment of high blood pressure involves reducing the blood volume by a low-salt diet and diuretics. (Incidentally, there are many subtle traps into which you may fall in trying to reduce your salt intake. Avoiding obviously salty foods is easy, but how is one supposed to know that Vichy water, for instance, is loaded with salt, or that many packaged foods are salt laden?) Arterial wall pressure must also be relaxed. Since the nervous system acts on the arterial wall to keep it tense, agents that neutralize these reflexes reduce blood pressure. These drugs may counter the nervous influences where they actually originate, that is, in the brain itself, or where they end up, in the nerves that supply the tiny muscles within the arterial wall which can constrict or narrow the vessel.

In some patients with hypertension, there is an excess of a hormone, called *renin*, that throws the arterial wall into spasm. This spasm can be neutralized by beta-blocking drugs, like Inderal and Lopressor. A new agent called captopril (Capotet), belonging to the family of drugs referred to as angiostensen converting enzyme inhibitors, prevents the formation of renin.

Combining Several Drugs in Small Amounts

We often use small amounts of several drugs in combination to modify the different mechanisms that may be raising the blood pressure. Using low doses of each agent reduces the incidence of side effects, most of which are determined by the size of the dose of any given drug.

Diuretics—No Wonder They're Called "Water Pills"

Unless you are diabetic or suffering from gout, the first drug your doctor is likely to give you is a diuretic. Most of the many available belong to a family of drugs called "thiazides." They lower pressure primarily by causing a loss of salt and water via the urine. As a result, you have to empty your bladder frequently. (These are not called "water pills" for nothing!) The "thiazides" increase the loss of potassium, as well as salt, in the urine. This doesn't create a problem for most people, if they take extra potassium in the form of orange juice, bananas or figs. It may, however, occasionally cause generalized muscle weakness. Also, if you are taking digitalis (Digoxin, digitoxin) too, low potassium levels do become important, because they enhance digitalis toxicity, which you will recognize by the onset of nausea and disturbances in cardiac rhythm.

The other consequences of the depletion of body sodium, potassium and other trace minerals like magnesium, is leg cramps. Diuretics may also raise blood sugar to diabetic levels; stopping them will usually result in a return to normal levels. (So, if you are told that your blood sugar is high, and you were recently started on a "thiazide" preparation, that may be the cause.) In addition to elevating the blood sugar, diuretics frequently increase the uric-acid content of the blood too. That usually doesn't amount to anything more than an abnormal value on paper. But if you have had gout in the past, it can precipitate an acute attack.

Some patients taking diuretics also develop higher levels of blood fats (cholesterol and triglycerides). As many as a third of the males taking them become impotent and fail to ejaculate. But before blaming the impotence on this medication or any other pill, remember that hypertension itself can cause sexual problems in men. Here is an important clue in helping to pinpoint the responsibility for the impotence, should it occur while you are taking diuretics. "Thiazides" may impair sexual function, but they do not diminish desire—an important distinction.

Aldactone and dyrenium, both diuretics (not "thiazides"), are sometimes used alone or in combination with other water pills, because they minimize the loss of potassium. Many men taking Aldactone become impotent and frequently develop large breasts as well. In women, the suspicion that it may cause breast cancer has also been raised. If you have been given Aldactone, discuss all these possible consequences with your doctor.

Anyone reading this list of side effects from the diuretics might easily conclude that they are horrendous drugs to be avoided and that it is preferable to take one's chances with the high blood pressure. That, of course, is nonsense, because most of their adverse reactions are mild and can be eliminated by adjustment of the dosage. One way to do that is to really cut down your salt intake. The less salt you eat, the less of the diuretic you will need.

When you complain to your doctor about any of these symptoms, he will either cut back the dose of the diuretic or eliminate it and go on to something else—probably a "beta-blocker."

My First Choice, the Beta-Blockers

In the United States, there are currently five available beta-blockers called Inderal, Lopressor, Corgard, Tenormin and timolol, with several more on the way. They are thought to neutralize the hormone *renin,* which is responsible for some cases of high blood pressure.

I prefer to initiate treatment of my hypertensive patients with beta-blockers because, in my experience, they have fewer side effects than do the diuretics. For example, they do not raise blood sugar, lower potassium, increase uric acid or keep you going to the toilet. You will, however, notice that they slow your pulse rate especially if you are also taking digitalis. You may feel somewhat more tired too, but only for the first few days. Bear in mind, however, that if you are asthmatic or have any degree of heart weakness or failure, these drugs may not be suitable for you.

There is no question that the beta-blockers can interfere with sexual function in men. When they do, before abandoning them, try switching to another "brand." For example, Tenormin is said to cause less impotence than do some of the others. Persons taking beta-blockers have also complained of nightmares; one man whom I was treating reported painful enlargement of his breasts; and others have had cramps and diarrhea. If you have been given beta-blockers for your hypertension and have angina as well, you should know that stopping the drug suddenly (as opposed to tapering it) may be dangerous and may induce a heart attack. But, all things considered, the beta-blockers are extremely useful, effective and well tolerated in the treatment of high blood pressure.

A third group of drugs sometimes used for lowering blood pressure is derived from an Indian herb called *Rauwolfia*. These are not nearly as popular as they once were. A purified form, reserpine, is available, either alone or in combination with other drugs. I have never liked it much, because it can cause serious depression, especially in older persons. I don't think this particular drug should be in your medicine cabinet unless you have no alternative.

Another agent still widely used, but which is not among my first choices either, is methyldopa (marketed as Aldomet). Although it lowers blood pressure effectively, it also causes impotence in at least 40 percent of men taking it, may produce retrograde ejaculation (during orgasm, the sperm is ejected back into the bladder instead of out of the penis), often makes the breasts larger and tender and may have other untoward effects on the blood. Never take it if you have any form of liver trouble. If this drug has been prescribed for you and you find that you have lost all interest in sex, or can't do much about it even if you still have the desire, ask your doctor to discontinue the methyldopa and give you some other medication. So many patients are afraid to make such suggestions to the doctor, especially when the side effects are in the sexual area. They suffer unnecessarily in silence, because they are too timid or ashamed to talk about it.

Clonidine, another blood-pressure-lowering agent, is chemically like methyldopa, but its side effects may include dizziness when you stand up suddenly, impaired sexual function and a rebound of blood pressure should you stop it abruptly. Do not take beta-blockers either. I use it only when nothing else works. (Like so many other discoveries in medicine, a very interesting, important and totally unrelated effect was serendipitously noted with this drug. It was found that when heroin addicts were given clonidine, the narcotic could be abruptly stopped ("cold-turkey") without the usual agonizing withdrawal symptoms. This may prove to be one of the most important pharmacologic observations in many years.)

Then there is guanethidine, useful in those cases of hypertension resistant to all other forms of therapy. I don't use it much anymore (unless I have to), because patients often suffer what we call "postural hypotension" when they change positions suddenly, as, for example, leaping out of bed in the morning. The blood pressure drops precipitously, leaving them very dizzy. Guanethidine may also be responsible for poor sexual function.

Your doctor may also prescribe prazosin ("Minipres") and hydralazine ((Apresoline"), both of which are very effective, especially when used in combination with beta-blockers or diuretics.

Whatever medications you take, if they give you disturbing symptoms that your doctor cannot seem to control, you should seek another opinion from an expert in this field.

Capotet (captopril) which blocks the formation of renin, is the newest of the anti-hypertensive agents. It was heralded as being effective with minimal side effects. The manufacturer and the Food and Drug Administration recommend, however, that it be used only when other medication doesn't do the job, or when side effects are intolerable. They warn against the possibility of running into kidney trouble with it. It can also reduce the number of white blood cells your bone marrow makes, rendering you more susceptible to infection. But these manifestations of toxicity are not common.

I have prescribed captopril according to the guidelines, and found it useful in some cases, but not revolutionary. I found it to reduce the elevated blood pressure only modestly when given alone, but much more effective in combination with a diuretic. Its greatest application in my own practice has been in men rendered impotent by other medication. If you have high blood pressure, and have such problems with your regimen, ask your doctor for captopril. There is not enough experience with this drug yet to warrant its use by pregnant women and nursing mothers.

What About TM and Biofeedback?

Can biofeedback, relaxation techniques or transcendental meditation reduce blood pressure? While I think these can all help you to relax and, in so doing, perhaps lower blood pressure slightly, I do not believe that used alone they are reliable or effective ways of treating high blood pressure over the long term.

Low Blood Pressure

Many patients complain of "nonspecific" symptoms whose causes are rarely identified. They have no energy, are always tired, nervous, weak and sweaty, and they are troubled by cold hands and feet. Even after we investigate them thoroughly, we often find no underlying disease. Thyroid function is normal, and there is no anemia. After such a negative work-up, there is a great tendency (and temptation) to ascribe these complaints either to low blood sugar (*hypoglycemia*, discussed elsewhere in this book) or low blood pressure.

Low Blood Pressure Is Not a Disease

If you learn nothing else about blood pressure, remember this: *Low blood pressure is rarely abnormal or a disease.* (That obviously does not refer to the low blood pressure [hypotension] induced by medication, shock or the drop that sometimes occurs in the course of a severe heart attack.) Those people with underfunction of the thyroid gland or Addison's disease (President Kennedy had it; it is an inadequate production of hormones by the adrenal glands) have low pressures, but then it is not a disease—only a symptom of another disorder. If you don't have such another condition, and your pressure is low, *leave it alone*.

The lower your blood pressure, the better off you are, so that even though 120/80 is excellent, 105/75 is still better. In our attempt to correct numbers or eliminate symptoms often due to other causes, we may be too vigorous and treat a perfectly good, but low blood pressure without reason.

So remember, if you have symptoms of weakness or dizziness and all your doctor can find is a "low blood pressure," ask for a second opinion if he recommends hormone treatment to correct the "disorder." Such therapy is rarely needed or justified.

KEY FACTS TO REMEMBER

High blood pressure is an important "silent killer." It is the major cause of strokes, and it may lead to heart failure, kidney malfunction, and other manifestations of arteriosclerosis. Although it sometimes is responsible for headaches and nosebleeds, more often than not it gives no symptoms and can be detected only by routine blood-pressure measurements. It tends to be more prevalent and severe among blacks.

The importance of treating all cases of elevated blood pressure has begun to be appreciated only recently. Because of the "free ride" for so many years, during which the patient experiences no symptoms, some doctors and many patients tend to be permissive about this serious disease. National educational and treatment programs relative to hypertension have already resulted in a 23 percent decrease in the incidence of strokes in the United States since 1972.

Weight loss, regular exercise and reduction of salt intake are all beneficial in controlling high blood pressure, but most people require drugs for the rest of their lives. When properly selected and in the right dosage and combination, these agents are well tolerated. Anyone who simply "can't take blood pressure pills" should ask for help from a specialist in this field.

Except in very rare circumstances, low blood pressure is not a disease but a blessing. Never agree to having it raised artificially without asking for a second opinion.

13

Thrombophlebitis, Varicose Veins and Blood Thinners

In an earlier chapter I described a hypothetical case of thrombophlebitis and the seemingly conflicting advice the patient was given for it. Let us now look at this disorder more seriously and in greater detail.

Thrombo means clot, *phlebitis* means inflammation of a vein. When the interior lining of a vein becomes inflamed, the blood no longer flows smoothly within it, and little clots form and stick to the vessel wall. Anything, therefore, that either injures the veins in your leg or causes the blood to flow more slowly through them can cause thrombophlebitis—an infection, a blow to the leg, prolonged bed rest or heart failure (when the blood stagnates within the vein), certain diseases in which the blood is more viscous than it should be, and various kinds of hormones (especially estrogens, which are used in the pill and in other situations). Also, when you develop phlebitis, first in one leg or arm and then in another, and for no apparent reason, we suspect the presence of a malignant tumor somewhere, most commonly the pancreas or the lung. Such cancers probably produce a substance that affects the circulation within the veins.

What Else Can This Leg Pain Be?

You wake up one morning with a "charley horse" or some other pain in the calf, foot, or other part of the leg. It hurts more when you stand on it or touch it. You think you may have knocked against some object—a table or other piece of furniture—without knowing it, and simply bruised the area. Or you think that maybe it's a muscle injury from too much jogging or tennis. You know that the diuretic you are taking may have thrown your muscles into spasm by causing a loss of magnesium or potassium (or both). You seem to recall similar symptoms when you were given Atromid-S for control of high cholesterol.

All these things may give you pain in a leg, and such pain is sometimes difficult to distinguish from phlebitis. But if you have varicose veins to begin with (through which the blood flow is slow) and have been sitting for long periods of time with your legs crossed or hanging down, as for example, on a plane trip (and the way the leg room and seats in economy class of airplanes are shrinking these days, or been confined to bed for days or weeks, this is becoming more and more of a problem), if you are taking the pill, have just had a baby or actually injured a vein in your leg by striking it accidentally, the likelihood that the pain is due to thrombophlebitis is somewhat greater.

The Dangers of Phlebitis

The danger of thrombophlebitis lies in the possibility that a piece of the clot attached to the vein wall will break off and travel along the circulatory pathway. Since blood coming from almost all the veins in the body (except from the brain and the heart) ultimately goes to the lungs, we worry about the clot ending up there. (A traveling clot is called an *embolus;* the organ in which it finally lodges is said to have an *embolism;* damage caused by the clot is called an *infarction*.) So, an embolus from a phlebitis in the legs, going to the lungs, gives you a pulmonary embolism with infarction. If the fragment is tiny and the size of the infarcted area is small, your symptoms will consist of nothing more than some pain in the chest when you take a deep breath, a little cough and perhaps some bloody sputum. You are sick, but you are not likely to die. On the other hand, if a big clot ends up in the lung, and obstructs a large blood vessel, you may be in serious trouble.

Pulmonary embolism is an important cause of death and

disability in patients with thrombophlebitis. Since we can never predict the size of an embolus, it is very important to diagnose the thrombophlebitis correctly and treat it properly —and in time. For some reason which I don't understand, phlebitis in the arms, the kind that sometimes follows intravenous therapy, rarely if ever sends clots to the lungs. It does not require the same treatment as does phlebitis in the legs.

How Phlebitis Is Diagnosed

When you show the doctor your painful leg, he must decide whether you have phlebitis. The diagnosis is often, but not always, obvious. The leg hurts; it is swollen, red, warm and tender to the touch. When the doctor abruptly jerks your foot up and back toward your knee, that worsens the pain in the calf of your leg. If, in addition, he can feel a swollen, tender vein in your leg, then you almost surely have phlebitis. But the classical clinical evidence that I have described is not always present, and the diagnosis based on that evidence is accurate in no more than about 50 percent of the cases. *Whenever phlebitis is suspected and the doctor is less than absolutely certain, objective testing is necessary.* Make sure you get it before making any commitment to therapy.

The need to be certain about the diagnosis is well illustrated in the following story. A fifty-eight-year-old man came to see me because of pain in the calf of his left leg. He had just returned from a trip to Europe. In the preceding few weeks he had done a lot of flying, walking and climbing—a perfect setup for thrombophlebitis. The sore leg looked a little larger than the other, and did, in fact, measure one quarter of an inch more around. But such minor variations in leg girth are not uncommon. It also felt a little warm, and it hurt, especially when I pressed on it. One fairly reliable test for thrombophlebitis was also positive—when I jerked the foot back toward his knee, the patient winced.

On Being Led Down the Garden Path—by Shingles

The diagnosis seemed fairly straightforward, and I sent the patient to the hospital for treatment of thrombophlebitis. Intravenous heparin, a potent blood thinner, was started immediately. The patient's family then asked for a consultant

whom they had used in another instance of vascular disease—
"just to be sure." The consultant examined the patient, and
he too was impressed by the findings. He nevertheless
performed a Doppler test to evaluate the blood flow in the
veins. It was completely normal. "How accurate is that
machine?" I asked. "Only about 60 to 80 percent," he replied.
"Well," I answered, "in that case, I think we should continue
the anticoagulants since the picture is so typical of phlebitis."
And we did. Some three or four days later, while reexamining
the leg, I noticed a few little pimples behind the knee.
Within the next twenty-four hours, the patient developed
shingles. This disease accounted for all the pain, redness and
warmth in the leg. I had been led down the garden path by
the herpes zoster virus. The Doppler test was right, and I
was wrong.

Treatment Depends on Diagnosis and Judgment

The basic treatment decision in any case of phlebitis
to use or not use anticoagulants depends on the veins
involved—whether they are deep or superficial. When the
phlebitis is superficial, it is easy to see, rarely embolizes, and
therefore does not usually require thinning the blood. Therapy involves resting the leg, keeping it elevated and applying
warm soaks. If pain is disabling, the addition of an anti-
inflammatory agent like phenybutozone (Butazolidin; Azolid-
A) will relieve symptoms. But never take it for more than five
consecutive days. It can cause serious injury to the bone
marrow. Symptoms usually subside in a few days. If they
don't, or if they appear to be getting worse, anticoagulants
may be necessary.

Sometimes, however, withholding anticoagulants in such
cases can be disastrous, when the deep veins, those that do
embolize, are diseased, too. Not long ago, another patient
came to me with a typical, superficial thrombophlebitis, and I
prescribed what I described above. I had her rest the leg,
elevate it, and apply moist heat. Two days later she called to
tell me that she was coughing, had a pain in the chest and
was spitting blood. She had, in fact, thrown a blood clot from
a coexisting deep-vein phlebitis, which had gone unrecognized.
The point to remember is that even when the phlebitis is

superficial, objective testing is a good idea, to make sure the deep, threatening form is not also present.

When Objective Testing Is Better Than Clinical Judgment

There are several diagnostic techniques to determine whether the deep veins of the leg are involved and, indeed, whether the leg pain is due to a vascular problem at all. The most definitive procedure is called a venogram, an X ray of the veins taken after a contrast medium has been injected into them. But most vascular specialists first evaluate blood flow in the leg noninvasively by the Doppler method described earlier, as well as by a procedure called venous outflow plethysmography. Don't hesitate to ask your own physician whether he needs to use any of these techniques in order to be absolutely certain about the diagnosis in your case.

When Phlebitis Strikes the Deep Veins

When the deep veins are inflamed, the risk of embolism is high and you will usually be sent to a hospital for several days to have your blood thinned. For an immediate effect, we start with intravenous heparin. Then, after a few days, we give you an oral preparation (warfarin). How long the anticoagulants are continued depends on several factors. If this was your first attack and was not complicated by a blood clot to the lung, anticoagulation is usually continued four to six months. If, however, you have varicose veins, suffer from recurrent phlebitis and have already had a plumonary embolism, you may well be kept on anticoagulants indefinitely.

Problems of Anticoagulation

Aside from the inconvenience (you need to have your blood tested at regular intervals [usually every three to four weeks] to make sure it is not too thin and hence vulnerable to bleeding) and cost, it is important that you not take anticoagulants unnecessarily. They can sometimes create their own problems. You may, for example, be allergic to them and develop a rash. If you have high blood pressure, anticoagulants put you at risk for a brain hemorrhage. And then there always is the danger of internal bleeding when the blood gets too thin, something that may happen spontaneously or after an accident. Remember, too, that the level of anticoagulation can be thrown off kilter by some other medication introduced into your regimen—a sleeping pill, antibiotic, or pain-killer.

Phlebitis and "Mainlining"

One form of phlebitis that we are seeing more and more these days results from the increasing use of illegal drugs by addicts. Because of improper sterilization techniques, the veins become infected by the contaminated needle, as is the clot formed within them. This gives rise to what is called "septic thrombophlebitis," a much more serious situation than is the sterile clot. Because now, instead of the embolus just blocking an artery in the heart, it spreads infection as well. Although septic phlebitis commonly occurs after illicit drug injection by addicts, it can also result from poor intravenous technique in hospitals.

Melting the Clot

There is an emerging form of treatment of phlebitis of which you should also be aware, although it is still mainly in the experimental stage and is restricted in its use to large medical centers. I am referring to "thrombolytic" therapy— the administration into the bloodstream of enzymes (streptokinase and urokinase) whose purpose it is to dissolve the clots. Their use at this time remains controversial, although the proponents are very enthusiastic. This treatment carries with it potential risks, mainly hemorrhage (in almost 10 percent of patients), but it should be considered in the setting of recurrent embolism despite anticoagulants. If decided upon, it should be done early, within five to seven days after symptoms appear, and it should be continued for 24 to 48 hours. You are not eligible for this treatment if you are a "bleeder," or have had a stroke recently. Thrombolytic therapy, however, should never be done except by an expert in its use, usually a hematologist (blood specialist) or vascular specialist.

Treating Varicose Veins

Before leaving the subject of veins, let us discuss the management of varicose veins. It is estimated that one in five Americans and half the population over fifty years of age have this condition. They often occur in various members of the same family and are seen most commonly in women who have had many children, or in persons who must stand a great deal at work. Varicose veins do not usually require surgery. If you keep off your legs whenever you can, avoid crossing your legs, elevate them when you sit (using an ottoman or footstool), raise the foot of the bed a little at night and wear support hose, chances are that you won't have any problem. Your legs may simply feel tired and ache at the end of the day.

In some women, varicose veins may become more tender during the menstrual period; in others, they are unsightly. Patients often ask for their removal for cosmetic reasons—a perfectly reasonable request. When the varicose veins are very small so that you see little red streaks in the legs but can't really feel them, operation does not usually help. The best thing to do in such cases is to wear an elastic stocking, many of which are now cosmetically acceptable. You can also help your varicose veins by a regular program of brisk walking, swimming as often as you can, performing simple leg exercises, and walking barefoot whenever possible.

The Expendable Vein

How can the blood continue to flow normally when a varicose vein is removed? There is a whole network of veins in the legs, and some pretty large ones can be cut away (as we do in coronary bypass operations, where we substitute a vein in the leg for the diseased artery) without affecting the venous circulation.

If you choose not to have surgery, the varicosities can be injected with a solution that closes them up. I am not sure that that is as safe and long-lasting as vein "stripping"—the operative approach. If you are advised to do it that way, make sure that your doctor is skilled in this technique.

KEY FACTS TO REMEMBER

Thrombophlebitis signifies the formation of a clot within a vein. This can result from a number of causes, ranging from simple injury to cancer somewhere in the body. Thrombophlebitis in the leg produces pain, redness and swelling, and it may be difficult to distinguish from several nonvascular causes. Correct diagnosis is imperative because, unless properly treated, phlebitis can result in a portion of the clot traveling to the lung (embolism—a dangerous complication).

When the possibility of phlebitis exists, a second opinion from a vascular specialist should be obtained. He will use several techniques, some of which are not invasive, to determine whether a clot is actually present. If the diagnosis is confirmed, anticoagulants will usually be given. In cases where, despite such treatment, phlebitis and embolism recur, some doctors are using "thrombolytic enzymes" to dissolve the clots. However, this technique is still experimental and is not without risk; it should be used only by experts (hematologists or vascular specialists).

In most cases, varicose veins can be managed conservatively, without surgery. If "injection" of the veins or an operation are recommended, consult a vascular specialist.

14

The Arteries and Your Circulation— From False Alarms to True Aneurysms

Sometimes but Not Always the Trouble

We are too quick to attribute any symptoms in the arms and legs, hands and feet, to poor circulation. "My toes are numb. They're probably not getting enough blood." Or "I know I have bad circulation, because of the terrible cramps in my legs that wake me up so often I spend half my nights walking around the room to get rid of them." The first complaint may be due to a circulatory disorder, the second probably is not.

Pain, weakness, cramps, numbness, tingling or coldness of the extremities, all can be due to many different causes only a minority of which reflect problems of blood flow. The long list of noncirculatory disorders that may result in these symptoms includes arthritis (of the limbs themselves or of the spine), other diseases that affect the nerves, making them irritable or interfering with their function (diabetes, syphilis), some medication you are taking (diuretics), and muscular injury, strain or spasm.

Mimicking Vascular Pain

You may not always know whether certain symptoms are due to circulatory causes, but your doctor will. Consider arthritis of the spine, for example, in which the nerves supplying the legs are either irritated by the diseased bone or displaced by a disc pressing on them. When that happens, despite a normal circulation, you may have pain in the legs, usually when you assume certain positions lying in bed, or sitting or standing. The trouble is in the spine, even though you perceive the pain along the pathway of the compromised nerve—in the toes, heels, buttocks, calves, shoulders, elbows, hands or chest.

In diabetes too the nerves are frequently diseased (diabetic neuropathy), not by mechanical pressure as in spinal arthritis or disc disease, but because of some chemical effect of the diabetes itself. These "sick" nerves cause pain in the legs (or elsewhere, depending on which nerves are affected). Again, these symptoms have nothing to do with circulation (although diabetics are, in fact, prone to vascular problems too).

You can suffer pain in the legs from muscle spasm due to any number of causes, including injury, strain, inadequate arch support, too soft a mattress, bad posture or excessive jogging.

"Feeling cold" in the hands or feet often reflects temporary constriction, spasm or narrowing of perfectly healthy arteries from which the blood has been shunted when the body needs it elsewhere. In this way, blood flow is temporarily diverted from relatively noncritical areas, like the hands and feet, to more vital organs, like the kidneys, heart, brain and liver. Finally, cold extremities may result from diseases that have nothing to do with poor circulation, as, for example, hypothyroidism. Such patients not only feel cold, they are cold. The beta-blockers, like Inderal, can also induce these symptoms. Switching from one of these drugs to another will often improve these symptoms.

When disease of the arteries does occur, it can involve many different areas—the brain, where it may result in a stroke; the eye, where it may cause blindness; the heart, where it may culminate in a heart attack; the kidneys, where it may end up as renal failure; and in the intestines where it causes severe pain after eating. The aorta, the large arterial trunk that leaves the heart and branches to all parts of the body, may also become arteriosclerotic, in which event, blood supply to the brain or legs may be reduced, depending on the site of obstruction. When the penis is deprived of its normal blood flow, the result is impotence.

How You Can Tell One Pain from Another

Symptoms of inadequate circulation, whether in the legs or in the chest, almost always occur with effort. When pain in the legs comes on at rest, during the night, or while you are standing or sitting still, it is not likely to be circulatory. But, if you suddenly feel a cramp or "charley horse" in the calf while walking (it may actually occur higher or lower in the leg, but the calf is the most common site), and it disappears within minutes after you stop, chances are that it is vascular. In angina pectoris—pain in the chest due to coronary-artery disease—there is a similar relation to effort. Angina occurs on exertion when the coronary arteries in the heart are narrowed and are unable to deliver enough blood to the heart muscle.

How Your Doctor Makes the Diagnosis

When you tell the doctor that you have pain in the legs on walking at a certain pace, he will do the appropriate tests to confirm the presence of circulatory insufficiency. He will first touch various parts of the leg, looking for temperature differences. When blood flow to any area is diminished, it feels cold, not only to you but to the examiner as well. It is not a very reliable way to establish the diagnosis, but it helps. He will also check the various pulses in your groin and legs, to see whether they are full, diminished or absent. He will look at the color of the legs to see whether either or both are blanched. Also, when blood supply is inadequate, men often lose the little tufts of hair on the top of their toes.

If your doctor is particularly interested or skilled in vascular disease, he will probably examine the circulation by the Doppler method, which employs an ultrasonic probe and assesses the blood mass flowing through the artery beneath it.

How Much Collateral Do You Have?

If the diagnosis of vascular disease is confirmed, don't worry about losing your legs. There are many thousands of people with this problem, only a very small number of whom eventually require amputation. Patients with arteriosclerosis are protected by the formation of a collateral circulation. The demand for blood in the muscles of the leg is increased by such exercise as regular walking. Since the narrowed arteries cannot supply the extra amount needed, the ever resourceful body forms new channels or widens smaller ones already there, providing "collateral flow." So, if you have pain when you walk, don't retreat to the armchair; the best way to improve your circulation is to keep moving as much as you can.

You Must Stop Smoking

There is something else that you will have to do, whether you like it or not. *You must absolutely stop smoking.* Not cut down, or change the brand, or avoid inhaling the smoke—all the old excuses—but never touch another weed, stogie or pipe. If you don't stop smoking, other treatment is almost meaningless. Moreover, most doctors, including me, will have nothing to do with you if you continue to smoke. Tobacco causes the arteries to go into spasm. This further constricts the already narrowed vessels, worsening your symptoms despite anything we can do for you.

But Don't Go Off the Wagon

According to tradition, a little alcohol at bedtime is good for you, because it supposedly dilates the arteries. That theory has been questioned recently, but it is such a pleasant form of therapy that nobody challenges it very seriously. If you have a problem with alcohol and have finally gone on the wagon, don't start drinking again in order to benefit your circulation.

I remember one patient with exertional leg pain to whom I recommended a brandy at bedtime. He never told me he was a recovered alcoholic. My well-meant advice, which he had accepted with great pleasure and alacrity, nullified the results of months of psychiatric treatment.

Whether you take that nip or two, there are other things to be done for the arterial circulation in your legs. Warm compresses or a heating pad applied near the groin or lower abdomen for a few hours at bedtime will reflexly dilate the vessels lower down in the leg and may improve your symptoms. But make sure that you don't burn yourself in the process, and never apply heat directly to the affected limb.

More advanced cases of circulatory disease in the legs sometimes benefit from the use of an oscillating bed which rotates a certain number of degrees very gradually, up and down, thus stimulating the circulation.

How to Waste Your Money

Too many doctors still indiscriminately prescribe the so-called vasodilator drugs for circulatory problems. I understand that the Food and Drug Administration is currently reviewing these agents to determine whether claims for their effectiveness are warranted. They may be when symptoms are due predominantly or solely to *spasm* of the arteries (Raynaud's disease) rather than obstruction by arteriosclerotic plaques. But most cases of arterial disease are due to blockage of the arteries, and here the vasodilator drugs are of little or no benefit whatsoever. As a matter of fact, at least theoretically, they can even make things worse. The blood vessels they end up widening are not the narrow ones that need it, because those are too rigid and diseased to respond. So they dilate the healthy ones. As a result, blood is shunted to them and away from the critically narrowed ones.

If you are being given medication to "improve" the circulation in your legs, ask your doctor whether he really thinks you need it. He may just be prescribing it to keep you happy that "something" is being done.

Is Your Cast Too Tight?

If you have diseased arteries in your legs, avoid tight or elastic stockings which only further compress already narrowed arteries. Also, take care to protect a limb with poor blood supply. Even a trivial blow, especially if it breaks the skin, may cause serious problems.

I remember an elderly lady who fell one day and fractured her knee cap. This required a minor operation to remove the broken fragments. After surgery, a cast was applied from the knee to the ankle. Shortly thereafter, she kept telling anyone who would listen that it was too tight, but was assured by her orthopedist that if it were any looser it would not support the injured knee securely enough. She continued to complain of burning pain under the cast until finally, a few days later, the pressure was relieved by cutting a little window in the cast. The skin thus exposed was found to be discolored and subsequently broke down, leaving a painful ulcer, which took many months to heal. This happened because the patient's circulation was poor to begin with, and it didn't take much compression by the cast to diminish the flow even more. Fortunately, in her case, the ulcer did clear up. I know of another elderly lady with vascular disease who lost her leg from having a cast applied too tightly; her pleas about it were ignored until it was too late.

Surgery Is Up to You

In most patients with vascular disease, such simple measures as stopping tobacco, regular walking, alcohol in moderation, reflex heat to the lower abdomen or groin, and weight loss if called for usually help somewhat. But what if you find that you can walk so little that your life style is really compromised? At this point, your doctor may propose an operation. But remember that surgery is really for your comfort and not usually because the arterial disease is a threat to life or limb. In other words, any decision regarding operation is up to you. If you are perfectly satisfied being able to walk only one or two blocks (and some people are, especially if they have some other physical problem that limits their activities) there is no point to undergoing surgery.

What Kind of Operation Is Best for You?

If you agree to surgery, an arteriogram must first be done. This is a special X ray performed in the hospital. Dye is injected into the arteries of the legs, usually at the groin, and outlines the portion of the vascular tree in question, indicating the site of narrowing or obstruction, how extensive it is and whether it can be corrected. Surgery involves either replacing the diseased artery with a dacron graft, or bypassing it by attaching the graft above and below the obstructed segment. In some cases, the artery can be reamed out (*endarterectomy*) and left in place.

A Newer Alternative to Surgery

There is a new technique that you should know about—*percutaneous transluminal angioplasty*—which may preclude surgery in some cases. It is done by a radiologist (with a vascular surgeon standing by in case anything goes wrong). An ordinary arteriogram is performed, except that the catheter through which the dye is injected into the blood vessel has an inflatable balloon at its tip. It is then threaded up to the obstructed area defined in the arteriogram. Then the balloon is blown up, compressing the material blocking the blood vessel against the walls of the artery. Several of my patients have had this procedure done in the legs. (It can also be occasionally used in certain cases of coronary-artery disease as well.)

The technique of angioplasty is still in its infancy and most vascular surgeons insist that conventional surgery is safer, more effective and longer-lasting. They worry about the possible complications of angioplasty, which include rupture of the arterial wall or the breaking-off of a piece of the obstructing plaque as the balloon is distended within the blood vessel.

Nevertheless, you ought to know that this procedure is available and is being used by a growing number of doctors proficient at it. Certainly, when arterial obstruction must be relieved, and the patient is a poor surgical risk, this alternative should at least be considered. And so, if it is recommended that you have vascular surgery, ask your doctor whether there is anyone in his hospital who has experience in angioplasty, and whether you might be a candidate for this procedure. You may possibly avoid an operation.

Heading for a Blowout

The popular term for arteriosclerosis is "hardening of the arteries." Its main effect is to narrow the interior channel of the vessel and so deliver less blood to whatever organ it is nourishing. But this "hardness" does not strengthen the artery. In fact, the reverse is true. The wall becomes progressively weaker, so that a portion of the artery may begin to balloon out. This happens most frequently in cases of long-standing, untreated high blood pressure. Such ballooning constitutes an aneurysm and renders you vulnerable to its bursting, or "blowing out," much like a damaged car tire.

Most aneurysms form in the aorta, anywhere between where that vessel originates (at the heart) and ends (in the lower abdomen). The most common site is in the abdomen. Aneurysms, however, can develop in smaller arteries, especially in the brain. Here the main cause is some congenital or developmental defect in the artery itself. The consequences of their rupture depend on their size and location, but death, often instantaneous, is a common result. So it is very important that any aneurysm anywhere be detected and treated in time.

Unless You Find and Treat It

An aortic aneurysm is not easy to discover before it causes any symptoms. It may be seen either on a routine X ray of the chest or felt when the doctor examines your abdomen. Once diagnosed, the critical question is whether and when to remove it surgically. Most specialists agree that when an abdominal aneurysm attains a size of 5 cm., or roughly 2 inches, across, it should be taken out, and the removed section replaced by a Dacron tube. This number was arrived at after years of experience revealed that almost half the patients with aneurysms greater than 5 cm. die from spontaneous rupture. And size has nothing to do with the presence, absence or severity of symptoms. There are some surgeons who recommend operation no matter what the size, but they are definitely in the minority.

A False-Negative Examination

I remember one man, sixty years old, who twenty years earlier had had a mild heart attack. His blood pressure had been "modestly" elevated, but came down nicely with treatment. One night he developed pain in his belly. It wasn't really too bad, but since the Memorial Day holiday was approaching, he decided to have it attended to. He went to the Emergency Room of our hospital, where he told the intern about some dietary indiscretion earlier in the evening. He was a great gourmet, and had had a "fabulous" meal with great wines at a famous French restaurant. The doctor performed a very careful examination of the abdomen, but found nothing unusual other than a little tenderness in its mid-portion. He concluded that the man had "gastritis," gave him a stomach sedative as well as a lecture about eating and drinking too much, and sent him home.

Two hours later the patient came back to the Emergency Room, feeling much worse. The pain was now agonizing. Again, a thorough examination gave no clues as to the cause. But the man was overweight, with a paunch, so that the belly was not easy to evaluate. In order to be safe, an X ray of the abdomen was done. It did not reveal any significant abnormalities either. Because the pain was so severe, a surgeon was called, and it was decided to "explore" the patient. When the abdomen was opened, we found a large aortic aneurysm, which had ruptured. It must have been there for years—silent and undetected—until it suddenly burst. The patient survived the operation and returned to his normal eating and drinking. He subsequently became very friendly with the intern, who is now a better diagnostician—and a gourmet.

So one can have an abdominal aortic aneurysm for a long time, yet feel perfectly well with it. But if it is found and is 5 cm. or greater in diameter, you should have the surgery if you are judged able to withstand it. Your chances of living another five to ten years are doubled if you do.

How Best to Determine Aneurysm Size

Since the size of an abdominal aneurysm is critical, it must be determined as accurately as possible. That is often difficult to do in the clinical examination, which at best affords only an approximation and is notoriously unreliable in fat subjects. X rays of the abdomen may give some indication of aneurysmal size, but this is not precise either. An arteriogram (injecting dye into the blood vessel itself) is not usually much help because the opaque medium so introduced tells us only how narrow the channel of the artery is, but nothing about the vessel *wall* or how distended it may be. The most accurate, safe and simple technique for assessing aneurysm size is the sonogram. This involves sending sound waves through the abdominal wall and analyzing the reflected echo. Be sure to ask for a sonogram if you are told that you have an abdominal aortic aneurysm, no matter how small it is estimated to be.

How Should Smaller Aneurysms Be Managed?

Abdominal aneurysms less than 5 cm. in diameter are usually left alone, but with this proviso: that they be watched very carefully for evidence of increase in size and for the onset of symptoms. The best way to reduce such progression is to make sure that your blood pressure is kept at a normal level.

Too conservative an approach—waiting too long to remove an aneurysm—can be disastrous. But so can premature surgery. That is why an additional opinion from a qualified vascular specialist is so important whenever an aneurysm is discovered.

KEY FACTS TO REMEMBER

Arteriosclerosis, or "hardening of the arteries," reduces the amount of blood delivered by an artery to an organ or tissue that it is nourishing. Symptoms of this disorder will depend on where this obstruction takes place. In the legs, it causes pain (usually in the calf) on walking quickly; these symptoms subside with rest. But there are many different causes of leg pain, which may mimic that due to vascular disease. When the latter diagnosis is suspected or made, it is wise to ask for a second opinion from a vascular specialist. He has at his disposal sophisticated tools that can measure blood flow in the legs.

Arterial disease in the extremities may severely limit your ability to walk any distance at a normal pace, but only infrequently does it progress to gangrene. This favorable course is the result of the natural development of a collateral circulation. "Dilator" drugs are usually a waste of money in such cases, exercise being the best stimulus for the formation of collaterals. But you *must* stop smoking.

If surgery is advised, despite the fact that you are willing to accept the limitations of the disease, ask for another opinion from a vascular specialist.

Should surgery actually be necessary, ask about percutaneous transluminal angioplasty. This is a new, nonsurgical method of relieving arterial obstruction. Still in its infancy, this technique can be used in a few selected cases.

An aneurysm is a "bubble" developing in the weakened wall of an artery. The most common cause is long-standing, untreated high blood pressure. If you are found to have one, consult a vascular surgeon. The best way to determine aneurysmal size is by sonography. Abdominal aneurysms that attain a diameter of 5 cm. or more should usually be removed.

15

Stroke—A Major Killer on the Wane

Ending Up a Vegetable

A major stroke is perhaps the one affliction that terrifies patients more than any other. It is perceived to be worse than cancer, which, for all the suffering it causes, is usually fairly short in duration. Nor does a heart attack generate as much panic as it once did. Many are so mild that they go unnoticed, undiagnosed and even untreated, and you may be none the worse after it. Even patients with severe heart attacks are, in the majority of cases, rehabilitated.

But the thought of a stroke and its effects—being unable to control one's bowels; having to be lifted from bed to chair or to toilet; sometimes being unable to communicate with one's environment, just lying or sitting there, hearing, seeing and usually understanding, but unable to respond—seems more frightening than any other in the layman's range of medical speculation.

The Fear is Justified

The fear of having a stroke is justified when you appreciate the fact that it is the third-leading cause of death and disability in the United States, following close on the heels of heart disease and cancer. There are about 750,000 new cases and 175,000 deaths each year. But even worse is the fact that

16 percent of survivors are destined to spend the rest of their lives in a hospital; another 20 percent will never walk again without help; 31 percent will remain dependent on others wherever they end up. Yet most of these victims were in good health just a moment before the catastrophe.

That's the bad news about stroke; here's the good news. The incidence is declining dramatically in this country because its leading cause—hypertension—is being so vigorously and successfully treated.

The Origins of a Stroke

There are three kinds of stroke. The first, *cerebral hemorrhage*, occurs when an artery in the brain whose walls have been pounded year after year by high blood pressure suddenly bursts. The key to its prevention is treating the hypertension as soon as it is discovered. Instead of rupturing, the cerebral artery may develop a clot (like rust in a pipe), which shuts off the blood supply to the brain (*thrombosis*). Some doctors think that keeping cholesterol levels down and avoiding cigarettes will reduce the incidence of this disorder. Finally, the vessel may become obstructed by an *embolus*, a traveling blood clot that usually originates in the left side of the heart or in an arteriosclerotic plaque in one of the larger arteries leading into or near the brain.

Embolism, Heart Rhythm and Strokes

Clots are most likely to form within the heart and end up in the brain when the cardiac rhythm is very irregular, a condition called *atrial fibrillation*. This disorder usually requires treatment with digitalis or some other drug. But, in addition, you can be further protected by having your blood "thinned." Despite the observation that strokes in patients with atrial fibrillation rhythm can be substantially reduced by taking oral anticoagulants, not all physicians institute this therapy. So, if you are a "fibrillator" due to whatever cause (and there are several), discuss anticoagulation with your doctor.

The "Strokelet"

There is a very common group of neurological symptoms called TIA (*transient ischemic attack; ischemic* means inade-

quate blood supply). A TIA is the result of a sudden, temporary reduction in blood flow to the brain. When it occurs,
patients abruptly develop any or all of the following symptoms: dizziness, or vertigo; double vision; numbness; tingling
or weakness in an arm or leg; and temporary slurring of
speech. These symptoms persist anywhere from a few minutes to several hours (but definitely not more than 24 hours),
then completely disappear, leaving you as well as you were
before. It is critical that a TIA be correctly diagnosed,
because it usually heralds a stroke. Indeed, 40 percent of
patients with such TIAs who are not treated, end up with a
stroke within five years. But classical as these symptoms
are, they can be confused with migraine, even without the
headache.

Aspirin, but Not for Women

How do we treat such warning symptoms? Not long ago,
there was little that we could do to avert a stroke after the
warning TIA. Today, one aspirin a day has been shown to
reduce the incidence of a subsequent stroke by about 50
percent in men. Strangely enough, it doesn't seem to work in
women or in diabetics. Remember, however, it must be
aspirin, and not a substitute like Tylenol. Aspirin affords this
protection by interfering with the blood-clotting mechanism.
And if you can't take aspirin because you are allergic to it or
have an ulcer, Persantine has similar properties. So use that
instead, although the evidence of its effectiveness is not quite
as convincing as that of aspirin's. I actually prescribe both to
patients with a TIA, even to women.

All TIAs Are Not Alike

If you are having TIAs consult a neurologist. It is important to determine their cause. These transient interruptions
in blood supply to the brain may occur in either of the two
major arterial trunks that supply the brain. One is the carotid
system, which goes up the side of the neck, and which your
doctor feels and listens to when he examines you. The other
is in the vertebrobasilar artery, situated in the back of the
neck, which cannot be examined except by X rays and other
procedures. Symptoms vary depending on the location of the
vascular problem, because these arteries supply different

parts of the brain. The carotids supply the retinal artery in the eye and the gray matter of the brain. The vertebrobasilar system supplies the back and undersurface of the brain.

When the carotid artery is involved, you may develop a constellation of visual disturbances in one eye, blackout for a few minutes, or develop weakness, numbness or tingling of a hand or a leg; you may drop something that you are holding, or lose coordination; or your speech may become slurred. Blockage of the vertebrobasilar artery, on the other hand, usually results in a graying of vision, or you see double or become totally blind for the duration of the attack. There may be weakness of all four limbs rather than only one arm, and you may lose your balance or suddenly keel over. Nausea, vomiting and speechlessness are also common.

How a Neck Collar Can Prevent a Stroke

The distinction between these two kinds of transient ischemic attack is important, because they may have to be managed differently. For example, when the carotid artery is involved, the arteriosclerotic plaque obstructing it can often be removed surgically. This affords an 80 percent chance of cure, assuming that the operation is done by an experienced surgeon. But the vertebrobasilar artery system is inaccessible to the surgeon. A clot there, especially in men, is best managed by aspirin. Make sure also that your blood pressure, if it is being treated, doesn't get too low, since a TIA may occur in patients with hypertension whose pressures drop too much—especially when they get up suddenly after lying down. When that happens, blood flow to the brain is decreased below a critical level. On rare occasions, too, the vertebral artery itself is narrowed by external pressure from arthritic changes in the bones of the upper spine, especially when you move your neck from side to side, extend it, or throw your head back. For that reason, I always order neck X rays in patients with vertebrobasilar artery symptoms. It is amazing how many "strokes" can be prevented with just a neck collar.

The Anticoagulant Controversy

Anticoagulants are required when a stroke has resulted from an embolism. Although there is no hard evidence that anticoagulants in fact reduce the incidence of stroke in patients with TIA, most doctors favor their use when aspirin doesn't do the job. They are usually prescribed for two or three months, but again, some experts advise taking them indefinitely. Remember never to take aspirin while anticoagulated, because the blood can then become too thin, and you run the risk of bleeding internally. It is a good idea to ask for a second opinion when long-term anticoagulation is recommended, especially if you have hypertension, bearing in mind that this form of therapy is still controversial.

The Question of Arteriography

When should you have an arteriogram (the injection of dye into the neck arteries to see whether there is a clot anywhere that can be removed)? This invasive X ray procedure is not without danger; it should be done only if the evidence points to obstruction in the carotid artery. If it is suggested to you, get a second opinion from another neurologist. But here again, remember that legitimate differences of opinion do exist about when this procedure should be done.

If you do have an arteriogram, and are found to have a plaque in the carotid artery that threatens to close off completely or break into little pieces that can end up in the brain, you may well need to have the artery "reamed out." Make sure that this operation, an "endarterectomy," is done by a neurosurgeon or a vascular surgeon in a hospital where such cases are frequently performed. In a neurological center, the risk of an endarterectomy is about 1 percent, but it may be twenty or thirty times that in a nonspecialized institution. So don't be shy about asking for another opinion before the surgery, and be sure to inquire about the performance statistics of the neurosurgical team that will be doing the operation.

Suppose that you develop a full-blown stroke either after a TIA or suddenly without any warning. You may now be paralyzed in one or more limbs; your speech may be impaired; your face may be distorted because of muscle weakness; or you may even lapse into coma. Whatever the symptoms, there is usually gradual improvement during the next few weeks in most cases. So, no matter how bad it looks at first, never lose hope. I have seen many people completely "stroked out" (to use a favorite phrase of interns) who have gone on to full recovery.

The Role of the Hospital

Every patient who suffers a stroke should immediately be admitted to the hospital—for two reasons. First, and most important, expert nursing care is needed in the early stages, while the stroke is still evolving. The biggest threat in the first hours and days is to the breathing and swallowing mechanisms, which may have to be assisted if the stroke has involved the muscles responsible for those critical functions. Tiding you over then may mean the difference between life and death. Second, every stroke patient should have a CT scan (the computerized brain X ray) to determine the kind of attack it was—hemorrhage, clot or tumor—and how to treat it. Sometimes a curable tumor may result in a stroke, as can various types of blood disease. Their outlook and management differ greatly from the more common hemorrhage or clot. Sudden disturbance of heart rhythm can also cause a stroke, and these can be identified by cardiac monitoring.

If you have suffered a stroke, you may also be given medication to prevent brain-tissue swelling that occurs immediately after a "cerebrovascular accident" (which is what doctors call a stroke). These drugs are called "osmotic agents," and the standard one is *mannitol*. Some neurologists prefer to administer steroids in high doses during the acute phase to reduce this swelling. You may also be given Dilantin to prevent seizures. (When the brain is damaged, it becomes irritable, resulting in epileptic like fits.)

Total Commitment Can Make a Difference

Always insist on total commitment in the medical and nursing care of a loved one who has had a stroke, especially during the initial phase. After the first week or two, we have a fairly good idea of what we call "residual disability," that is, how much of the damage is permanent. But even if it appears to be substantial, do not "pack it in." Today's sophisticated physiotherapy and rehabilitation techniques using newer electronic appliances are able to effect miracles on paralyzed patients. What seems like only insignificant improvement to someone in good health, may, in fact, make a major impact on a stroke patient's life style. If he can be equipped with some device, or have his muscles reeducated by exercises so as to permit greater independence at toilet, eating, walking or even turning the pages of a book, life becomes more bearable. The stroke patient should not be allowed to vegetate and die like a wounded animal.

After the first two weeks, when the stroke is "completed," the aggressive, optimistic doctor may recommend angiography to see whether the attack was caused by plaques in the carotid arteries. Reaming them out, even at this late stage, may prevent further extension of the paralysis. If he doesn't make the suggestion, ask him about it.

Occasionally, in the course of a routine physical exam, your doctor may detect a murmur or "bruit" (the French word for "noise") in one or both sides of your neck when he places his stethoscope over the carotid arteries. This sound may be transmitted there from a narrowed heart valve, or it may originate in the carotid artery itself. In the latter event, it represents an area of narrowing in that blood vessel. You may be entirely without symptoms, or you may be experiencing TIAs. In the former event, some doctors will want to pursue the investigation to see if the blockage is significant. (The extent of narrowing isn't related to the intensity of the "bruit," since a minor narrowing can create a great deal of noise.) Other physicians will choose to ignore it, especially if the pulse itself is good and strong. If neurological symptoms are present, however, the cause of the "bruit" must be investigated.

Until quite recently, the decision to proceed with testing or not was an important one, because the only way to do so was with "invasive" techniques such as an angiogram. Today, blood flow in vessels suspected of being narrowed can be determined by several sophisticated methods which are painless, noninvasive and without risk. In view of the fact that the carotid artery is usually accessible for necessary surgery, there is no reason to perpetuate the debate. If you are told you have such a "bruit," and the finding is not pursued (especially if you have symptoms suggestive of interference with the blood supply to the brain), ask for a second opinion from a neurologist.

KEY FACTS TO REMEMBER

Interference with the blood supply of the brain causes stroke. That can happen when an artery to or in the head ruptures and hemorrhages, or is obstructed by a clot or arteriosclerotic plaque. *The most important cause of strokes is untreated high blood pressure.* Certain disturbances of cardiac rhythm can result in embolism to the brain—and stroke. Predisposition to the latter usually requires anticoagulants.

A stroke may occur suddenly or may be heralded by warning symptoms referred to as "transient ischemic attacks." When premonitory evidence does occur, treatment with aspirin may reduce the likelihood of a full-blown stroke by about 50 percent. This protection seems to be afforded only to men.

Most strokes, unless massive, usually clear up or their symptoms improve after a few days. When they do not, aggressive management and imaginative rehabilitation techniques are required.

Decisions about how to investigate stroke patients so as to prevent recurrences and whether to operate should be made only in consultation with an expert neurologist.

16

Parkinson's Disease—
A Triumph of Treatment

Trembling with Fear

Not a week goes by but that I get a panic call from one of my patients complaining that "my hands are trembling and I can't control them. I think I have Parkinson's disease." It doesn't usually turn out to be so. Tremor can result from a host of other conditions, and it is only one of many symptoms of Parkinson's disease. So, if you are given that diagnosis, consult a neurologist to be sure. If you are chilled, excited or have just participated in some very strenuous physical exercise, you may develop a transient, residual shaking. That's normal. Tremors may also run in families, and may have nothing to do with Parkinson's disease. Since alcohol often eliminates such a tremor, patients so affected may develop a drinking problem over the long term. Certain kinds of liver disease, multiple sclerosis, chronic alcoholism, drug addiction (especially during the withdrawal phase) and overfunction of the thyroid gland can all produce a tremor. So can certain medications, like thorazine (a tranquilizer) and reserpine (used mostly in the treatment of high blood pressure). Remember, just shaking a little bit or even a lot, doesn't necessarily mean that you have Parkinson's disease.

The slight tremor that older persons sometimes develop is usually of no consequence except that it worries them. It is

most apt to occur when they do something with their hands—
try to reach for an object, to write or perform some fine
movement. It is very important that you know this, because it
is completely different from the tremor of Parkinson's disease,
which occurs mainly at rest. The moment the Parkinsonian
patient reaches for something like a knife or fork, the tremor
improves markedly in most instances.

You Need Good Contacts

Parkinson's disease develops when a specific area within
the brain is deprived of a chemical called dopamine. It is the
substance responsible for nerve impulses making the proper
contacts, so it's called a *neurotransmitter.* For some reason,
whatever causes Parkinson's disease reduces the supply of
dopamine. That can happen in middle-aged people as well as
in the elderly. One form of the disease followed the worldwide pandemic of encephalitis in 1919 and occurred in young
persons. For this reason Parkinson's should not be considered
a disease of aging—that is, an inevitable or integral part of
getting old. Neither is it always due to hardening of the
arteries, although it sometimes occurs after a stroke.

How to Recognize It

Like most other diseases, the severity of Parkinson's
varies widely. It is most always insidious in its progression
and may not cause real trouble for many years. For example,
you may initially become aware of just a slight tremor, or
perhaps some difficulty in your coordination; there may be
some slowing of your muscular activity or a tendency for your
limbs to be stiff. When full-blown, however, Parkinsonism is
fairly typical. Patients have a "dead-pan" expression; they
don't blink their eyes very often; the mouth drools at the
angles and remains slightly open; they have trouble walking,
and they seem to lurch forward, slightly bent at the trunk, as
if running after their center of gravity; the arms do not swing.
Such patients have a characteristic tremor of the thumb,
making it look as if they are rolling a pill. When they reach
for an object, the tremor is markedly reduced, and it disappears during sleep. The tremor may involve one arm or both;
and as the disease progresses, the legs, jaw and neck may
begin to shake too. The speech is either slow and monoto-

nous or it may sound like gibberish. One of the more troublesome symptoms of this disease is a tendency of the blood pressure to drop precipitously when the patient suddenly stands up. This can result in a faint.

A Happier Outlook

Although it is usually a progressive disease, the treatment and outlook of Parkinson's have changed so dramatically in the last few years and are continuing to improve at such a pace that anyone with this disorder has reason to be optimistic. Before the recent advances in drug development, death from Parkinson's was three times that of the general population. Today, it's just 1½ times greater. At least five years of better life have been added to the average patient's survival, a significant figure in the elderly.

What shortens the life of patients with Parkinson's is not any specific aspect of the disease itself, but some injury resulting from it. For example, because they have difficulty getting about, due to spasm, tremor, rigidity of the muscles and poor coordination, they often fall and fracture a hip or some other bone. In old age, that spells trouble. Other Parkinsonian patients have difficulty swallowing, so that the food "goes down the wrong way"—into the lungs instead of the stomach—and may result in an aspiration pneumonia. That used to be fatal, but with today's new antibiotics and pneumonia vaccine, the number of such deaths has been very much reduced.

How Treatment Started

About a hundred years ago, atropine (belladonna), a drug that had been around a long, long time even then, was found, almost accidentally, to help patients with Parkinson's disease. (It is the same antispasmodic, anti-cholinergic, given to patients with duodenal ulcers and the drying agent administered before anesthesia). Because drooling is one of the symptoms of Parkinson's disease, a French physician decided to use it for that purpose. He noted, however, that it not only dried the mouth but, more important, it also reduced tremor and rigidity. And so for the next hundred years, until quite recently, various kinds of belladonna preparations (as well as antihistamines) formed the mainstay of treatment for Parkinson's disease. (Antihistamines are mild sedatives and have a drying effect—which is why we use them for a cold and runny nose.) The anti-cholinergics (Artane, Kemadin, Parsidol, Cogentin, Pagintane and Akineton) and antihistamines are still the first line drugs. They help relieve rigidity and tremor. They do, however, make your mouth dry and cause constipation or diarrhea. If you have heart trouble, as some elderly patients do, check with your doctor about the advisability of taking these agents.

A Revolutionary Treatment

The introduction of L-dopa (levodopa) in 1970 totally revolutionized the treatment of Parkinson's disease. Today, most patients respond well to this drug or one of its derivatives. In 50 percent, the improvement is so great that those formerly bedridden can now feed themselves, dress and move about without help. About 20 percent are so strikingly benefited that they can barely be recognized as having the disease.

How L-Dopa Works

L-dopa corrects, at least partly, the chemical defect in Parkinson's disease. The original preparation has been succeeded by a new generation of drugs called Sinemet (in the United States) and Madopar (in Europe). These contain not only L-dopa, but another agent (carbidopa) as well and are more effective and cause fewer adverse symptoms. The addition of the carbidopa permits a 75 percent reduction in the dosage of L-dopa.

Although levodopa is the wonder drug of Parkinson's disease, like any powerful medication it has its problems—and you should know about them. First of all, its effect begins to wear off anywhere from three to five years, so the later you start it the better. (Actually stopping the drug for one or two weeks, and then re-starting it may restore some of its efficacy). If you're given the drug as soon as the diagnosis of Parkinson's is made, ask for another opinion from a neurologist. It also has significant side effects, the most troublesome of which is the "on-off" phenomenon. You take the pill, it works fine, and then abruptly, and without reason, there is a sudden reappearance and worsening of the symptoms. If this happens while you're driving a car, for example, it can be disastrous. L-dopa can also cause nausea and vomiting and a variety of psychiatric or behavioral disorders, including paranoia (persecution complex).

One useful tip that doctors do not always give patients is to avoid Vitamin B_6 (pyridoxine), which is found in so many over-the-counter multivitamin preparations. Pyridoxine blocks the action of L-dopa, so that if you take it, your Parkinson's symptoms may become worse.

Active research for new drugs to help the Parkinson's patient continues. Three are two new products now in clinical trials but not yet released; fergolide (Eli Lilly Co.) and lesuride (Schering). Ask your doctor if they are available to him, if you are no longer benefiting from the levodopa-carbidopa combination.

Serendipity in the Soviet Union

Another drug developed for use in Parkinson's disease has an interesting history. It is called amantadine (marketed in the United States as Symmetrel) and was used primarily in the treatment and prevention of influenza.

The Russians were using amantadine fairly widely during their flu epidemics. In so doing, they noticed that, among those patients who also happened to have Parkinson's, symptoms of that disease were improved by the flu treatment. So they analyzed the properties of this drug and found that it acts very much like L-dopa (less effectively, perhaps, but with fewer side effects). When they reported these observations, neurologists here took a second look at amantadine and have since confirmed the Russian observation that patients, particularly those with early, mild Parkinson's disease, do benefit from this drug.

The practical implications of this discovery are that if you have been on the antihistamines or belladonna-type drugs like Artane and now require something more effective, ask about amantadine since it is better not to "graduate" to L-dopa before you really have to. Also, if you can't tolerate L-dopa in any form, amantadine may be a useful alternative.

More Drugs on the Way

Bromocriptine is another new agent now being used in the treatment of Parkinson's. Like L-dopa, it affects the chemical environment in the brain. It is said to have an interesting side effect to which I cannot personally yet attest—increasing sexual potency in men and sexual desire in women. I have many patients (and friends) *without* Parkinson's disease, who are anxiously awaiting confirmation of that claim. Unfortunately, large doses of Bromocriptine can cause psychiatric disturbances.

The Key to Successful Treatment

There are several important facts for anyone interested in Parkinson's disease to appreciate. Many of the symptoms associated with it are either emotionally induced or worsened by anxiety, depression and stress. So, an important part of treatment is to convince the patient that it *can* be controlled, is not fatal, and is worsened by worrying about it. Drug manipulation so as to give the best possible results in Parkinson's disease often requires that you consult an experienced neurologist. If things aren't going well, do not hesitate to do so.

The Role of Surgery

In the days when drug therapy for Parkinson's disease was really inadequate, several operations were devised to help control the tremor and muscular rigidity that made life so miserable. They were of help in many cases, particularly when tremor was the major complaint. But such surgical procedures now are rarely necessary. It is not likely that they will be recommended to you. If they are, ask for a second opinion.

KEY FACTS TO REMEMBER

Parkinson's disease is only one of many different causes of tremor. The diagnosis should always be confirmed by a neurologist. Patients with this disorder (it is not a disease of aging) have rigidity and spasticity of their muscles in addition to tremor.

Treatment and outlook of Parkinson's disease have improved greatly in recent years, since the discovery of L-dopa. But patients using this drug may develop side effects from, and become intolerant to it. It should, therefore, not be prescribed before the several other available medications have been tried. The combination of L-dopa and carbidopa (Sinemet) represents a major advance. In any patient not responding to therapy, a second opinion from a neurologist experienced in the management of this disease, should be obtained.

17

Myasthenia Gravis—
New Hope for an Old Disease

An Important Disease—Statistics Notwithstanding

In medicine, statistics have very little immediate application to a specific patient. For example, if you are told that the risk of dying from a heart bypass operation is now well under 2 percent and you lose a loved one during such a procedure, the excellent figures for the rest of the population are of little comfort to you. So, by the same token, although myasthenia gravis affects only one person in twenty thousand or thirty thousand and is not a common disease, I have encountered at least fifteen cases in recent years (without having examined the 450,00 people that, the statistics say, are necessary to find that number). So, numbers notwithstanding, I am including a short discussion of this disease for those of you who either have it or who care about somebody who does.

A Serious Disease of Muscle

Myo means muscle, *asthenia* means weakness, and *gravis* means serious. So, *myasthenia gravis* is a "serious disease of muscle." The clinical scenario may vary in patients with this disorder, but it commonly goes something like this. You notice an unusual weakness after some activity with which you never had any trouble before—swimming a length or two

235

in the pool, or going for your usual morning walk. You don't worry at first, because you bounce back after resting for a while. But then the fatigue recurs, and in time even after less effort. It seems to involve the muscles of your head and neck more than other parts of the body. Eventually you may find that you tire just brushing your hair; you prefer not to have to chew a steak and opt for softer foods. One day, you look in the mirror and find one or both eyelids drooping.

The Diagnosis May Not Be Obvious

Some of these symptoms can, of course, be caused by other disorders, like a stroke or even an hysterical reaction. Early in the disease, unless your doctor thinks about the possibility of myasthenia gravis, he may tell you that you are overworked. Even a thorough checkup may be normal at this stage. He will then reassure you, give you a stronger vitamin and if you continue to complain, possibly send you to a psychiatrist. I know of one man in his seventies, who was told that his profound, generalized weakness was due to premature aging and "softening of the brain." Before making arrangements for custodial care in a nursing home, his son asked for a second opinion from a neurologist, who made the correct diagnosis of myasthenia gravis. The patient was given the proper medication and is now living a virtually normal life.

We are just beginning to understand what myasthenia is all about. Remember that muscle fibers contract in response to stimulation by nerves. At the site of the nerve ending in muscle, a specific chemical is released, which enables that contraction to take place. For some reason—probably because of the production of an antibody against it—the necessary chemical substance loses its ability to function normally in myasthenia gravis.

Who Is Vulnerable?

This disease affects three different age groups—newborns (especially those whose mothers have the disease); persons under forty, mostly women, and including teen-agers; and finally, adults of both sexes over the age of forty. In a typical case, a patient will consult the doctor because of weakness, usually of the eye muscles. He may have double vision or difficulty in keeping the eyelids open. Later, as other muscle groups become involved, there may be trouble swallowing, speaking and, finally, breathing. Although most untreated patients gradually become worse in time, some young women do improve spontaneously. Such remission, however, is rarely permanent.

When your doctor suspects the possibility of myasthenia gravis, he can confirm it very easily by injecting a medicine called Tensilon into the veins. This instantly cures the disease—for a few minutes.

Your Treatment Options

There are several treatment approaches to myasthenia gravis. The first is a pill marketed in this country as Mestinon, which replaces or simulates the action of the critical chemical at the nerve-muscle junction. This drug permits many patients to lead normal lives for years. Unfortunately, in others, as the disease progresses, a tolerance develops to it, so that more and more medication is required until some other form of treatment finally becomes necessary.

Removing the Thymus—Benefit versus Risk

An alternative form of therapy has an interesting history. In 1938, a patient with myasthenia gravis happened to develop a tumor of the thymus (a gland in the lower part of the neck, not to be confused with the thyroid gland). When the tumor was removed, the symptoms of myasthenia gravis virtually disappeared. That led to the conclusion that malfunction of the thymus was responsible for at least some cases of myasthenia gravis. As a result, many patients with this disease have had this gland removed. The operation itself is not a risky one, provided that it is done by an experienced surgeon. But we now know that, while thymus surgery may benefit persons at any age, the operative risks for those in their seventies or eighties usually outweigh the advantages. In patients under fifty years, however, there is noticeable improvement in almost 75 percent of cases, although it may take as long as five years for it to become apparent. The earlier the operation is done, the better the results. Also, if, after it is taken out, the thymus is found not to have a tumor within it, the outlook is better than when it does. So, if you are under fifty, have myasthenia gravis, and are *not* offered thymus surgery, ask for a second opinion from a qualified neurologist. Also, if you are over fifty and surgery *is* recommended, you should ask for another opinion. In short, always solicit input from a specialist who has particular expertise in this disease.

Steroid Hormones

The third major approach to the treatment of myasthenia gravis is the use of steroid hormones. These substances often improve patients dramatically. Other drugs that suppress the immune response—the kind we administer to patients with heart or kidney transplants to prevent rejection—may also help in myasthenia. If you are not doing well and have not been given steroids, ask another neurologist for a second opinion.

Now In Research—For The Worst Cases

Finally, in the handful of cases of myasthenia gravis who have failed to respond to the anticholinesterases, or removal of the thymus gland or high-dose steroids, there is yet another option—plasmapheresis. It is still in the investigational phase, which means you can't just go to any doctor or any hospital and ask to have it done. But there are several institutions across the country studying the effects of this procedure, and there is optimism, even enthusiasm, that it may help. Basically, it involves removing from the blood by filtration those substances thought to be responsible for causing or aggravating the disease. Plasmapheresis, in itself, is not a new technique. It has been used in a variety of conditions where some toxic substance, chemical or protein, needs to be taken from the blood. Its application in the management of myasthenia gravis, however, is new.

Skip the Gin and Tonic

In addition to knowing about what treatments help, you should also be aware of drugs that may worsen the condition. These include four commonly used heart medications— Quinidine, Pronestyl, Lidocaine and Inderal and other beta blockers.

There are other substances that can aggravate myasthenia gravis which are often taken unknowingly and unnecessarily. Quinine is one. If you have this disease and take a gin and tonic (the latter contains quinine) your symptoms may worsen. Certain antibiotics, particularly the "mycins"—Gentamycin, Kanamycin, Neomycin, Streptomycin, Achromycin—should also be avoided.

We have come a long way in our understanding and management of myasthenia gravis. It is no longer the dread disease it once was. Today, because of modern treatment ranging from long-acting medications to thymus operations, steroids and other immunosuppressant agents, most patients can lead virtually normal lives.

KEY FACTS TO REMEMBER

Myasthenia gravis is not a common disorder. It is characterized by the interference with the response of muscle to the stimuli of nerves which normally make it contract. The result is poor muscle function and weakness. When untreated, this disease becomes generalized over a varying period of time and ends in death. Most patients can be managed by the expert use of certain drugs and cortisone. In others, removal of the thymus gland results in great improvement. The decision concerning medical or surgical treatment or both should be made only after consultation with a neurologist experienced in this disease.

18

Infertility, Contraception and Abortion

When You're Impregnable, Inconceivable and Unbearable

Birth control gets all the publicity, be it the pill, the promise of a contraceptive to be taken the "morning after" sex (perhaps in a nasal spray), reversible vasectomies, thinner condoms and better diaphragms. Our society is also deeply immersed in the debate about abortion. So it is ironic that while much of the world struggles to attain zero population growth, and millions of women worry about how to avoid pregnancy, there are still so many among us who yearn to have at least one child of their own—but can't.

The large and growing number of adoption services from coast to coast, unable to keep up with the demand for babies, attests to the fact that between 10 and 20 percent of married couples in the United States are unable to conceive. They spend much of their time at fertility clinics, where they are tested, retested and treated, often without results. If and when the cause of the infertility is eventually identified, there is the additional frustration of learning that there may be nothing to do about it anyway. So the barren couple, sad, anxious and vulnerable, is ripe for exploitation by quacks whose stock in trade is false hope and expensive, unnecessary testing and therapy. If you are among those who run from doctor to doctor and from clinic to clinic because you have been persistently infertile, you owe it to yourself to know when to stop, and when *not* to ask for yet another opinion.

The Sterile Male Chauvinist

Traditionally, at least as far back as Biblical times, a barren marriage was always blamed on the woman. But we now know that in as many as 40 percent of couples who cannot conceive, the problem lies, not with the female, but with her mate. Whereas it is usually time-consuming, complicated and expensive to evaluate a woman's fertility, it is relatively quick, cheap and easy to check her partner. All it takes initially is a look at his sperm under the microscope. So it makes good sense for any woman to demur if she is advised to have exhaustive fertility testing before her partner is evaluated.

Get It to the Lab on Time

How you obtain your sperm for study is your affair. Whichever way you do it, the ejaculate must be examined within two hours. First we measure its volume. A fertile man produces between two and five cubic centimeters of fluid per ejaculation—but not, of course, when it's the third time round in one day. We then determine how much of this volume is fluid and how much is actually sperm. You need a minimum of twenty million sperm in every cubic centimeter of ejaculate in order to be fertile. But there is more to it than numbers alone. When we examine the sperm under the microscope, we look to see if they are normal in appearance. Also, more than half of them should be moving about actively. If we are sure that the volume is adequate and that there are enough energetic sperm of normal shape, then and only then should the female partner of the sterile couple undergo a fertility evaluation.

Sexuality versus Fertility

Gloria Steinem was probably right. Men *are* chauvinists at heart. I have never yet met one who has graciously accepted the fact that his deficient sperm were responsible for the barren marriage. I remember one young man who was told that he would never be able to father a child. His initial reaction was to bemoan all the time, money and worry he had expended over the years, during which time he was unnecessarily preoccupied with techniques of contraception. He had missed a "free ride" all that time. Another more typical reaction to this kind of news is indignant rejection, followed by tales of sexual prowess and the inevitable conclusion: that there must have been some mistake in the analysis.

It is often hard to convince men that potency (the capacity to engage in sexual intercourse by virtue of being able to achieve and maintain an erection) is not the same thing as virility (the ability of the sperm to fertilize an egg). I know many men who have each fathered several children, despite chronic, premature ejaculation and an organ that was rarely ever more than semierect. Although they hardly qualify as great lovers, they are fertile, because they can deliver the right amount of healthy sperm to a waiting ovum. And that is what counts when you want to make a baby. By the same token, a Don Juan may find himself in the anterooms of fertility specialists—because, despite the magnitude of his potency and sexual appetite, his sperm are inadequate. I know one such man who was so outraged when told that he was infertile, he set about to disprove it. Unfortunately, he was right—and his girl friend, not his wife, became pregnant! His sperm concentration was probably just borderline, not quite enough to impregnate his wife, but adequate for a lucky strike with his girl (who was younger than his spouse and probably more fertile to boot). His wife never learned about his success, and she wonders to this day why, so many years later, he still remains confident that "we will one day have a family of our own."

"Healthy" Men with Sick Sperm

What can render the sperm of an otherwise healthy, sexually active young man deficient? Some obvious causes are direct injury, infection (mumps in adult life is the classic example), or other damage to the testes, whose function it is to make vigorous sperm in adequate numbers. Such insults may be only temporary, in which case the testes (balls) bounce right back. But sometimes the injury is permanent, in which event there is not much to be done about it. Occasionally, at birth, one or both testes remain in the abdominal cavity instead of descending into the scrotal sac. When that happens, these glands don't make sperm. They can sometimes be brought down surgically, more for cosmetic reasons than any other, because, unfortunately, a testis that didn't get there on its own hardly ever works right. Also, since an undescended testis sometimes becomes cancerous, it is frequently removed. If you are told to "leave it alone," get another opinion. Many doctors think that you should have it "biopsied" at an early age to detect any cancer that may be developing there.

Several drugs, including some used in the treatment of cancer, ulcerative colitis and peptic ulcers (cimetidine) can interefere with sperm production too. If your sperm count is low, review with your doctor the medications you are taking before you submit to a more sophisticated investigation of the problem.

The testes make the healthiest, most active sperm in a cool environment, so that chronic fever may result in an abnormal analysis. If your sperm production is borderline, avoid taking hot baths before you try to make a baby.

In addition to local trouble in the testes themselves, you may have a hormonal disorder elsewhere that affects them secondarily. For example, when the thyroid gland (in the neck), the adrenal glands (which sit on top of both kidneys) or the pituitary (in the brain) are not working right, sperm production in the testes may be defective, because the hormones produced by these other glands influence testicular function.

Although the focus of the consequences of (diebylstilbestrol) DES has been on the daughters of women who took this "fertility" vitamin, it is now apparent that their sons may also have been affected. In one study, infertility, at least temporary, was noted in 14 of 17 young men whose mothers had taken that medication when pregnant.

Finally, it appears that some 5 percent to 10 percent of the men have antibodies against their own sperm. These circulate in the bloodstream causing otherwise healthy sperm to clump together, thus immobilizing them. Although it is not clear why such antibodies are formed, some researchers claim to have developed a blood test to identify their presence.

Where infertility is due to such anti-sperm antibodies, treatment with steroids may be helpful.

Good Sperm with No Future

A man may be infertile even though his testes and sperm are healthy if some mechanical problem interferes with the delivery of the sperm. For example, an obstruction anywhere in the various ducts through which the sperm must pass en route out from the testes, may prevent their arrival in adequate numbers to the vagina. Chronic infection and scarring of the genital organs can result in such blockage. In such cases, a simple operation may solve the problem. Varicose veins of the scrotum (*varicocele*) are also associated with an increased incidence of infertility. So, if your sperm are normal, but you are nevertheless unable to make a baby, it is a good idea first to be checked out by your urologist, who can evaluate all the possible mechanical factors, and *then* by an endocrinologist (gland specialist) for an assessment of your hormonal status.

Retrograde Ejaculation—"Wrong Way Corrigan"

There is an interesting situation in which you may fail to deliver sperm "on target" despite normal hormone function, adequate sperm production and an intact physical delivery system. In this condition, called *retrograde ejaculation,* the sperm, instead of coming out of the urethra, go backward from the testes and empty into the urinary bladder. This reversal of flow sometimes happens after prostate surgery, but certain drugs, particularly Aldomet (widely used in the treatment of high blood pressure), can also cause it.

No Magic in Hormones

What can be done for the infertile man obviously depends on what's causing the trouble. If he is lucky and his problem only a mechanical one like a varicocele, surgical repair is easy and will do the trick. Also, if the testes have been injured physically or by some infection, the condition may clear up on its own. Some doctors and many patients think that hormones are the magic cure-all for infertility. That's usually true only when the hormone (testosterone) is shown to be lacking. But its indiscriminate use will rarely benefit the infertile male if glandular function is normal—with one exception. Occasionally, for reasons that are not understood, testosterone injections may increase the motility or activity of the sperm. If this treatment is going to work at all, it will be apparent after three months. There is no point in continuing the injections beyond that time. If you are advised to do so, ask for a second opinion from an endocrinologist.

Common Sense May Be All You Need

If you are told that your sperm count is borderline and not "all that bad," a few simple procedures may improve your chances of making a baby. First, be sure to take advantage of the best times (from a fertility, rather than a social, point of view) to have intercourse. Try to deliver the sperm when the egg is right there, waiting to be fertilized—approximately mid-cycle. Then, make sure that your mate remains in bed for a while after intercourse with her knees slightly bent and her hips on a pillow, giving the sperm the best chance to get where they should go. Finally, remind her not to douche for several hours.

If a complete analysis of your sperm reveals that they are just not up to snuff and there is nothing to be done, think positively. You may want to adopt a child. You can have enormous fun trying to prove that your doctor is wrong. Your mate(s) will be grateful to you for having liberated her (them) from the pill, IUD, jellies and all that mess—and you will save a small fortune on condoms.

But if you are really determined to have your very own child, despite the fact that you have no sperm of your own, the following late news will interest you. In 1980, a man who was born without testes received a testis transplant from his brother. The following year, the recipient's wife gave birth to a normal child!

The Effect of Environment on Your Sperm

The inability to produce healthy sperm may be due, not to any disease or disorder of your reproductive system, but to environmental pollution. In 1929, average sperm counts in the United States were 90,000,000 per cubic centimeter (remember, you need at least 20,000,000 to impregnate an egg). By 1974, the median sperm count had dropped to 65,000,000. In a study of 132 students at Florida State University in 1975, the average value was 60,000,000, with 23 percent of the men having fewer than the critical 20,000,000 value. And every one of these samples contained an abnormally high concentration of chemical contaminants from the environment (DDT, hexachlorbenzenes and polychlorinated biphenyls, or PCB). In addition to being carcinogenic, PCB reduces sperm count in experimental animals.

The Barren Woman

Let us suppose that in our barren couple, the male has been found fertile. It is now the woman's turn to be evaluated. Infertility in the female is usually due to any of the following causes: (a) hormonal imbalance (one third of cases), in which a gland somewhere—the pituitary, adrenal, thyroid or the ovaries themselves—is not working right; (b) mechanical problems (half the cases) which, as with the sperm of the male, may interfere with the passage of the egg and prevent its rendezvous with the sperm (typical examples are a scarred Fallopian tube, an abnormal position of the uterus, or the angle at which the cervix projects into the vagina); finally, (c) about 15 percent of women have what is called a "hostile" cervix—the portal through which the sperm must pass in order to get into the uterus is "shut" by chemical changes.

Evaluation of the infertile woman consists of investigating these three major obstacles to pregnancy. However, there is no point in testing the patency of the tubes or the chemical environment of the cervix if you are not ovulating to begin with. So, first make sure that your ovaries are producing eggs. This is something you can do yourself—simply by taking your temperature. Finding it elevated for four or five days at mid-cycle is presumptive evidence that you are ovulating. If there is a temperature rise, then presumably you have the egg, but there is some fault in its physical or chemical environment.

If you are ovulating normally, the sequence in which I would suggest that you investigate your infertility is as follows: (1) check out the possibility of a "hostile" cervix; (2) look for mechanical problems interfering with egg transport; (3) have your hormones analyzed.

The Hostile Cervix

The *postcoital* test is used to check the mucus around the cervix in order to see whether it is hostile—that is, impenetrable—thus preventing the sperm from reaching the uterus. Here is how it's done. First, you must have intercourse while you are ovulating. Then go to your gynecologist anytime in the next two to sixteen hours. The doctor will then collect a specimen of the mucus from your cervix, examine it under the microscope and look at the condition of the sperm it contains. If the mucus is clear, and the sperm within it are moving about normally, then your cervix is "friendly." But if, on the other hand, the mucus is cloudy and the sperm are clumped together and sluggish, they have been trapped and can go no further. This "barrier" is likely to be the reason for your inability to conceive. If so, there are medical measures that can modify the chemistry of that environment. Ask your gynecologist about them.

Mechanical Causes of Infertility

As we work our diagnostic way up from the cervix in the search for causes of infertility we may find various different structural abnormalities in the uterus and tubes that can interfere with the passage of the sperm. These can often be detected in the routine gynecological examination without the need for complicated tests, and they are frequently amenable to surgical correction.

If the uterus itself is normal, we check whether the Fallopian tubes, down which the egg passes from the ovary to the uterus, are open. For even if you ovulate normally and your partner's sperm are healthy and able to enter the uterus without trouble, you still won't become pregnant if the egg can't get down from the ovary to meet them because the tube is scarred. The patency of these tubes can be determined in several ways. The simplest is with an X ray (unless you are allergic to the dye)—a procedure with the tongue-twisting name *hysterosalpingography*. Another technique, devised many years ago and still widely used, involves blowing carbon-dioxide gas into the tubes and then taking X rays to see if they are open (Rubin Test). There are other methods, but they are more complicated, uncomfortable and invasive—as, for example, looking directly into the tubes through a lighted instrument (culdoscopy), or into the pelvis (laparoscopy). Have those done last.

Medicines Against Infertility

Sometimes low-grade gynecologic infections are responsible for infertility, and these usually respond to antibiotic therapy. But if such is not the case, and if the cervix mucus is normal and there is no physical barrier to pregnancy "higher up," you should then undergo a battery of blood and urine tests to determine whether all your glands are working properly. Hormonal imbalance often can be corrected. Recently, Bromocriptine, used in the treatment of painful female breasts that secrete too much of a hormone called prolactin, has also been found to increase fertility. Vitamin B_6 suppresses prolactin too, and in one study, when the vitamin was given to fourteen previously infertile women with high levels of prolactin, twelve of them were able to conceive. Ask your doctor about it. Another drug called Danazol, which has been available for the treatment of a painful gynecological condition called endometriosis, has also been found effective in some cases of unexplained infertility. So help is on the way.

Commonsense Home Remedies

If your entire gynecological workup reveals nothing abnormal, collect all the data that have been accumulated and consult one more gynecologist who specializes in infertility. If he can't help you, then call it quits. But try some commonsense, home remedies. Assume the optimal position(s) during intercourse. Afterward stay put with the knees up for a little while, and never rush to douche. Although douching is not a reliable contraceptive, it can interfere with fertility, especially when the sperm count is borderline.

Maybe It's All in the Mind

Before you abandon hope and decide that you simply "cannot" have a baby, look into the possibility of some psychological, rather than physical, explanation. I don't profess to understand how emotional problems interfere with conception, but many experienced obstetricians and gynecologists tell me it's possible. I know of several couples who tried for years without success to have a baby and finally adopted one. Then, a few months later, perhaps because of the pleasure this gave them, or the absence of the tension and frustration during their infertile years, they were able to conceive. So, it is a good idea, after you have consulted the urologists, endocrinologists and gynecologists without success, to talk with a psychiatrist.

Recreation Without Procreation—Sterilization Techniques

Sterilization techniques in women include either *hysterectomy* (removal of the uterus), or *tying off the Fallopian tubes* (so that the egg cannot get from the ovary, where it is produced, to the uterus, where it is fertilized). Don't confuse sterilization with contraception. The latter is temporary—effective only as long as you want it to be. Sterilization, on the other hand, is usually permanent, although procedures like vasectomy and tubal ligation can sometimes be reversed.

Why Remove a Healthy Uterus?

I believe it is unnecessary and undesirable to remove a perfectly healthy uterus to effect sterilization. I have discussed this question with several gynecologists whose opinion I value, and few of them consider it an acceptable procedure for that purpose. A hysterectomy, after all, is real surgery—with all the risks, pain and cost of any important operation. But, more than that, the uterus is also a symbolic organ for most women. Its extirpation has a psychological impact that perhaps is not always fully appreciated by men, be they husbands, lovers or gynecologists.

Why perform a hysterectomy when sterilization can be achieved just as effectively by cutting or tying the tubes? The answer offered by those doctors who still recommend it is that, once done, it is final, it is irreversible, and it prevents pregnancy forever. It also eliminates the possibility of ever developing uterine tumors and cancers in the future. Removing the uterus, they argue, permits you to take estrogen-replacement therapy after the menopause without fear of getting cancer later on. The final decision about how to be sterilized, if that's what you want or need, should be up to you. But, if hysterectomy is advised for that purpose, ask for another opinion.

The Sometimes Reversible Vasectomy

Of course, some women prefer their mates to have any sterilization surgery that is to be done. *Vasectomy* is the male equivalent of tying the Fallopian tubes. Sperm, which are produced in the testes, make their way via a system of tortuous tubules up from the scrotum and out through the penis. One of the ducts through which the sperm must pass is called the vas deferens. In a vasectomy, the vas is cut and divided, so that the sperm have no access route out. About one million such male sterilizations are being done every year in the United States. It is a simple procedure and is often done right in the urologist's office. It is effective, but to what extent is it reversible? Urologists with whom I have discussed this question tell me that in about 50 percent of cases the vas can be restored. However, some surgeons claim much higher success rates.

It's Simple, but How Safe Is Vasectomy?

A word of caution about the vasectomy. Questions have been raised about the safety and long-term consequences of cutting the vas deferens in healthy men. Although no harmful effect has thus far been observed in humans, some disturbing changes have been noted in monkeys and other animals. These consist mainly of what we call "autoimmune responses." Every one of our tissues and organs has the capability of being "rejected" by the rest of the body. This occurs when natural defenses, which normally are directed against a foreign body or invading organism, inappropriately attack a perfectly innocent native tissue. The result is a "disease," and new "autoimmune diseases," involving virtually every organ of the body—the blood, thyroid, heart and lungs—are being recognized all the time.

What happens with vasectomy (at least as far as animals are concerned) is that when the vas deferens is tied off so that the sperm can no longer get out, the body regards those left behind in the testes as "hostile," and it tries to "reject" them. The consequences of this reaction are not yet clear, but one real possibility is that when the vasectomy is surgically restored, the sperm now able to emerge will be altered in some way and will have lost their ability to fertilize an egg. My advice, therefore, if you have *any* intention of ever having children again, however remote the likelihood, is not to have a vasectomy. I have known several men who, although ostensibly "finished with raising a family," years later either divorced or became widowers and ended up marrying younger women who wanted to have children. An earlier vasectomy made that possibility much less likely.

Fertile but Unwilling—The Art of Contraception

Although some of us choose to be made sterile, surgically and permanently, for many millions, *contraception*—temporary and reversible—is the preferred technique of birth control. The method you select is usually, but not always, a matter of personal preference.

The combination of sexual abandon and ignorance among teen-agers has resulted in an enormous and growing number of unwanted and unexpected pregnancies in this age group. Part of the answer to this problem surely lies in more effective education and parent-child communication. If you belong to your PTA, press for such sex education to be made available in your child's school.

Choosing a Contraceptive

Contraceptive techniques—believe it or not—include total abstinence (unacceptable), withdrawal of the male organ just before ejaculation (coitus interruptus—enough to make a nervous wreck out of any man and woman) and natural family planning (if you are religiously inclined). But most couples rely on the pill, the intrauterine device, the condom, the diaphragm or barrier contraceptives. Chinese scientists have come up with gossypol, an oral contraceptive made from cotton seed oil, for men. It is apparently very effective, dropping the sperm count to zero in about twelve weeks. Its safety is still being evaluated, but of some concern is the fact that when it is stopped, some 20 percent of the men taking it failed to make sperm again. American investigators testing it think that it has promise—but it is still years away from release here. Another new contraceptive, this one for women, administered in a nasal spray, is being evaluated in Sweden, where it was developed. Effective and convenient, it must be taken every day—but it should never be confused with nasal decongestants used for colds and stuffy nose.

The effectiveness of each of these contraceptive techniques varies somewhat, and you should know about all of them before committing yourself to any one. The stakes, if you miscalculate, can be high, especially if pregnancy can endanger your life because of some cardiac disease, blood disorder, kidney trouble or other serious medical problem.

When to Go to a Movie Instead

If you definitely don't want a large family, but your religious beliefs do not permit medical or mechanical means of contraception, you should practice natural family planning. Physicians are, of course, unenthusiastic about this method from the scientific viewpoint, although we realize that there are many persons who choose to rely on it. The available statistics indicate that if you do, the failure rate with the method may be as high as 27 percent, depending on how careful you are and how regular your periods happen to be.

I hadn't referred to this method in the first edition, for which I was criticized by questioners in the audience during several TV interviews. So here goes. There are two techniques that couples who follow planned family planning must learn. The first is the ovulation method. Here, the woman comes to recognize the appearance of the mucus from the vagina and cervix as an indicator of ovulation. The second aspect of this kind of birth control is called sympto-thermal. In addition to watching the mucus, the woman records daily temperature readings to determine the time of ovulation. The trick is to identify the days in mid-cycle when one is most fertile and avoid sexual relations at that time. Keep track of your last ten or twelve cycles. See how long each lasts. Then subtract eighteen days from the shortest cycle and eleven days from the longest. For example, if your periods vary between twenty-seven and thirty days, subtracting eighteen days from the shortest puts you to day nine; eleven days from the longest cycle would be nineteen. Between those two dates, watch TV, read, or go to the movies—but abstain from sex. The problem with this method of birth control lies in those last few words.

An Interrupted Affair

Coitus interruptus is probably the oldest form of contraception. It is commonly used in a chance encounter, when sexual union was not expected, and neither participant came "prepared." Under these circumstances, the male has no alternative but to withdraw. This decision, made at peak passion, takes tremendous will power, determination or, to be honest, fear. Even if you act in time, the risk of pregnancy is still about 15 percent for the casual encounter, and 30 percent in couples who practice coitus interruptus regularly. Although you withdraw before ejaculating, there is always some prior sperm leakage—and that's often enough, Dad. Coitus interruptus is no way for an affair or a marriage to be consummated and continued over the long term.

Condoms—What the Well-Dressed Man Should Wear

Condoms have been around for centuries and are an acceptable, popular form of contraception. In fact, they are now the most widely used form of birth control after the pill. The rise in the popularity is probably the result of increased attention to sexually transmitted diseases. They would be more widely used were it not for the reduced sensation experienced by the male wearing one. Originally, they were made from sheep's gut; later thin rubber was used; and today they are mostly plastic (even though they are still called "rubbers"). Not unlike a new suit, condoms are advertised in a selection of colors and fabrics.

Patients come for advice about various contraceptive techniques, especially the pill, but no one has ever yet asked me how to use a condom. Men think there is nothing to it—just slip one on, and away you go. But when using a condom, you must be sure to leave about ½ to 1 inch free at the tip in order to accommodate the pressure and volume of the ejaculate. If you put it on too tightly, it may burst. Also, don't let your ego get the better of you. Use it only if you are an "achiever" with substantial erections, so that the condom is tight and leakproof at the top. Remember, too, not to dally after ejaculation, because as the penis shrinks, the contents of the condom may escape into the vagina. Hold on to it when you withdraw after coitus, otherwise it may slip off, a reasonably good way of ensuring a pregnant partner. For all these reasons—breakage, leakage and improper use—regular condom users, especially careless ones, run a 5–15 percent risk of inducing pregnancy.

The condom should be used by every man on the move, not only as a contraceptive, but also for protection against venereal infection. This is especially important if you go from partner to partner, including some whose credentials are uncertain.

No Protection from a Douche

There are still some women who believe that *douching* immediately after intercourse constitutes effective contraception. In practical terms, "immediately" usually means five to ten minutes. That's too late, because within two minutes, the sperm are well into the cervix on their way to uniting with the egg. So if you want to douche for purposes of hygiene, that's fine. As a contraceptive, forget it.

The Diaphragm—What the Well-Dressed Woman Should Wear

The *diaphragm* is about as safe as the condom. When properly used, it is 95 percent effective. But just as the condom can slip off, leak or break, so the diaphragm will not protect you if it is fitted incorrectly or you don't insert it properly. And even when it is the right size, and is put in as directed, it may become dislodged by a vigorous thrust during intercourse.

A diaphragm is somewhat inconvenient in that it must be inserted *before* intercourse. That's acceptable for a couple living together, but not the ideal contraceptive for the unpredicted sexual encounter. For example, if you are being coy, or are "surprised" to find yourself in a vulnerable situation, the presence of a diaphragm on your person will expose you for the "fraud" you are. The diaphragm also requires the use of a spermicidal preparation, which some couples may find distasteful, especially those who indulge in oral sex. What's more, should you decide to have another go at it, you should get up and apply a second coat of jelly. Remember to leave the diaphragm in place for at least six hours after its last use.

If the diaphragm concept appeals to you, but you find it inconvenient for some of the reasons described above, you should know about the cervical cap. It's not formally available at this time in the United States, but is under study as an "investigational device." It has been widely used in Europe for two or three years. It is a thick rubber cap, like a thimble, which fits over the cervix, so that the sperm have no access to the uterus. And the great thing about it is you can leave it there for several days. If, for some reason, none of the other contraceptive techniques is available to you, ask your gynecologist if he or she has access to the study so that you can be a "guinea pig."

The Pill—Fifty Million Women Can't Be Pregnant

The *pill* has had a profound effect on our life style, the role of women in our society, our social standards, our economy and our politics. Some fifty million women throughout the world are currently taking it; they were preceded by the same number beyond the childbearing age who no longer need it. There have been substantial changes in the composition of oral contraceptives since their introduction, and they continue to be more than 98 percent effective when used properly. Despite all the adverse publicity concerning the pill, it remains the number one method of contraception among married couples in this country.

No Egg—No Baby

The basic ingredient of the pill is estrogen, the female hormone, which prevents the release of the egg from the ovary—and without an egg, you can't have a baby. But estrogens, especially in large doses, can produce side effects. Thus, they may raise the blood pressure, predispose to clotting within the veins (phlebitis) or arteries (resulting in heart attacks and strokes), increase the blood sugar (diabetes mellitus), and elevate the amount of fats like cholesterol in your blood, perhaps making for greater vulnerability to hardening of the arteries (arteriosclerosis). In addition to these fairly major potential consequences, estrogens often give troublesome "minor" symptoms. For example, if you take them in large doses you may develop nausea and suffer migraine headaches (if you have had these headaches before, they may become worse). Estrogens may also injure the liver (although stopping them will result in return to normal function); they may make you vulnerable to fungus infections of the vagina (this has recently been disputed), foul up your normal menstrual cycle and, finally, increase your risk of getting cancer of the uterus.

You might wonder, looking at this list, why on earth anybody would take such a medication. The fact is that all these adverse effects occur in a really minuscule percentage of cases in relation to the total number of people taking the medication, and even then, they are very much dose-related—the less you take, the fewer and milder the side effects. For this reason, the pills currently being manufactured contain less estrogen than did earlier preparations, and more of another hormone, *progestin*. There is a dosage level, however, below which one cannot reduce the estrogen without substantially compromising the contraceptive effect.

Contraceptive pills now being made range from those with a relatively high estrogen content and little progestin, to the "minipill," which contains only progestin and no estrogen at all. There are some thirty-five different formulations of the pill currently marketed in the United States. When your doctor prescribes one for you, ask about its composition. The dosage schedule (and side effects) for each pill depends on its composition. For example, if it consists predominantly of estrogen, it is taken for twenty or twenty-one days, then stopped for the next seven or eight days. The minipill, however, must be taken without interruption, and it is not as reliable a contraceptive. There is also less satisfaction among women on the minipill than those using a preparation with estrogen in it, as judged by the drop-out rate. Despite the fact that it has fewer potential side effects, it may cause considerable irregularity in menstrual bleeding. A particular variation of pill contraception, recently banned in the United States, was the "sequential system," in which you took pure estrogen for two weeks, then progestin for one week and nothing at all the fourth week. It was withdrawn from the American market because the concentration of estrogen in this schedule gave unacceptable side effects; moreover, it was implicated in at least twenty cases of subsequent cancer of the uterus.

When It's Better Not to Use the Pill

What other information should you have about the pill? What information should you volunteer to the doctor when he prescribes it? What should he bear in mind when you both select the pill as your contraceptive?

If you are thirty-five years or older, you are better off using some form of contraception other than the pill—especially if (a) you smoke cigarettes, (b) you are overweight, (c) you have high blood pressure (or a tendency to it), (d) your cholesterol level is very abnormally elevated, (e) you have fibroids of the uterus, (f) you suffer from migraine headaches, or (g) you are epileptic. It has been observed that women with these "risk factors" in this age group who take the pill have a slightly higher incidence of heart attacks, strokes and other complications than those who do not. Mind you, the risk is statistically small, but it is better not to take the chance anyway.

When You Absolutely Mustn't Take the Pill

There are certain women who should not take the pill *at any age*. This includes those who have had cancer of the breast (or in whose family there is a strong history of breast cancer), suffer from any kind of circulatory or liver problem, or are prone to undiagnosed vaginal bleeding. Many doctors also feel that diabetes and the pill don't mix, but more and more are prescribing it for their diabetic patients. If you are black and have sickle-cell anemia or sickle-cell trait (3 percent of the black population in the United States are affected by this disorder), taking the pill may also cause clotting problems. If you have had bad varicose veins and/or have suffered attacks of phlebitis in the past, your chance of developing either phlebitis or some other clotting abnormality of the blood is increased some five to ten times over the 3 per 100,000 in normal women.

An area we sometimes forget about is emotional vulnerability. If you are prone to depression or are being treated for it with medication, the pill may make you worse. Prolonged bed rest itself predisposes to blood-clot formation, so if, for example, you have gone skiing, broken a leg and are going to be off your feet for any length of time, stop the pill temporarily. (Besides which, in bed with a broken leg, you don't have too much use for a contraceptive. If you do, use a diaphragm.)

One other caveat. Soon after a pregnancy, you are quite naturally eager to resume sexual relations after the long, enforced period of abstinence. It is best not to use the pill at that time if you plan to breast-feed, because not only do the hormones reduce the quality of the milk, they are also consumed by the baby. Finally, should you be scheduled for any surgery in the future, it is best to stop the pill about two weeks in advance, in order to reduce the possibility of clot formation or embolism, either during the operation or in the post-operative period.

Intrauterine Devices (IUDs)

Some 2½ to 3 million American women now use an *intrauterine device* (IUD). Unlike the pill, the IUD does not require the discipline of a dosage regimen, and it also lacks the inconvenience of the diaphragm or the mess of vaginal jellies, foams or suppositories. Once in place it is about 96 percent effective, according to the latest estimates.

Despite these advantages, the IUD is less popular than it was ten years ago. That's probably because of the concern some women have that it may lead to infertility after it is discontinued, or that it may result in a tubal pregnancy. If you are offered an IUD by your gynecologist, discuss with him whether this is the best contraceptive for you if (a) you've never had children (because women with IUDs are at three times the risk of developing pelvic infections which may jeopardize future pregnancies), and (b) if you have many sexual partners (again, because of the increased risk of infection).

Modern IUDs cause less cramping and bleeding than earlier models because they are smaller and are impregnated (unfortunate word) with metal, usually copper. Some also contain a built-in hormone, progesterone, which is released very slowly over the months, and which reduces the chances of cramping and bleeding. But remember that the medicated ones must be replaced yearly. The others should be changed every two years. Most IUD's are usually in the form of a T or an L, but the French make one that is heart-shaped and a

Japanese model is in the form of a rising sun. I suppose we may expect the next-generation American IUD to resemble an eagle—or a dollar sign.

When to Have It Inserted

If you have decided to use an IUD, your gynecologist will find it easier to insert while you are having your period. The orifice of the cervix into which the device is placed is more open then to permit the outflow of menstrual blood. Also, if it is fitted at any other time, there is a possibility that you may already be pregnant (which you are not likely to be if you are menstruating). It is not safe to have an IUD in a pregnant uterus because of the greater risk of bleeding, infection and abortion.

The IUD works as long as it stays in place. But it can fall out without your knowing it, especially if the device is a small one. In order to protect you against that possibility, most IUDs come with a little tail that you can feel for at the crucial moment. Never forget to do that. (Recently it was suggested that the tail can provide a route of infection from the outside. So ask your gynecologist to cut it as short as he can before inserting the device.)

We used to think that the IUD acted as a contraceptive by irritating the wall of the uterus and thus preventing implantation of the fertilized egg there. Also, in its constant efforts to expel the IUD, a "foreign body," the uterus thus rids itself of any fertilized egg that did manage to settle within it. These are probably oversimplifications. Most gynecologists now believe that the presence of the loop or copper T in the uterus sets up a low-grade infection of the lining of the uterus, creating an inhospitable climate for the fertilized ovum.

After the IUD Is Removed

Suppose that you have been using the IUD for months or years, and then decide that you want a baby. You have the loop removed. Are you immediately as fertile as you were before it was inserted? We used to think so, but some new evidence suggests that the lining of the uterus remains inhospitable to the products of conception for several more months thereafter, during which time you may have trouble conceiving. So be prepared for some delay. Or, as I mentioned earlier, don't use an IUD if you don't already have at least one child.

Abortion—What Could Have Gone Wrong?

You have been watching the calendar with some anxiety. You are worried because you have always been regular in the past—periods every twenty-nine days, like clockwork. But suddenly you are almost three weeks late. How could you possibly be pregnant? You have never missed using your diaphragm when necessary (although you didn't coat it a second time one night). What other explanation could there be? You are not on the pill or any other hormone that might interfere with your cycle. You have not been taking any tranquilizers or sleeping pills (they can upset your menstrual rhythm). There has been no recent illness or emotional shock. You do remember that once, a long time ago, when you went on a crash diet and lost a lot of weight quickly, you missed a period. But nothing like that has happened this time. What's more, you had your routine checkup only a few weeks before, and everything was just fine, including your thyroid tests.

So now you are almost sure you are pregnant. You think of buying one of those do-it-yourself pregnancy-testing kits in the drugstore, but decide that this is too important a decision for an amateur to fool around with. And you don't want to go through the experience your girl friend had. One of these kits indicated that she was "positive." She worried herself sick for weeks until she went to her doctor, who found it was all a mistake.

After waiting a few more days in the hope that something will happen, you finally summon the courage to visit your gynecologist. He uses a new technique called the radio-receptor assay, which can tell him in just a few hours whether you are pregnant—as early as ten days after your last missed period. He takes some blood (or collects some urine), and before long you get the results. You are pregnant.

Is It Ms., Miss or Mrs. Jones?

Even if you are *Mrs*. Jones, if your religious and personal principles permit, you may want an abortion because you already have enough or more children than you can cope with—physically, emotionally or financially. Also if you are *Miss* or *Ms.* Jones, becoming a mother at this particular time may not be convenient for a host of other reasons. Then again, married or single, you may actually want a baby very much, but have been advised against it by your doctor. He may think that the stress of a pregnancy and delivery are not advisable at this time because of some underlying illness—physical or emotional. Perhaps, too, there is a strong possibility that your child will be born seriously deformed because of some genetic abnormality in your family or an infection contracted during pregnancy (toxoplasmosis, German measles).

For whatever reason, then, you may begin to think about how, when and where to have an abortion. Happily for you, despite all the marches and protests these days for and against, it is the law of the land that a woman may terminate her pregnancy on the basis of her own wants, needs and preferences. In fact, more than one million women have been doing so every year in the United States since 1973, when the Supreme Court made it legal, and there are more abortions being performed in this country (and in England) than appendectomies. Remember, making it legal doesn't guarantee its safety.

Your Abortion—Where, When and How?

Now what's involved? Must you go into a hospital? Can the procedure be done safely in your doctor's office? (That would save you the cost of hospitalization—an important consideration, since some states and insurance policies don't pay for abortions.) Does it have to be done as a "scraping," using a sharp instrument, or can the unwanted contents of your uterus be "sucked out?" And suppose that you really haven't yet decided about having the abortion and you need more time to think it over, how long can you safely wait before you have it done? I have known many women, married and single, who were in a rush to terminate a pregnancy and later regretted having done so. Unmarried couples sometimes discover later that they too would like to have had the child.

The Key Factor Is Timing

Let us go through the decision-making processes that you and your doctor will face in the next few weeks if you should decide to have the abortion. Remember, the key factor is time. Think of the ten lunar months or forty weeks of pregnancy in terms of three 13-week periods, each of which is called a *trimester* (three months). The safest and easiest time to have an abortion is during the first trimester, or twelve weeks. After that, the procedure becomes more complicated to do and the risk increases. Also, abortion is illegal in the third trimester, or after the twenty-fourth week, at which time the fetus can survive in the outside world. Abortion at that point, according to the law, involves killing a human being that has a legal right to life. Of course, the pregnancy may legally be terminated at any time if it is determined that the fetus is already dead or if continuing the pregnancy constitutes an unquestioned risk to the life of the mother. In the latter circumstance, every effort must be made to save the prematurely born infant.

The First Twelve Weeks—Suction or Scraping?

In the first trimester, there is not much choice about how an abortion is performed. In order to empty the contents of the uterus, the doctor can either *scrape* them out, or he can employ *suction curettage*. In the latter technique, the tip of a syringe is inserted through the cervix into the lower part of the uterus, and the contents are aspirated. In either method, you need not be put to sleep. The surgeon freezes the cervix with a local anesthetic before he inserts the instrument.

Most doctors prefer the suction method for the following reasons. Curettage with a metal instrument may perforate the uterus, which, since it is pregnant, is now softer than normal. (In the diagnostic dilatation and curettage [D and C] done to determine the cause of bleeding, the risk of perforation is much smaller, because the wall of the nonpregnant uterus is firm and thick.) Also, the pregnant uterus is congested with blood in order to nourish the fetus, so there is always the chance that the instrumentation will result in a hemorrhage. Since bacteria thrive in an environment rich in blood, poking about a pregnant uterus can cause infection too. Finally, the possibility of adhesions (scar tissue) forming within the uterus is also greater after frequent metal curettage.

Although most gynecologists use suction in the first twelve weeks, some—usually because of habit or convenience— still prefer to scrape. Discuss with your doctor what method he plans for you. But remember, even suction is not without complications, and it too can cause hemorrhage. More important, however, is the possibility that the contents of the uterus will be incompletely evacuated with this technique. There is a gynecologist now being sued by a woman on whom he had performed a suction abortion. Eight months after the procedure she delivered a healthy baby boy. She had attributed her weight gain after the curettage to overeating! I heard of another woman who had a congenital abnormality—two uteri, no less. One was pregnant, the other was not. The gynecologist emptied the wrong one. (As one "pro-life" reader wrote to me after reading the first edition, in her opinion, the *right* one was emptied.) So if you have a suction curettage, insist that what is removed be examined carefully to make certain the pregnancy has not been left behind.

The Second Trimester—the Risk Increases

The risks to the mother are somewhat greater when the abortion is done in the second trimester, that is, between the twelfth and twenty-fourth weeks. Unfortunately, about 15 percent of pregnancies are still terminated that late in the United States; only 3 percent are done in the second trimester in Denmark and Japan, where there is a more sympathetic view of the problem. No woman who has decided to have an abortion should have to wait until the second trimester. But some still delay because of ignorance, failure to accept the facts, or the hope that the pregnancy will somehow "go away." For others, philosophical or religious torment prevents them from going through with it during the first three months. The poor have other problems. Abortion services they can afford are not always easy to find, and some legislators have succeeded in making it more and more difficult for the indigent to have an abortion safely, easily and inexpensively. Economic factors account for at least one quarter of the abortions that are done in the second trimester. Finally, a few are performed late because the medical reasons for doing them in the first place did not exist or were not apparent earlier. If no abortions were undertaken after the twelfth week, the number of deaths in the United States from this procedure, small as they are, would be halved.

So here you are, really pregnant—fifteen or more weeks along—and you still want out. If, when you are examined, the doctor can hear the fetal heart beat, you can be sure the fetus is at least eighteen weeks old, no matter how carefully you have calculated. Although some doctors will abort you by means of a curettage as late as fifteen or sixteen weeks, this technique should rarely be used at that late stage, even by a very skilled surgeon. By that time, and certainly beyond sixteen weeks, metal curettage is hazardous, because the pregnant uterus is now very soft. What about suction? This far along, the products of conception are often too large to be sucked out but not yet really big enough to warrant a surgical approach through the abdominal wall. To be absolutely sure that the fetus is in fact too big to be aspirated, a sonogram (echo test) can be done on the pregnant patient. If the pregnancy is small enough, then suction can still be used. It is somewhat safer than the alternative techniques described below.

When It's Too Late to Aspirate or Scrape

In most cases, this late in the game, abortions are performed by injecting a drug or solution into the sac that contains the fetus (the amniotic sac). The substance used will depend on your doctor's preferences, your own physical condition and what is available. You have the choice among a simple salt solution, a hormone called prostaglandin, and urea.

Injecting Salt

Injecting salt into the amniotic sac is the method currently used in about two thirds of cases after the sixteenth week of pregnancy. We are not sure how or why this brings on the abortion, but it does so in about a day and a half. It is a proven and effective technique, has few failures and rarely results in a living fetus—something that can occur late in the second trimester. However, salt injection, despite its widespread use, may produce some undesirable side effects and is not entirely without risk. You will see why in a moment.

Prostaglandins—Now and in the Future

Your doctor may inject *prostaglandin*, rather than salt, into the amniotic sac. Prostaglandins are a large group of naturally occurring hormones produced in different parts of the body and affecting the function of many organs and systems. They not only initiate labor, they also have something to do with causing high blood pressure, heart attacks, inflammation, resistance to infection, and a host of other processes. As a matter of fact, aspirin, with its myriad effects, ranging from pain control and fever reduction to anticoagulation, appears to work through the prostaglandin system. New prostaglandins are being identified all the time, and the more we learn about them the more fascinating they are.

For purposes of inducing an abortion, a specific prostaglandin (in this instance PGF2a) is injected into the amniotic sac after the sixteenth week. It results in the pregnant contents being expelled in twenty to twenty-six hours. This method has fewer side effects than salt and is safer. However, it does occasionally permit the birth of a live fetus—something that rarely happens with saline.

Urea—More Than a Waste Product

A more recent development than salt and prostaglandin injections is the introduction into the amniotic sac of a substance called *urea*. This is a naturally occurring chemical found in varying amounts in everyone's blood. It is a waste product of liver metabolism and is excreted into the urine by the healthy kidney. When injected into the amniotic sac, it terminates the pregnancy safely and effectively. Furthermore, it almost never results in a live fetus. All things being considered, this is probably the best way now available, for women with normal kidneys and liver, to have a late abortion.

There are several additional techniques of inducing abortion now being developed and tested, some of which may soon be available. The most promising is a vaginal suppository containing prostaglandin. It will eliminate the need for any procedure, operation or injection; you'll simply insert it and wait for things to happen. Another method involves getting an injection of prostaglandin not into the amniotic sac but into your backside, just like a penicillin shot.

Time for a Good Going Over

In order to decide which injection technique to use in the second trimester, your doctor should give you a thorough medical evaluation. Be sure to disclose to him all the pertinent facts in your medical history. For example, if you have high blood pressure or a tendency in that direction, it is not a good idea to have salt injected, because some of it may be absorbed and raise your blood pressure even further. The same is true if you have a cardiac condition, in which case the added salt may result in fluid retention and heart failure. If your kidneys are not functioning properly, neither urea nor salt should be used (elimination of urea from the body requires a healthy kidney). If you are asthmatic or have emphysema, prostaglandins are to be avoided, because they can induce spasm of the bronchial tree and throw you into an acute wheezing attack.

You see, then, why abortion is not a matter to be taken lightly, and why it is important to avoid having it done in an abortion mill. You need a doctor who will examine you carefully and assess your overall physical condition before he performs the procedure, especially in the second trimester.

In Hospital or Doctor's Office?

Where should abortions be performed—in the hospital, outpatient clinic or in your doctor's office? While it *must* be done in a hospital after the first trimester, you do have a choice in the first twelve weeks. Most states, however, have regulations concerning the minimal requirements of a legal abortion facility. For example, in New York, abortions may be performed only where blood transfusion is immediately available (because of the risk of hemorrhage or perforation of the uterus). The same law also states that your blood type must be determined *before* the abortion is done. It must then also be cross-matched, that is, the actual blood you may need in an emergency is earmarked for you and held in readiness.

Now, think for a moment. Does your own doctor have that capability in his office? Probably not. So for that and other reasons he is more than likely to recommend that you come into the hospital, perhaps overnight, even if you are still in the first trimester. That usually is good advice, although more and more doctors are terminating pregnancies in their offices before the *eighth* week, using the suction technique. In any event, it is a good idea to double-check and get a second opinion if you are advised to have your abortion done anywhere but in a hospital.

Don't Join the "Underground"

Unfortunately, there is a large group of doctors who used to do abortions "underground" before legalization. If you should happen to visit such an "old-timer," he may urge you to have the procedure done in his private facility. In the old days, you had little choice but to do so; today you do. While it is true that some of these abortionists are experienced and capable surgeons, they may nevertheless not meet modern legal and medical standards. So, if you choose to go into one of their private clinics, make sure that it is equipped to handle the kinds of emergency that occasionally occur, and is clean and well staffed. Remember that infection remains a risk in any abortion despite all the antibiotics at our disposal. While it is true that there are only some five deaths (due to infection, hemorrhage, rupture of the uterus) for every 200,000 abortions performed in the first trimester, that statistic does not tell the whole story—the complications short of death, the suffering, pain, prolonged hospitalization and sterility—when an abortion is done improperly or in the wrong place.

After the Abortion

After abortions became legal, there were set up in many communities reputable clinics, where the procedure could be done properly, easily and at reasonable cost. These centers are usually run by trained professionals who are able to perform abortions on an outpatient basis. After the uterine contents are aspirated, you rest for an hour or two, and if everything is all right, you may go home. Most women can resume their usual regimen the next day, but they should avoid douching, tampons or intercourse for at least one week. Also, you may expect to have some bleeding for a week or so after the abortion, very much as you would in the last few days of a normal menstrual period. An abortion can be physically and emotionally stressful, so it is a good idea to get plenty of rest and to take iron supplements to prevent anemia due to the blood loss.

Amniocentesis—Pros and Cons

If you are over thirty-five years of age, and certainly if you are beyond forty, the chances of your giving birth to a mongoloid or some otherwise deformed baby are increased, especially if there is a bad genetic family history in that respect. Your doctor should then recommend *amniocentesis*, which involves obtaining some of the fluid from within the products of conception and studying the cells under the microscope. We can often tell by this technique whether your baby will be normal. (In New Jersey, not long ago, two gynecologists were held liable for not advising amniocentesis for a thirty-eight-year-old expectant mother. She subsequently gave birth to a child with a serious congenital abnormality, and she was awarded compensation for mental anguish.)

Amniocentesis is not entirely without risk—of infection or improper interpretation. I know one unfortunate forty-year-old woman who had it done safely and without incident and was assured that she would have a normal baby boy. She had a boy all right, but he was a mongoloid. Another woman of forty refused to have the amniocentesis because of its potential risk and because no one in her family had ever given birth to an abnormal infant. She ended up with a seriously deformed baby. What is one to do, especially since the risk of amniocentesis can approximate that of having an abnormal infant? Have it done, but make sure that the procedure is done by an expert and interpreted by a geneticist working in this field. They can be found by asking your local society or closest university hospital for their names.

KEY FACTS TO REMEMBER

Between 10 and 20 percent of married couples in the United States have an infertility problem. They are often the victims of repeated and unnecessary testing and quack remedies.

When a couple is unable to conceive, the fault lies with the male in almost half the cases. Since evaluation of male infertility is much simpler and less costly than that of the female's, no woman should undergo such testing until her mate has been checked out first.

Male infertility may be due to defects in sperm quantity or quality, hormone imbalance, or some mechanical problem that interferes with the passage of the sperm en route from the testes to the egg. The latter condition frequently can be corrected surgically. You should be aware of several medications and substances in the environment that may interfere with normal sperm production. When male infertility is suspected as the cause of the failure of a couple to conceive, a urologist should be consulted first and then, if necessary, an endocrinologist. If you are found to have an undescended testis, remember that it has the potential for becoming cancerous. If you are advised to "leave it alone," a second opinion should be obtained. If you continue to be given testosterone shots for infertility for longer than three months, without results, ask for a second opinion from a urologist or an endocrinologist.

Infertility in the female is usually due to hormonal imbalance, mechanical problems due to scarring or chronic infection of the reproductive organs, or abnormal chemical changes in the cervix. Your gynecologist should be consulted first for any unexplained difficulty in conception and then, if necessary, see an endocrinologist. Simple diagnostic measures should be exhausted before more painful and costly tests are done. There is a new and growing group of medications becoming available for infertility due to hormonal abnormalities. When no apparent cause for the inability to conceive can be found after appropriate testing of both partners, a psychiatrist should be consulted, since emotional factors may play a role in infertility.

If *sterilization* procedures are recommended for a woman, a second opinion should be sought from another gynecologist, especially if a hysterectomy is planned. Tying the tubes is less complicated, cheaper and equally effective. Removing a healthy uterus is not usually desirable. In males, vasectomy is simple to perform, but this procedure is not always reversible.

There are several different *contraceptive techniques* available. Their efficacy depends on proper use. Selection of the appropriate technique should normally be made by you and your gynecologist. However, the family doctor or internist may need to be consulted if the pill is being considered, since there are several medical circumstances in which this method should be avoided.

Abortions are either voluntary or medically necessary. In the latter event, if you want the baby, but have been told that the pregnancy must be terminated for your own good, get a second opinion. There have been major advances in management of pregnancy in the presence of diabetes as well as certain cardiac and other abnormalities that now make it possible for such women to have their babies.

The best technique for performing an abortion depends on how soon—or late—it is being done. During the first twelve weeks, suction or scraping methods can be used, but suction is generally preferred. If suction is not recommended to you, discuss it with your gynecologist or get another opinion. If the suction technique is selected, make sure that what was removed is examined to determine that the pregnancy was, in fact, removed by the procedure.

At some point between twelve and twenty-four weeks it becomes too late to suction or scrape. There are then three different methods of aborting, each with certain advantages or disadvantages. Discuss with your gynecologist which one is best for you. The technique finally selected should be discussed with your internist, to make sure that it is safe. There are certain medical disorders that might lead you to favor one procedure over another.

Most abortions should be done in a hospital or a clinic. If it is suggested that you have it performed in a doctor's office, make certain that legal requirements are met. You may want to have another opinion to see if it is indeed the best way to go about it.

If you are over thirty-five years of age and are pregnant, you should have an amniocentesis to determine whether the unborn child is abnormal. Since this procedure is not entirely without risk and requires expert interpretation, it should be performed by a specialist and perhaps be double-checked by an experienced geneticist.

19

Impotence—It May Not Be All in the Head

When Nothing Happens

The reasons for Richard Nixon's resigning the presidency and the Shah of Iran's renouncing his throne are no secret. But did you know that King David abdicated because he could no longer achieve an erection? Mind you, he didn't quit without trying. It was only when, as a last resort, a fair young virgin was prescribed by the wise urologists of Biblical times and when the King tried, nothing happened, that he decided it was time to go.

And You Couldn't Care Less

Impotence—the inability to achieve and/or maintain an erection and sometimes not caring whether you do or you don't ("frankly, I'd rather play golf")—is one of the most common problems a physician encounters in daily practice. For example, a forty-seven-year-old man came for a checkup the other day. He was dynamic, vigorous and healthy, and he found his wife as attractive as always. So he was puzzled by the fact that, whereas he had formerly enjoyed intercourse three times a week, he could now "take it or leave it." And when he decided to "take it," it didn't often work out. In otherwise healthy men, such complaints may begin in the middle to late forties or not until the eighties.

But before you search your own memory, and begin to panic, remember that male sexual performance is rarely effective on command. In normal men, there are occasional failures due to variations in mood, interest and energy. But if, over a period of several months, you fail to come through two or three times in every four attempts, you should consult your doctor. One of the first questions he will ask is whether the impotence occurs only at home. I remember one man who complained of failure to achieve erections. When I asked him if this was also true if and when he "cheated", he looked at me incredulously and answered, "Of course not!" That's a simple way to distinguish psychogenic from organic impotence.

Many commonly used drugs may cause impotence. These include Aldomet, Inderal, various diuretics, Aldactone, reserpine (all used in the control of hypertension) alcohol, antidepressants and sleeping pills.

Even smoking has been implicated.

Impotence may also be the first clue to the fact that you are diabetic. If you've always functioned normally in the past, and gradually begin to lose your sexual vigor, have your blood sugar level checked. Normal erections depend not only on an intact blood flow to and within the penis (see below), but also on the integrity of the nervous system to coordinate and deliver all the complex messages involved in the sexual act. Diabetes can impair the vascular supply and also affect critical nerves.

After a pharmacological cause has been excluded, most doctors do a routine physical exam. If they find nothing wrong, they simply tell the patient it's all psychological and that he'll be "all right"—eventually. But such evaluation and advice may not be enough, so don't stop there. Ask to see a urologist. In order to determine whether there is a physical or hormonal basis for your complaints, he will do special tests and measure the testosterone (male hormone) level in the blood.

One of the procedures now being done is evaluation of "nocturnal penile tumescence." This usually permits the doctor to differentiate between psychological and physical causes of impotence. In the former, but not the latter, erections do occur during rapid eye movement (REM) sleep, and can be assessed by a variety of recording techniques. But remember too, despite all the media hype about the splendor of old age, that performance and libido do taper with the years. Don't expect to perform at sixty-five as well as you did at thirty.

When You Pass the Physical—but Still Can't

If you are obviously fatigued, overworked, depressed, worried or bored, most urologists will offer reassurance that the impotence is not physical and that altering your life style is all that is necessary. And sometimes they're right. Such impotence is especially common after business reverses, disappointments, difficult decisions or crises. "Workaholics," totally preoccupied with their life's goals, may also find no capacity for or interest in sex. We encounter it too among men who have had a heart attack and who worry that sexual activity may damage their heart.

If simple reassurance is not enough, then—from a practical point of view—the doctor will, in most cases, prescribe testosterone injections or pills to help solve the problem. That may work at least for a while.

The patient may then be referred to a trained psychologist, psychiatrist or sex-counseling clinic, where any psychological problems can be probed intensively and in depth. There are various treatment techniques ranging from short-term psychotherapy or counseling to analysis or hypnotism, any of which may be successful.

It May Not All Be in Your Head

But if you have gone that far without results, ask for a second opinion. It has only recently become apparent that the time-honored methods for evaluating the physical causes of impotence are not sensitive enough. In many cases, patients have been shortchanged when they have been told there was "nothing wrong." We now believe that there is a real basis for impotence in men of all ages and that in many cases, it is treatable. Current emphasis on the psychologic approach may, therefore, not always be warranted.

The Deprived Penis

Recent research indicates that about half of the men who can't "perform," especially those with diabetes or high blood pressure, have a *measurable* decrease in blood flow to the penis. These data were obtained by using the Doppler technique, which measures blood flow in small blood vessels such as those found in the penis. A tiny blood-pressure cuff is wrapped around the [limp] organ. A Doppler probe on its surface determines the volume of blood flowing into it. Remember, erection is the result of *more* blood to that organ. Even if you are emotionally stable, without that extra penile blood supply, you'll never "get it up."

In addition to reduced blood supply *within* the penis itself, the larger blood vessels that deliver the blood to it may be arteriosclerotic, further decreasing the circulation to that organ. However, whether the problem lies in the penis itself or in external arteries that supply it, the important fact is that vascular insufficiency, not psychological problems, may be the cause of impotence. This new information may save you lots of time and money, spare you indefinite weekly testosterone injections, and get you off the analyst's couch.

Effecting an Erection

If the problem lies in vascular obstruction within the large arteries, such as the aorta, that supply the penis, it can be corrected surgically. This is being done all the time. If the trouble is local, within the penis itself, a "bypass" operation (similar to that performed in the heart for coronary-artery disease) theoretically can be done, but this particular approach has not yet been very successful. If it is recommended to you, get another opinion.

The most innovative, imaginative approach to erection failure when blood supply cannot be increased, or when the problem is, in fact, hopelessly psychological, involves the insertion of a rigid or semistiff prosthesis into the penis itself. Several different such devices are now available and widely used. There are essentially two different types. The first is a rigid rod, which functions like a gooseneck lamp. Although it does make intercourse possible, the trouble is it keeps the penis in a state of near-erection at all times. That is not as good as it sounds. Think what you would look like in your bathing trunks! One way to deal with this problem is to hold the penis up against the abdomen with a "jockstrap" and release it at the appropriate time.

Most urologists recommend the rigid prosthesis, but some prefer to insert two cylinders, one on each side of the penis, which can be inflated (surreptitiously) at will and deflated when the job is done. The pump that supplies the cylinders usually is inserted into the scrotum, while the fluid is stored in a reservoir just under the abdominal wall. One good squeeze results in the release of fluid into the rods rendering the penis erect. The entire maneuver, when skillfully done, can be unobtrusive. In fact, in one survey, some of the female partners were not even aware that their mates had been surgically endowed. Unfortunately, in about one case in three, this system breaks down because of some trouble in the pump, valves or tubing, and reoperation is required.

Interest in penile prostheses is expanding. They are now among the most important topics at national and international urological conferences. If you think you may be a candidate for one, ask your doctor about it. If he is not aware of work in the field, get a second opinion from a urologist who is. Don't be shy about it, either. After all, we use prosthetic joints, prosthetic limbs, prosthetic heart valves and implanted pacemakers all the time. There is no reason why the phallus should be excluded from consideration. But if you are offered such a device, consider it very carefully, get a second opinion, and be sure that you are made aware of the possible complications. For example, there is the risk of infection—not great, but ever present. Also, if you are one of these men who still happily awakes from time to time with an erection, and you have an implanted prothesis, the combination of the natural and artificial erection may give you a lot of pain. But that will soon disappear, because when a rod is inserted into the erectile tissues of the penis, it usually permanently destroys those tissues, together with your ability ever to get a natural erection in the future. So, before having a prosthetic device inserted, make sure that you have exhausted all the other possibilities for treating your impotence.

KEY FACTS TO REMEMBER

Impotence is not to be confused with *infertility*. The former refers to the inability to obtain an erection, the latter to failure to father a child.

Impotence used to be attributed almost always to psychological problems. While these are, in fact, very important, we now appreciate the role of hormonal and circulatory factors. Every apparently healthy male complaining of impotence, should be checked by a urologist to rule out local disease in the genitourinary tract and deficiency in testosterone (the male hormone), and to determine the adequacy of blood flow to and within the penis. When real trouble is found, it frequently can be corrected. Thus, local infection can be treated, testosterone can be given orally or by injection, and interference with blood supply to the penis can be surgically corrected. When these measures either cannot be done or fail, or when psychological problems are paramount and cannot be resolved, there is now the alternative of prosthetic penile devices.

20

The Hysterectomy—
Our Most Unnecessary
Operation

Unnecessary—Like the Tonsillectomy?

Whenever and wherever the subject of unnecessary surgery is raised, the operation most likely to come to mind is the hysterectomy (removal of the uterus). We are leaving more and more tonsils and adenoids alone, because the alleged benefit from their removal has been seriously questioned. But despite the evidence that hysterectomies are too often performed without good reason, they are still being done as frequently as ever.

Is Your Gynecologist a Male Chauvinist?

I don't consider myself either a "feminist" or a "male chauvinist." However, I do believe that too many gynecologists (the great preponderance of whom are men) are insensitive to the psychological impact of removing a uterus from any woman, particularly one who still is in the childbearing age. We joke about it by saying "a hysterectomy removes the baby carriage but leaves the playpen." That's cute, but it does not allay the anxiety of the prospective surgical patient, who, incidentally, never finds it funny.

The Symbolic Uterus

Unlike the tonsils, appendix or even gallbladder, the uterus is a symbol of fertility and femininity to most women. Its necessary extirpation may have profound psychological implications to which the doctor is not always attuned. For example, although some women are relieved at the new sexual freedom that a hysterectomy confers, many view their sexuality as having been compromised. It also signifies the end of child-bearing, a fact in itself almost synonymous with aging. It is one thing to engage in contraceptive techniques that you can discontinue when you decide you want to have a baby; it is quite another matter to have your fertility so drastically, completely and permanently terminated. For all these reasons, this operation should never be done without a very good reason.

Looking Over Your Gynecologist's Shoulder

In the absence of public pressure and awareness, and when their peers aren't monitoring them either, how often do gynecologists perform hysterectomies without justification? This crucial question was studied a few years ago by representatives of the medical profession itself in Saskatchewan, Canada. Review committees there redefined the circumstances under which the operation *should* be done. Using these new criteria, they concluded that 23.7 percent of all hysterectomies were unnecessary. They then publicized the new standards and indicated that henceforth all such operations would be monitored for compliance. In the first year alone, the percentage of unjustified hysterectomies dropped to 7.8 percent. So, if you are living in an area where such formal guidelines have been neither enunciated nor enforced and you are advised to have a hysterectomy, it goes without saying that you should get a second opinion from another gynecologist.

The Advice May Be Right or Wrong

In most cases, your doctor will advise you to have a hysterectomy when it is an absolute must. But from time to time, as we know from the statistics, you will be sent for surgery when you really shouldn't be. Let me illustrate for you a few typical situations in which the operation is, and isn't, necessary.

When the Uterus Must Come Out

Suppose that you consult your doctor because of vaginal bleeding or pelvic pain. After he performs the necessary studies (pelvic exam, Pap smear, sonography) he finds a cancer of the uterus. The uterus then almost always *must* come out. But remember, ask for a second opinion to make sure that the diagnosis of cancer was correct in the first place.

You are also better off having the uterus removed if it contains a large fibroid (a benign uterine tumor) pressing on neighboring organs in your pelvis. Most gynecologists will recommend such surgery when they estimate the weight of the uterus at greater than 200 grams (normal weight is 60-80 grams). However, if it produces uncomfortable symptoms a hysterectomy should be done even if the fibroid is smaller than that.

If your Fallopian tubes are scarred by chronic infection, giving you constant pelvic pain, and antibiotics don't help the situation, hysterectomy is usually the best recourse.

If you wet your pants whenever you cough or sneeze because repeated pregnancies have left your vaginal walls or muscles too weak to control urination, your doctor will then need to repair and strengthen the flaccid structures. If you are beyond childbearing age, he will quite properly recommend hysterectomy at that time too because unless the uterus is removed, it will continue to exert pressure on the lax vaginal walls, bladder and rectum, and the operation will not be entirely successful.

Finally, if you have an ovarian tumor that needs to come out, and you are over forty-five years of age, the uterus should also be removed. It has no physiological function without the ovaries and can develop cancer later on, especially if you are taking estrogens; so, there is no point in retaining it. (We also recommend removal of the *unaffected* ovary at the same operation, since cancer of the ovary is second only to cancer of the breast as a cause of death from malignancy in women.)

When to Say No

Some doctors recommend hysterectomy when they find small uterine fibroids in the course of a routine examination.

If you have no pain, bleeding, pressure or other symptoms, don't allow it. Even if the fibroids are large enough to cause some discomfort, if you plan to have children in the future, do not agree to the operation without at least a second opinion from another gynecologist.

The "Useless Uterus" Syndrome

An "abnormal" Pap test per se is not usually cause for removing the uterus. It tells us only that something is amiss; it does not always indicate with complete certainty whether the cause is inflammation, infection or cancer. Even if some malignant cells are found, the problem usually can be managed by surgery or radiation limited to the cervix, without removing the entire uterus. Yet there are doctors who tell their patients in this situation that "You might as well have *all* of the uterus taken out." This "might as well" psychology is to be deplored and should always be rejected.

In some women who have chronic pelvic infection, or whose periods are always very painful, some gynecologists are too quick to whip out the uterus instead of first trying medication and hormones. Never submit to such surgery until the medical alternatives have been considered and tried, although occasionally, you may elect hysterectomy rather than endure chronic pain and prolonged treatment.

There are other circumstances too under which the uterus should definitely not be removed, one of which is *unexplained* vaginal bleeding. Such bleeding, if not due to tumor, is probably the result of a hormonal imbalance. This is often resistant to treatment, taxing the ingenuity and patience of the gynecologist, who, in frustration, may recommend a hysterectomy in order to "be done with it." That is bad medical practice and equally bad advice. If it is given to you, don't hesitate to get a second opinion.

You don't need to have the uterus taken out in order to be made sterile—if that is what you want. Although some doctors still recommend it, most don't. The objective of sterility is to prevent an egg from mating with sperm. That can be done just as effectively by cutting or tying the Fallopian tubes (where the ovum travels from the ovary to effect its rendezvous with the sperm.) Tubal ligation is a lot easier for you and makes more sense than undergoing a major operation to remove a perfectly healthy organ.

I know patients who have had the uterus taken out simply because it was "retroverted" (tilted backward), or because they complained of backache or persistent vaginal discharge. One wonders whether they would have been so advised had the gynecologist been a woman.

Much as I deplore the needless hysterectomy, I must say, in all fairness, that the blame does not always lie solely with the doctor. Too often, the patient herself (or her husband) will insist on having the operation and so avoid repeated office visits for the control of bleeding or other symptoms. It is essential that both *you* and your doctor appreciate the undesirability of the unnecessary hysterectomy.

KEY FACTS TO REMEMBER

Surgical removal of the uterus is too commonly done without good reason. The statistics suggest that whenever this operation is recommended, another opinion should be obtained. In addition to unnecessary pain, risk and cost, casual hysterectomy often has profound psychological impact. However, the operation must be done when there is cancer of the uterus, or benign fibroids that are causing pressure symptoms and/or bleeding. Chronic infection of the Fallopian tubes, resulting in pain that is otherwise unmanageable, may also justify hysterectomy. When cancerous ovaries are removed, the uterus is also frequently excised as well. However, hysterectomy should be resisted when done solely for purposes of sterilization, bleeding due to hormonal imbalance, or for treatment of "backache."

21

Peptic Ulcers—Down with the Diet?

The Changing Scene

The word *peptic* is derived from the Greek *peptein* ("to cook, to digest") and is applied to the substantive "ulcer" to signify its location in either the stomach (gastric) or the duodenum.

Back in the 1940s, when peptic ulcers were much more common in the United States than they are today, one American in ten was expected to develop an ulcer sometime before the age of sixty-five. But this very common malady may be on the wane, and no one knows why. For example, in the decade of the 70's, hospitalization for duodenal ulcer dropped by 43 percent and for gastric ulcer by 10 percent. Ulcer deaths are declining too at the rate of 5 percent every year. But these figures may simply mean that diagnosis of peptic ulcer is more accurate, and its treatment more effective, while the true incidence of the disease is actually unchanged. Nevertheless, even now ten thousand people die every year in this country from ulcers and their complications— hemorrhage (the ulcer erodes a blood vessel), perforation (it bores a hole in the wall), obstruction (the intestinal tract is scarred from repeated ulceration and healing), or penetration (the ulcer burrows through the wall of the gut to involve an adjacent organ like the pancreas).

You Don't Die from Indigestion

Ulcers are too often blamed for far more serious problems. Attributing a bellyache to an ulcer you don't have can be dangerous. For example, we so often assume that any discomfort in the upper abdomen or lower chest after eating—heartburn, pressure, fullness or heaviness—is due to chronic "indigestion." Sometimes, however, these complaints are the result of heart disease, not stomach trouble, and the failure to make that distinction can be disastrous. I remember one patient who frequently developed chest pain when walking soon after he ate. It was typical of angina and I told him so. But he refused to believe the symptoms were cardiac, because he experienced them only after eating. He could walk to "his heart's content" any other time. He decided, on his own, to have X rays of his upper intestinal tract (GI series) to prove to himself (and to me) that he did, in fact, have either an ulcer or a hiatus hernia. During the test itself he suffered a massive heart attack—and that finally convinced him. So remember, if you have any upper-abdominal or chest pain or pressure, especially if it is worsened by emotional stress, walking or some other physical activity, check with your doctor to make sure that the trouble is not in your heart even though the symptoms occur only after eating.

A Hole in the Wall—Stomach versus Duodenum

An ulcer is an erosion or hole in the lining of any organ. You can develop one in your eye if you injure it or on your skin if you burn it. In this chapter we will discuss ulcers of the stomach and the duodenum. They are not quite the same disease. Symptoms, complications, outlook and, most important of all, treatment differ substantially in the two. A brief review of anatomy will help you appreciate why this is so.

The stomach is a J-shaped organ that narrows at its end to lead into the small intestine (duodenum) where three quarters of all ulcers occur. The first major difference beween stomach (gastric) and duodenal ulcers is that the latter are never malignant, whereas the former can be. In practical terms, that means that the result of treating a duodenal ulcer can be judged more or less by how you feel and how much pain you have. Repeated X rays, in the absence of bleeding are neither necessary nor desirable. On the other hand, if you have a gastric ulcer, you should be under the care of a specialist (gastroenterologist). Regardless of symptoms, he will be watching it very closely until he has *proved* that it is completely healed. That requires X rays at regular intervals, and/or gastroscopy (also called endoscopy), wherein you swallow a thin, very flexible tube with a light at the end of it that is then passed directly into the stomach. This permits the doctor actually to see the ulcer and if necessary, biopsy a piece to be examined under the microscope for evidence of malignancy.

Symptoms of gastric and duodenal ulcers are also different. For example, food relieves the gnawing hunger pain of a duodenal ulcer, but may aggravate one in the stomach. Nor is their treatment the same. Antispasmodics (no longer widely used because of their side effects, and because there are newer, better agents) are generally of greater benefit in duodenal ulcers than in gastric ulcers. Patients with duodenal ulcers are usually between twenty and fifty, while those with gastric ulcers are likely to be older, in the middle sixties.

Sex Differences Too

Interestingly enough, as in arteriosclerotic heart disease, women who are still menstruating develop duodenal ulcers much less commonly than do men. We assume that men are more vulnerable to both diseases because they lack some protective factor that is present in women, perhaps a female hormone. This theory was the basis for some trials, a few years ago, in which men suffering from severe and recurrent duodenal ulcers were given female hormones. But, as in heart disease, this intervention made no apparent difference.

Acid Is Bad—Mucus Is Good

Most normal people secrete acid in the stomach to help the process of digestion. But in some vulnerable individuals, this acid eats away the lining of the gastric and duodenal walls, creating ulcers. Why this doesn't happen to everyone is not clear. The answer may lie partly in the amount and kind of *mucus* secreted by the intestinal and stomach walls. Mucus coats the lining and thus helps prevent erosion by acid. Also, acid-resisting properties of the cells lining the stomach and intestinal walls may vary from person to person. The stomach also secretes a substance called pepsin, an excess of which also contributes to ulcer formation. Finally, the *amount* of acid produced by the stomach is critical too. This is very much influenced not only by the food we eat, but also by the activity of a certain nerve called the *vagus*. An overactive vagus results in greater acid secretion by the stomach. That is the reason we try to suppress it with antispasmodic medication and cut the nerve when all else fails.

Anxiety and Frustrated Anger

We can all recognize the "ulcer-prone personality" (in someone else)—the harried, high-powered executive (or doctor), the tense television producer, the anxious stockbroker, the aggressive, angry, frustrated politician. But, although these "types" develop ulcers, so do many of us who don't fall into that category. Some of the quietest, withdrawn, placid patients I know have ulcers. I suppose that is because different stresses affect each of us in different ways. What is unnerving for you may be handled in stride by your neighbor. Many persons doing "stressful" work—surgeons performing delicate operations every day (and worrying about the results the night before and the night after), combat personnel, key executives, hostages—do not, in fact, have a greater incidence of ulcers than do the rest of the population. So, in addition to emotional stress, which obviously plays some role, there must be other responsible factors.

How to Make an Ulcer

If, for any reason, you would like to have an ulcer of your own, you can improve your chances of getting one by excessive cigarette smoking, too much alcohol, and the chronic use of certain medications, including aspirin (the most common offender), the many newer antiarthritic and painkilling drugs like Indocin, Butazolidin and Motrin, cortisone (when used in large doses for weeks or months) and reserpine (a substance sometimes prescribed for the control of high blood pressure). A strong family history of ulcers, as well as certain other diseases—as, for example, cirrhosis of the liver, emphysema of the lungs and rheumatoid arthritis—may also leave you more vulnerable.

Tums versus Rolaids

Suppose, then, that you complain to your doctor about a chronic "hunger pain" in the mid-portion of the upper abdomen, relieved by food, milk or some antacid that you heard about on TV. Two or three hours later (after the food has passed through the stomach and is no longer buffering the acid) the pain starts up again. You also remember having similar symptoms last spring, but they cleared up on their own. The pain has begun to interfere with your sleep, and it awakens you between midnight and three o'clock (but never, curiously enough, just before you would normally get up, like six or seven in the morning).

Making the Diagnosis

As you describe these symptoms, your doctor will immediately think "ulcer." When he examines you and presses hard on the abdomen just above the belly button, it will hurt. After the physical, he will ask for a stool specimen and analyze it for the presence of blood. As I wrote in *The Complete Medical Exam*, blood from high up in the intestinal tract—that is, originating in the stomach or the duodenum—is usually black by the time it appears in the stool, because it has been chemically altered as it traveled down the gut. (But remember, if you happen to be taking Pepto-Bismol, or iron supplements for "tired blood," your stool will be black too). Finally, to establish the diagnosis (which he already strongly suspects from your history and physical exam), he will send you for an X ray following a barium drink. This will usually reveal the ulcer. If it is in the duodenum, you are free and clear as far as cancer is concerned; but if it is in the stomach, it may be malignant. Sometimes even if the history, physical findings and blood in the stool all suggest an ulcer, the X ray may not show it because it is tiny or buried in one of the folds of the stomach wall. In that case, your doctor will recommend a gastroscopy. He will also do so if a gastric ulcer is found by X ray, so that he can take a biopsy to make absolutely sure that an early, curable cancer is not being missed. What's more, even if the first biopsies taken with the gastroscope show it to be benign, you should still be re-X-rayed or gastroscoped again in six to eight weeks after treatment—just to be sure.

If you have a gastric ulcer the key sequence for you to remember and to insist upon is (1) X ray; (2) endoscopy with biopsies; and (3) repeated evaluation until the ulcer has been shown to have disappeared.

Antacids—Very Effective but Not Harmless

Since ulcer disease involves erosion of the lining of the gut, the first step in treatment is to give you something to neutralize the acid that is doing it. Many people believe that *antacids* are inert and that it is safe to take as much of them as you want—indefinitely. We have all seen the ulcer patient who walks around with pockets full of antacid tablets, swallowing or chewing them every few minutes, while under stress or after drinking in excess. Too much antacid is neither harmless nor inert, and there are significant differences among the various brands available. Some contain calcium, which in large doses can eventually cause heart and kidney problems. Others, like baking soda, contain large amounts of salt which is bad for people with high blood pressure and heart failure. Some antacids will constipate you or, if they have magnesium hydroxide, give you diarrhea. Finally, if you're taking antacids containing aluminum over the long term, you may suffer demineralization of your bones due to loss of calcium and phosphorus. Post-menopausal women are particularly vulnerable to this complaint.

Because of these varied potential untoward effects, commercially available antacids are frequently made up of several different ingredients, each of which offsets the side effects of the other. For example, they may contain equal amounts of substances that will constipate you and give you diarrhea, the net result being neither. The most widely advertised antacids are Maalox, Gelusil, Mylanta, Di-Gel, Titralac and Riopan—not to mention Tums and Rolaids. Although the tablet is more convenient, the liquid is better for an active ulcer, because it neutralizes acid more effectively than do tablets. Also, for the most prolonged effect, be sure to take antacids *after* meals, when they act for as long as four hours; when taken on an empty stomach, they work for only twenty to thirty minutes.

Do you remember when patients with peptic ulcer consumed large quantities of milk and cream to relieve their pain? If they happened to believe that too much cholesterol causes arteriosclerosis and heart disease, they had a lot to worry about. You'll be happy to know, if you have ulcers, that milk and cream are not even as effective as most other foods in buffering stomach acidity, and there's no reason for you to keep taking them.

Antispasmodics Are Not for Everyone

If you have a duodenal ulcer (and, less often, a stomach ulcer) you may also be given an *antispasmodic*. There are many such preparations available and are marketed as Robinul, Donnatal, Probanthine, Daricon, Valpin (and at least twenty others). Most contain atropine or one of its derivatives, and they depress the vagus nerve, which, as I mentioned earlier, stimulates the stomach to secrete more acid. Antispasmodics, however, have certain side effects of which you soon become aware. They leave your mouth dry. If you are a middle-aged or older man, or if you have some prostate trouble, you may have difficulty emptying your bladder because of the action of the antispasmodics on the muscles controlling urination. This can create an emergency situation in which your bladder is filled with urine that you can't void. That means that a catheter may have to be passed through the penis into the bladder—painful, inconvenient and occasionally the cause of subsequent urinary infection. So, if you've had any indication of prostate trouble (getting up several times at night to void, trouble starting the stream, dribbling when you are finished) tell your doctor about it when he prescribes antispasmodics. Also, avoid these drugs if you have glaucoma, since they increase pressure within the eye and can worsen the condition. If you have any irregularity of the heartbeat or palpitations, remember that antispasmodics tend to increase the heart rate. So, antispasmodics aren't the first line drugs they used to be. Cimetidine (Tagamet) and antacids are more effective and have fewer side effects.

You May Eat Whatever You Want (Well, Almost)

Not too long ago the most important part of ulcer treatment was a very strict diet. You were allowed to eat only bland food, forced to drink lots of milk and cream, and forbidden everything else, especially if you really enjoyed it. But that is all a thing of the past, just like prolonged physical inactivity or forced retirement after a heart attack. Now you eat virtually anything you want. *A diet limited to bland foods does not promote healing of the ulcer.* Despite this, most hospitalized ulcer patients are still being prescribed severely restricted diets. If your doctor also does so, discuss it with him. If he insists on it, which he is not really likely to do, you may have to get another opinion from a gastroenterologist.

The facts are that you may safely and comfortably eat what your heart desires as long as you avoid alcohol (which stimulates the formation of acid and irritates the raw ulcer); certain medications mentioned earlier, especially aspirin; cigarettes (which promote acid formation); and all caffeine (coffee, tea and cola drinks), which increase gastric acidity. Incidentally, decaffeinated coffee, popularly thought to be permissible, has the same adverse effects on an ulcer as does regular coffee. And it's not only the caffeine, but also something else in coffee that irritates the ulcer.

Ulcers, Tranquilizers and Psychiatrists

It is almost a reflex act for doctors to prescribe tranquilizers for ulcer patients to "help you relax." A sedative is helpful if you are nervous, apprehensive and on edge, but not otherwise. Tranquilizers do not in themselves promote ulcer healing. By the same token, don't consult a psychiatrist simply because you have an ulcer. Psychotherapy is of no help to the ulcer itself and may provoke more anxiety and make things worse. In fact, it is better not to get started with a psychiatrist during the acute phase of the disease unless there is some obvious, compelling reason to do so.

Cimetidine—a Major Breakthrough

In recent years, a new antiulcer drug, cimetidine (Tagamet), has been developed that works in a totally different way. Most doctors prefer it to antacids as the mainstay of tretatment, because it is so effective and so much easier to take. This new agent, available since 1977, actually *prevents* the formation of acid by the stomach—and "no acid" means "no ulcer." Patient compliance with this drug has been excellent, especially because it successfully controls pain during the night.

It is still too early to be absolutely certain that cimetidine is completely safe when taken for many months or years. For example, as discussed in an earlier chapter, there is evidence that it reduces the sperm count in otherwise healthy men. It may also enlarge their breasts. There is speculation that it may lead to certain chemical reactions in the stomach and thus may be carcinogenic over the long term. The theoretical possibility exists too that it may cause some adverse effects in the brain when taken for prolonged periods. But for the acute phase, it has been shown to be safe and extremely effective.

Heart Trouble and Ulcers in Tandem

I had a recent experience with cimetidine that impressed me very much. One of my patients, a sixty-five-year-old man, previously in good health, was admitted to the hospital because of severe cardiac pain. His electrocardiogram was very abnormal, but all the other tests indicated that though he might well be on the verge of having a heart attack, he had not yet sustained one. Despite treatment, he continued to have chest pain, some of which suggested the possibility of a noncardiac source. So, very gingerly and cautiously, we X-rayed his upper intestinal tract and found a large duodenal ulcer.

Now we had two problems—the heart and the ulcer. Because his pain persisted and was often accompanied by ECG abnormalities, we performed a coronary angiogram (that is, dye was injected into his coronary circulation to determine the location and extent of any blockage there). We found one of his major arteries to be 99 percent occluded) and presumably about to close. Two others were also severely narrowed. In my judgment, he was heading for a serious, life-threatening heart attack and needed immediate bypass surgery. I was concerned about the added stress of a major heart operation on his already "hot ulcer." However, we gave the patient cimetidine intravenously and sent him to the operating room. The operation was successful, and ten days later he went home. His heart was fine, the obstructed arteries had been bypassed with vein grafts, and—thanks to the cimetidine— his ulcer was almost healed, despite the surgery.

I think it is a very useful drug, but if your doctor tells you to take it indefinitely, get another opinion from a gastroenterologist. I don't think we have enough evidence yet to justify that position.

Research and development in antiulcer treatment is ongoing and very active. There are some promising new agents of which you should be aware. For example, the makers of cimetidine (Tagamet) are working with a new preparation, ranitidine, which acts the same way as cimetidine, but has greater potency, and its effect is longer lasting. So, it needs to be taken only twice instead of four times a day. It may also cause fewer side effects than cimetidine, and be safer over the long run.

There is a group of drugs called tricyclics. You know all about them if you've been taking anti-depressive medication. One of them, Surmontil, has a cimetidine-like effect, and is useful in the treatment of ulcers because it reduces acid secretion. Another tricyclic, pirenzipine, (this one not an antidepressant) is still in research, but is also said to be at least as effective as cimetidine.

Yet another agent used in Japan for ten years, is now available. Called sucralfate (Carafate), it coats and protects the ulcer crater and also reduces the secretion of pepsin by the stomach cells; most important, it is not absorbed. You may think of it as a "Band-Aid" for the ulcer, which it covers for five hours.

The prostaglandins, naturally occurring substances that are present in virtually every organ system in the body, (and which I have discussed briefly in the chapter dealing with abortion) have generated great excitement in the potential treatment of peptic ulcer disease. They are, however, some years away from clinical use.

KEY FACTS TO REMEMBER

Ulcers of the stomach (gastric) and duodenum are on the wane, but they still account for several thousand deaths each year in the United States alone. Anyone with recurrent "indigestion" should make certain that the symptoms are not due to heart disease.

Duodenal ulcers are virtually never cancerous; gastric ulcers frequently are. Treatment of an uncomplicated duodenal ulcer is simple and straightforward. Gastric ulcers, however, require sophisticated diagnostic follow-up and should be managed by a gastroenterologist. Most gastric ulcers require gastroscopy and biopsy.

Stress frequently but not always contributes to ulcer formation. Psychiatric care is usually not necessary for ulcer patients, unless there are specific unrelated emotional problems. Such treatment is particularly undesirable in the acute stage of the ulcer.

The mainstays of ulcer treatment are cimetidine, antacids and antispasmodics. Diet restriction, except for cigarettes, caffeine and alcohol, is usually unnecessary.

22

Viral Hepatitis—Avoiding a Jaundiced View

The Seat of the Soul

The ancients called the heart "the seat of the soul." Most people think the brain should have been so designated. I take exception to both nominations. In my mind, there is no question that the liver deserves this signal honor—for it is at least as complex as the brain, as vital as the heart, and is responsible, to boot, for a multitude of body processes. No wonder then that a Frenchman, whenever he is feeling sick or just out of sorts, invariably blames his liver.

It Gives You Hepatitis

Ask any child what the heart does, and he will answer, quite properly, that it sustains life by pumping blood to the rest of the body. Who doesn't know that the brain controls our every movement and thought? It is common knowledge that the kidneys make urine in which the waste products of the body are excreted. But when I asked several people recently what the liver does, none of them really knew— except for one woman who answered, "It gives you hepatitis."

The liver, of which incidentally we have only one, performs a staggering array of very sophisticated functions. It is important that you know what they are, because, only then will you appreciate what can go wrong with you when your liver is sick.

Albumin and Globulin—Key Proteins

Let us begin with the synthesis or manufacture of scores of different kinds of proteins. The liver, using as its building blocks the basic elements in the foods we eat, reconstitutes them into complicated proteins like albumin and globulin.

Albumin is fundamental to our survival. Attached to this protein and transported by it is an array of minerals and hormones, each of which is discharged by the albumin wherever and whenever needed. Albumin also maintains the balance of pressure between the fluid within the blood vessels (veins and arteries) and that in the surrounding tissues. When there is not enough albumin around, as happens in severe liver disease, fluid seeps out of the blood vessels and results in swelling of the body.

Globulins are the cornerstone of our body defenses, making all kinds of antibodies, which help us resist infection and possibly even cancer.

There are scores of other less-well-known proteins, all of which are extremely important to the maintenance of our health and biological status quo. For example, have you ever considered what prevents you from hemorrhaging internally? It is the many proteins that are made by the liver which maintain the exquisite balance between the clotting and bleeding mechanisms—fibrinogen, prothrombin, and a host of other "factors." A deficiency of only one of these factors can be responsible for a serious bleeding disorder, as for example, hemophilia.

The liver also builds up, rearranges and breaks down many other protein molecules, like a child with his Mechanoset or building blocks. Most important in its function as molecular architect in this regard is what the liver does to amino acids, a large group of essential body proteins—constantly changing their composition from one to another.

The liver also converts ammonia, an end product of protein metabolism, into harmless chemicals. Unless this is done, ammonia, derived from the protein in our diet, accumulates in the body. Enough of it will render you unconscious. That is the mechanism by which chronic alcoholics and others with severe liver disease go into coma and die.

Fifty Million Frenchmen Can't Be Wrong—Can They?

The liver is involved in literally hundreds of other chemical reactions, many of which are mediated through enzymes. These are responsible for everything from digesting the food we eat to making sure our blood clots and flows properly. It makes bile which it sends to the gallbladder for storage and to the gut for digesting fat. How much cholesterol and triglycerides you have, whether you develop "low blood sugar" or not, the fate of so many of the pills you take (why they just don't keep accumulating as you take one or two every day)—all this is determined by the liver. It stores substances, detoxifies them, eliminates them, or changes their chemistry so that they don't poison you. You name it, the liver does it. As I reflect on this myriad of functions, I'm beginning to think that the French are right about their "mal de foie."

Just as the liver has so many critical roles to play, so is it vulnerable to a wide variety of disorders ranging from physical injury to viral infection. You can poison your liver with alcohol or cleaning fluid; some disease process or other can interfere with its blood supply; the bile-carrying ducts that interconnect it with the gallbladder and intestine can become obstructed by stone or tumor giving you jaundice (the bile backs up into the liver and bloodstream); it may develop a cancer of its own or play host to one originating elsewhere in the body. These are just some of the major things that can go wrong with the liver. Fortunately, this complex organ has a large reserve for the jobs it does. With the exception of cancer, native to it or "imported," and a few of the more serious infections and toxic agents, the liver can take a lot of abuse before it really gets its back up.

Different Kinds of Hepatitis

Hepar means "liver," and *itis* "inflammation" or "infection." *Hepatitis*, therefore, refers to any of a wide variety of insults—chemical, bacterial, parasitic (such as when a worm gets to it from the gut), alcohol, and viruses, which end up inflaming or infecting the liver. In this chapter, however, I will limit my discussion to viral hepatitis, a group of very common disorders that affect many thousands of people each year. You should be aware of the new and important information about their diagnosis and treatment.

The liver is made up of several different kinds of cells, each involved in its own particular way in the many functions of this organ. When attacked by the specific viruses that cause hepatitis, these cells stop working properly, and you begin to feel sick. You will likely develop a fever, start to itch all over, lose your appetite, experience continual nausea for a few days and even vomit. You find yourself tired, have a feeling of soreness over the liver (in the right upper portion of the abdomen) and become yellow (jaundiced). Smokers completely lose their taste for tobacco. It is not unusual, especially in one of the forms, Virus B hepatitis, to have aches and pains in all the joints—a form of arthritis. These symptoms may come on abruptly, in a matter of a few days, or insidiously, over a period of weeks, depending on the particular virus infecting you. Symptoms may last for about four to six weeks in uncomplicated cases. But how sick you get and how quickly you recover depends, in part, on your age (older, fragile persons tolerate the infection less well) and the severity and the nature of the infection itself.

A, B, and Non-A, Non-B with More on the Way

We currently recognize three different types of viral hepatitis at the present time—in terms of how they are transmitted, identified, treated, their outlook and their prevention. (Actually, more and more subgroups of these major viruses are being identified all the time, but for purposes of simplicity, I will limit my discussion to three.) They are called Virus A (formerly called infectious hepatitis), Virus B (the old designation was serum or transfusion hepatitis) and a newly recognized one (or more) that is neither A nor B, and which most doctors call Non-A, Non-B (NANB), though a few traditionalists have defiantly named it Hepatitis C). Although there is some overlap, the basic differences among them are as follows: Virus A is primarily harbored in the gut, and is transmitted by that route (fecal-oral). For all practical purposes you contract Virus A hepatitis from food (usually shellfish) or water contaminated by sewage. Therefore, this type of hepatitis is found in largest numbers where public-health measures are primitive or inadequate and sanitation control poor, and where there is overcrowding such as occurs in jails or army barracks. It occurs most commonly among the young, is rarely fatal, and hardly ever ends up giving you chronic liver disease. Its symptoms tend to develop rather quickly, and you are most contagious to others during what is called the "prodromal state"—after you have been infected but are still not feeling sick with the disease. This incubation period usually lasts between twenty and forty days, and patients remain infective to others for about twenty-one days after symptoms begin. The hallmark of hepatitis is jaundice. Once the yellow hue appears, the patient is usually no longer infective. So, if you are close to someone who has developed jaundice and worry about whether you too will get hepatitis, think back on the nature of your contact *before* the jaundice became apparent.

Hepatitis B and NANB are very much alike in most respects and so are generally considered together. They have a similar mode of transmission, which differs from that of A virus. They also have more serious potential consequences than does hepatitis A. (Both A and B viruses can be identified by tests or "markers" in the blood.) The existence of NANB hepatitis (which may actually be due to more than one virus) was assumed when the B virus could not be identified in cases where that diagnosis was made on clinical grounds. If it was neither A nor B, what was it? Obviously Non-A, Non-B. What else?

How They're Transmitted

While Virus A inhabits the intestinal tract and is transmitted primarily by contamination from it, Viruses B and NANB are found in the blood. You "catch" their diseases from someone else's infected blood. How might that happen, assuming that you are not a vampire? The most obvious way is via a transfusion with blood donated or sold by someone who has the disease. Such blood can be screened to eliminate infection by B virus, but we cannot detect NANB virus, which causes 80 or 90 percent of all *transfusion hepatitis*. In addition to transfusions, you can also get B or NANB hepatitis when your skin is broken (transcutaneous route) by a needle that was used in drawing blood from someone with the disease and was not properly sterilized. (Unfortunately, disposable needles are not yet used everywhere.) And that can happen in such respectable places as your dentist's chair, or in questionable situations like tattoo parlors. Another obvious reservoir of infection, one that is of great and growing concern, is the drug addict. If he is a Virus B carrier or incubating the disease, he will give it to everybody with whom he shares syringes or needles. Medical and paramedical workers, who are in contact with scalpels, other instruments, patients' blood (as for example, in dialysis units) and tissues of various sorts, are especially vulnerable to this disease and have a high incidence of it. Finally, Hepatitis B (but strangely enough not NANB) is also spread by the venereal route. The incubation period of Hepatitis B is longer (usually 60 to 110 days) than that of A virus, while the incubation of NANB is somewhere between the two (35 to 70 days). Virus B, because of the way it is transmitted (blood, needles and the venereal route), is more apt to involve the elderly and homosexuals.

Although Virus A is transmitted differently than B and NANB, the clinical distinction among all three forms is not always clear-cut. From time to time we encounter patients who have B or NANB virus hepatitis in whom we simply cannot elicit any history of infection by the needle or blood route. It is more than likely that in these cases, the viruses were spread some other way. This is supported by the finding of the B virus in mother's milk, in semen, gastric juices and, even, in urine and feces (usually the hunting ground of the A virus). So, from the point of view of prevention, the nursing care of a patient with Virus B or NANB hepatitis should focus primarily on the sterilization of any needles involved in testing or treatment, and normal hygienic attention to the disposition of stool and urine as well. Oral and other intimate contacts should also be avoided during the infectious stage in all patients with any hepatitis.

Whereas the A type (which, incidentally, is the least common form of hepatitis) is almost always benign, Virus B and NANB hepatitis can lead to prolonged illness, chronic hepatitis and death. According to the most recent experience, the death rate in B and NANB may be as high as 15 percent, while the chances of developing chronic liver disease is 10 percent in B cases and between 10 and 40 percent for NANB infections. So if you get "hepatitis" make sure to ask what type it is. That is determined by analyzing a specimen of your blood.

Too Much Rest

Despite the differences between virus A hepatitis and the other two forms, the treatment for all three is basically the same—supportive. There is no cure for any of them, no medicine or antibiotic you can take to destroy the viruses. We simply recommend plenty of rest and nutrition until the disease runs its course. It is often very frustrating to remain at home and "do nothing" until it is all over. But too much of a good thing is not desirable either, and that's what we used to do in the treatment of hepatitis. Patients were advised to stay in bed until all liver tests had returned completely to normal and/or until the jaundice had disappeared. Also, the diet was very restrictive—no fats, limited proteins and lots of carbohydrates—a very boring menu, which didn't help to ensure the necessary nutrition or stimulate an appetite that was poor to begin with.

The Army to the Rescue

We are indebted to the military for the modern treatment of viral hepatitis. As you might expect, the Army is not keen on pampering its personnel, tucking them into bed for months and feeding them special diets. So they decided to see whether prolonged bed rest really made any difference to patients with hepatitis. They found, after very careful studies, that it did not. Neither did special diets. On the basis of these and other later studies, we now recommend that if you get hepatitis, rest in bed only as long as you have fever and the liver tests are getting worse. You may safely get out of bed and even return to work while you are still slightly jaundiced—as soon as you feel better, your temperature is normal and your liver-function tests begin to return *toward* normal. And from day one you may eat whatever you like if it agrees with you, as long as you abstain from alcohol in any form.

Suppose someone with whom you have had close contact (roommate, lover, parent or child) comes down with jaundice.

Can you do anything to prevent getting it yourself? If the hepatitis was due to Virus A, a gamma globulin shot will reduce the risk some seven- or eightfold, provided that you take it early enough. Even if you do develop it, the disease will be less severe if you take the shot. Gamma globulin also affords two- to threefold protection against NANB hepatitis, but it is of no use in type B. For the latter infection, a new immune globulin, marketed in the United States as HEP-B-Gamma Gee, protects you about three- to tenfold and the protection lasts for two months. If you have been infected accidentally—by a needle scratch, as might occur in a hospital worker—you will need two shots of this immune globulin, the first as soon as possible, but no later than seven days after exposure, and the second in about one month. This vaccine is made from the blood of patients who have had Hepatitis B and, therefore, contains natural antibodies against that virus. Unfortunately, it is still very expensive, about twenty times the cost of standard gamma globulin.

Prophylactic Gamma Globulin

If you are going to a country with poor hygiene, where you run the risk of contracting virus A hepatitis from the food or the water, get a shot of gamma globulin before you leave the United States. It will protect you for up to six months. In some countries, the gamma globulin supplies themselves have been reported to be contaminated with virus B. In that event, you may end up getting a shot that protects you from virus A but gives you the potentially more serious virus B!

Hepatitis B Vaccine—Finally

The most exciting development in the field of hepatitis is the availability of a vaccine to prevent the virus B infection. It is the first new vaccine in ten years. Make sure you get it as soon as possible if you are a practicing homosexual (in whom 48 percent of all cases of B hepatitis are found) or if you do the kind of work that exposes you to infected needles or blood, or if you are a drug addict.

After the Acute Attack

If you get sick with hepatitis A because you ate some contaminated raw clams, you will be fine once the acute illness is over; you are not likely to develop chronic liver trouble. But it is a different story with hepatitis B or NANB. In Hepatitis B 10 percent go on to a chronic form of the disease. In NANB cases, the incidence is even higher. The chronic hepatitis may be either *persistent* or *active,* and there is a world of difference between the two, in terms of both outlook and treatment.

If you should develop chronic, *persistent* hepatitis, you will be mildly sick, but you will recover. Just keep away from alcohol. In a few months your symptoms will disappear and your liver tests will return to normal no matter what life style you follow.

In contrast, chronic, *active* hepatitis is a serious illness that often causes progressive liver destruction and, in about 50 percent of patients, death within five years. It requires vigorous treatment—which, however, is not always effective. We administer steroid hormones and a group of medications called immunosuppressive agents (used also to control the rejection phenomenon in patients receiving organ transplants). Interferon is now in the testing phase for possible use in the treatment of chronic, active hepatitis. (Interferon, a normal constituent of the body found in certain types of white cells, is also being studied as a potential antitumor agent.) Although it is too early to predict its effect in the management of chronic active hepatitis, initial reports are encouraging. Ask your doctor about it. The diagnosis as to which form of chronic hepatitis you have can really only be made by a liver biopsy. That means sticking a needle into the liver through the abdominal wall. It takes only a few minutes, and it is relatively easy to do—provided that it is done by an experienced gastroenterologist.

If you are being given potent medications because you have "chronic hepatitis," ask what kind you have. The chronic *active* form is the only type that warrants such treatment.

KEY FACTS TO REMEMBER

The liver is one of the most complex and important organs of the body. It is vulnerable to a host of disorders, including poisoning from chemicals and alcohol, bacterial infections, parasites, tumors, injury and viruses. *Viral hepatitis* is a common and important worldwide disease, with three important forms thus far identified. They all have similar symptoms—jaundice, weakness, low-grade fever, lack of appetite and "malaise." The mode of transmission differs among them. One variety is basically food-borne, the other two are transmitted primarily by infected blood. Homosexuals and drug addicts have an especially high incidence of hepatitis. Most cases clear up spontaneously, without specific treatment. A few of the blood-borne types, however, may result in serious liver damage and death. The major pitfalls of therapy, for the mild, garden-variety hepatitis, are over-treatment and unnecessary dietary restrictions. A vaccine to *prevent* Hepatitis B is now available and should be taken by anyone chronically exposed to the disease.

23

Gallbladder Disease—A Variety of Treatment Options

The Five F's and the Thin Spinster

As a medical student, I was taught that patients most likely to have gallstones are characterized by the five F's—fat, female, fertile, fortyish and flatulent. Over the years, I have found that to be true. The fatter you are, the more vulnerable. The incidence of gallstones among women, especially those who have had children, is twice that among men. It is a disease of adult life, and its major symptom is gas. So much for the five F's. But if I had suspected the diagnosis *only* in those persons, I would have missed an awful lot of gallbladder disease over the years—in men, even children, and thin spinsters.

Who Else Is Vulnerable?

Gallstones are very common in this country; present in some 15 million women and 5 million men. There are one million new cases discovered and 500,000 cholecystectomies (gallbladder removal) each year. If you are an American Indian, your chances of getting gallstones are 7 out of 10! If you have rheumatic heart disease, especially of the mitral valve, or take the pill, you are also more prone to have them than is the rest of the population. Also, if you are on Atromid-S (clofibrate) for the reduction of your cholesterol and triglycerides, you should know that it too is associated with a higher incidence of gallstones.

Squirting on Demand

Bile, which is required to digest the fat in your diet, is made in the liver and stored in the gallbladder. The fat you eat passes from your stomach into the small intestine, where its arrival signals to the gallbladder to send down some extra bile. The normal gallbladder then contracts, and squirts out the amount necessary to digest the fat in the gut. A sick or nonfunctioning organ fails to do so, and the undigested fat leaves you feeling full, bloated and gaseous.

The Gallbladder X Ray

A gallbladder X ray not only reveals any stones within it, but also indicates whether the organ itself is working properly— that is, squirting on demand. So, in addition to the dye pills taken the night before, the procedure involves giving you a fatty drink, to see whether the gallbladder contracts normally. Although stones indicate disease or inflammation of the gallbladder, their presence is not always associated with poor function. By the same token, we may find the gallbladder free of stones, but not working as briskly as it should.

Sonography, the Modern Alternative to the Gallbladder X Ray

Now here's some useful advice. Sonography of the abdominal contents, including the gallbladder, represents a great advance in diagnostic medicine. It is accurate, relatively inexpensive, painless, noninvasive, can be done in the radiologist's office, and does not expose you to radiation. Whenever there's a question of whether or not you have gallstones, and a gallbladder X ray is advised, indicate your preference for the sonogram. It has many advantages. The obvious one is that it spares you two or three doses of radiation. Also you don't have to take the dye pills the night before, and that will avoid diarrhea and nausea the following morning. You don't have to fast for six hours, and the whole procedure takes only five minutes when done with the newer real-time scanners. But traditions die slowly in medicine, and most doctors still, almost instinctively, opt for the X ray first. There is no real justification for your doing it that way.

The usual symptoms of gallbladder disease are the feeling of fullness, bloating, discomfort or pain in the right upper portion of the abdomen or under the lower part of the breast-bone after eating cabbage, fried or fatty foods. But every now and then, in the course of a routine checkup, we find gallstones in persons who have no symptoms whatsoever.

Silent Stones

What should you do if you are incidentally found to have gallstones in the course of a routine examination? (They can often be seen in X rays taken of other organs such as the bowel or kidney.) Before you make any decision, there are some facts of which you should be aware. About 65 percent of persons, including those who have already had one gallbladder attack, will have no subsequent trouble. Among those who do have symptoms, most will improve if they simply follow a low-fat diet. So, there is no need to rush to surgery. Even if the gallbladder flares up, there is usually time enough to act. Remember that in every operation, no matter how trivial, there is some risk—the anesthesia, an unforeseen complication during the operation itself, a blood clot afterward, or infection.

When to Operate—Under the Sword of Damocles

What do I advise my own patients with gallbladder disease? If you keep suffering attacks of gallbladder pain despite your best attempts to adhere to a diet, you should have the gallbladder out. This is especially true if the X ray shows many very small stones (as opposed to one or two large ones). A tiny stone can pass from your gallbladder into one of the ducts carrying the bile into the intestine, blocking it and leaving you jaundiced. If you have such small stones, you may be sitting on a keg of dynamite or under the sword of Damocles should you suddenly develop "biliary obstruction" in some remote area, hours away from good surgical care. If you have had a heart attack recently, it is better to postpone the operation if you can. We have found that *any* surgery done within six months of a heart attack carries with it significantly greater risk.

It is only fair to tell you that some doctors disagree with my position. They believe that, since the presence of stones means disease, you are going to need surgery sooner or later, and so, regardless of symptoms, it is best to have it done "sooner," while you are still in good health. If you find yourself in a gallbladder "situation," consult a gastroenterologist, not a surgeon, about what to do.

Dissolving the Stones

Since 1972, we have known that certain pills can actually dissolve gallstones in some cases. They are called *chenodeoxycholic* and *ursodeoxycholic* acid.

In order to determine how successful and safe these treatments really are (the dosage of medication required, how long it takes to work, whether the stones recur and when), a large nationwide study was launched in the United States. Over 900 patients with gallstones were followed at ten clinical centers for a period of two years. The results of this investigation, published in mid 1981, were somewhat of a disappointment to me. It turns out that although the drugs are safe, (for at least two years), they were successful in dissolving the stones completely in only 13.5 percent of patients. These agents worked best in women and in thin people, when the gallbladder contained many cholesterol stones (so that there was a large surface area in contact with the drug), and when the cholesterol level was on the high side. Administration of these drugs seemed to have no effect on attacks of pain or the need for surgery.

If this therapy is recommended to you, get a second opinion. It would, at the moment, appear to be most appropriate for those who need surgery but in whom the operative risk is high.

KEYS FACTS TO REMEMBER

Gallbladder disease may exist with or without the presence of gallstones. But the finding of stones, even in the absence of symptoms, bespeaks a diseased gallbladder. Sonography represents a more desirable method of diagnosing gallstones than the traditional X ray.

Gallstones are very common in the United States, particularly among American Indians. Certain drugs and diseases also predispose to their formation.

Doctors disagree about how to manage "silent" stones, incidentally discovered. Many recommend early prophylactic removal of the gallbladder even in the absence of symptoms. Others advise a wait-and-see attitude. Before making a final decision, consult a gastroenterologist.

In a small percentage of patients, gallstones can be dissolved chemically. If you have gallstones, and surgery is not urgently required, ask your doctor about this treatment, especially if you are female, thin, have many stones and your cholesterol level tends to be high.

24

The Bowel—When and How to Treat Its Symptoms

Bellyachers—Young and Old

If you were to take a poll every time you sat in your doctor's waiting room, you would almost certainly find at least one patient there with symptoms originating somewhere in the gut. You name it, most Americans have bowel trouble some time or other—indigestion, bloating, cramps, constipation, "gas," diarrhea, mucus or blood in the stool, or the TV catch-all of "irregularity".

When your elimination "acts up," and you consult the doctor for help, he will listen to your symptoms, examine you and then arrange for whatever tests he thinks are necessary. The workup will almost always include a rectal exam in which the doctor feels for growths in the anal area. You will have to provide a stool specimen to be analyzed for blood, bacteria, parasites, mucus or chemical composition. Sometimes proctoscopy (in which he looks through an instrument inserted into the rectum for tumors or other evidence of disease) or colonoscopy (using a thinner, more flexible tube, which goes up much higher) needs to be done. Frequently, a barium-enema X ray is necessary for a better assessment of the large bowel.

An upper gastrointestinal series (in which you drink the

barium instead of having it inserted into your rectum) is required to clarify any problems in the esophagus, stomach and small bowel. A sonogram (sound waves are directed into the abdomen and the reflected echo reveals the presence of fluid or a growth) may also be ordered. A CT (CAT) scan (the computerized X ray that visualizes the abdominal contents without barium) may be helpful. The doctor may also want to perform endoscopy (you swallow a thin tube with a tiny light at the end, which permits him to look directly at all parts of the upper intestinal tract from esophagus to stomach, and to snip off any suspicious piece of tissue).

After any or all of these tests have been completed, your doctor will almost always have the answer to your problem. If you are unlucky, he may find that your symptoms are due to a growth (either benign or malignant) somewhere in your bowel. Or, more likely, he will conclude that you have picked up a virus or some other infection. Again, you may turn out to have "inflammatory bowel disease," a term used to denote a chronic condition called "ulcerative colitis," or a disorder called "regional ileitis" (Crohn's disease, named after the doctor who first described it).

Man May Not Be Able to Live by Bread (and Milk) Alone

One particularly common cause of diarrhea, cramps, gas, bloating and discomfort of which you should be aware is "*lactose intolerance*." Many "normal" persons are deficient in lactase, the enzyme that breaks down lactose—found in milk and milk products. Failure to digest the milk products we consume causes all these symptoms, which clear up the moment you eliminate lactose from your diet.

Nor is lactose the only substance that can "upset" your digestion and elimination. There are several foods to which one can be "allergic" and which, when eaten, cause an array of intestinal complaints ranging from cramps to diarrhea. A common one is gluten, found in grains. As with lactose, when the offending substance is eliminated, symptoms usually disappear. So, even foods that are symbolic of healthy nutrition, like bread or milk, may be harmful to some of us.

The Growling Bowel

But most people with indigestion end up with the diagnosis of *irritable-bowel syndrome*, a catchall for a variety of "functional" disorders of the bowel. By functional, I mean that there is really no apparent structural abnormality—nothing to see on the X ray, no infection, no trauma, no anything. All you have is symptoms, chief among which is chronic constipation.

Movements are usually "hard," little pellets accompanied by lots of gas. At other times, they are loose, with mucus on the stool (but never blood). You may experience lower-abdominal pain after eating, and the "gas" is perennial. As many as 70 percent of people who go to a gastroenterologist with bowel complaints of one kind or another suffer from the "irritable bowel."

You're Not Necessarily Neurotic

Most patients are relieved when told that all they have is an "irritable bowel" (synonyms are "nervous stomach" and "spastic colitis"), and not cancer. Such reassurance alone will leave them feeling a whole lot better. But given this diagnosis, with the words "irritable," "nervous" and "spastic," both you and your doctor may now conclude that your trouble stems from your personality "type." While it is true that tension may aggravate a "nervous" bowel, there are many people who have an irritable bowel despite their apparent ability to cope adequately with their problems. I am further impressed by the fact that the increase in the incidence of this disorder in the United States seems to parallel our greater consumption of refined sugar since 1900; that it is most frequently seen in countries where the diet is similar to our own, and that eating bran helps the situation a great deal, no matter what the personality pattern happens to be. So, don't buy the "neurotic" diagnosis as the sole and most important cause of your "spastic colon."

"Relax"—The Impossible Prescription

Anyone with an irritable bowel is immediately told to "relax." That's more easily said than done. There is no more frustrating advice a doctor can give a patient. There are, however, real and tangible things you can do, *practical* measures that will make you feel much better. For example, avoid laxatives when you are constipated. They will only further aggravate an already irritated bowel, which needs a rest, not stimulation. Take antispasmodic medications when necessary to reduce intestinal spasm; never ignore the urge to move your bowels; schedule a regular time for elimination, and stick to it—no matter what.

Avoid Old-Fashioned Dietary Warnings

The key to management of the irritable bowel lies in the kind of food you eat. We have learned a great deal in recent years about what is good and what is bad for you. We used to prescribe bland, puréed diets. That was wrong. What you need is *bulk,* which you can get in a high-fiber diet that includes lots of bran, other cereals, fruit and vegetables. I grew up thinking that bran was good for constipation but made diarrhea worse. That too is wrong. Diarrhea, which is part of the irritable-bowel syndrome, may actually be improved by the high-fiber diet. Also, eating bran regularly will give you a more definite urge to "go" when the time is ripe because the increased bulk stretches the rectal wall and makes the signal to empty it stronger and more difficult to ignore. Soon after you start eating bran, you may have a lot more "wind." This will pass (no pun intended) with time. And if such a diet alone doesn't do the trick, you may use stool softeners (wetting agents), some of which come with additional bulk in them, like Metamucil, Konsyl, Colace, Surfak and Modane. Prunes or prune juice in the morning may also help.

The "Musical" Foods

What *shouldn't* you eat if you have an irritable bowel? Certain foods like cabbage, beans and cauliflower can ferment, giving you lots of gas. Avoid them. Tea and coffee may also aggravate diarrhea in some patients. (That may surprise your grandmother and Maria, my South American housekeeper, both of whom believe that hot tea is the best treatment for whatever ails you.) Exercise is good for the gut and for your own sense of well-being. Long walks especially will make you feel better—even jogging, if you've been given cardiac and orthopedic clearance.

Some doctors simply don't have the time or patience to give you the practical advice you need for coping with the "spastic bowel." Instead, they may send you for psychotherapy. Unless you have some other reason to go, don't head for the couch because you occasionally have to rush to the head. If your doctor treats you like a psychological misfit, simply because you have a "spastic bowel," seek a second opinion from a gastroenterologist.

Remember that the irritable bowel is a chronic problem, something that you may just have to live with. Resist *repeated* X rays to make sure that there is nothing else going on. Excessive dependence on the X ray is the crutch of an insecure doctor, and one that may be dangerous to you.

Diverticulitis—As Common as Hiatus Hernia

Let us consider now another common condition in the lower intestinal tract—*diverticulitis*. As is the case with hiatus hernia, if I were to accost a hundred people over fifty years of age on the street at random and invite them in for a barium enema, I would probably find *diverticula* in more than half. These are little outpouchings from the bowel—fingerlike projections—which usually don't cause symptoms. When we find them incidentally on an X ray, and they are not giving you any trouble, we say that you have *diverticulosis*. But if and when they become inflamed (which, by the way, doesn't always happen), you develop a painful, tender belly, constipation and fever. When that occurs, your diverticul*osis* has become diverticul*itis*. This used to be attributed to irritation or infection of the little sac by a seed or piece of nut. I'm not sure that that theory is correct. According to current thinking, the acute pain of diverticulitis may be due to irritation or, in some cases, even perforation of the diverticula resulting from simple infection.

Diverticulosis is a relatively "new" disorder in our society, but one that is becoming more and more common. The records of Mayo Clinic are a good place to look for changing trends in disease in the United States. "Mayo" is synonymous with the "checkup," which at least until recently often included routine X rays of the bowel. In 1930, only 5 percent of persons above forty years of age so X-rayed at Mayo were noted to have diverticula. Today, in the same age group, the incidence is 30 percent. (In persons over seventy years, the figure may be as high as 60 percent.) Something in our environment is giving us these diverticula. I think the culprit is our diet.

Diverticulosis—A Matter of Thoroughly Modern Milling?

What change in the American diet may be responsible for the increase in diverticulosis? Is it the greater quantities of fat and sugar? These foods now provide twice the amount of calories they did in the diet of the 1800s. We are also eating more meat, but at the same time fewer potatoes and less bread, both of which contain fiber. What's more, the bread we do eat has had 99 percent of its wheat fiber removed by modern milling processes. One hundred years ago, that undigested fiber was left intact. If we compare our incidence of diverticulosis with that of other populations, we find that in Africa, for example, where the natives eat six or seven times the amount of fiber that we do, diverticular disease (and "spastic colon" too) are very uncommon. But when Africans move from the jungle to live in the cities and begin to eat like we do, the incidence of both these disorders begins to approximate our own.

For more than fifty years we prescribed a low-residue diet for patients with diverticulosis. Old myths die hard. Many patients (and some doctors) still follow this treatment. As with irritable bowel, it is wrong. The key here too is roughage. The richest sources of high fiber are cereals, whole-grain flour or bread, green vegetables, nuts and berries. Fiber makes the stool heavier and more bulky, requiring less pressure for it to be moved along the bowel. It also distends the wall of the gut, which further reduces the pressure within it. This decreases the chance of the little pouches or fingers (diverticula) from forming as a result of herniation through weakened areas of the bowel wall.

If you are having repeated attacks of diverticulitis, try adding two teaspoons of unprocessed bran to your soup or your usual breakfast cereal. This may well give you relief. Roughage can, however, make for some gas. That is not bad for you physiologically, but is socially embarrassing. (But who knows? Perhaps as our diet becomes richer in fiber, expelling gas may become an acceptable custom, just as belching was the thing to do after a Roman feast.)

Turista or Travelers' Diarrhea

A major challenge to travelers, doctors and pharmaceutical manufacturers is how to prevent diarrhea when you visit "exotic" lands. You may be offered the time-honored advice, "Don't drink the water, avoid raw fruits and vegetables, and don't let the bartender put any ice in your drink," or be given certain medications during and after your visit.

You should be aware of several recent interesting observations apropos this problem. The first is that Pepto-Bismol, which has been around since 1906 for the treatment of heartburn, is effective in the prevention and management of travelers' diarrhea. We thought it was because of the bismuth it contains, but that can't be the whole story, since if you take bismuth alone in some form other than Pepto-Bismol, it is not nearly as effective. Well, why don't we all simply load up with Pepto-Bismol on our next trip to diarrhea country? Because the amounts necessary to do the job would require your taking a suitcase full of it.

Another observation is that the antibiotic doxycycline (marketed in the United States as Vibramycin) can prevent travelers' diarrhea, and this protection lasts for about five weeks after you stop the drug. You take it just before you arrive at your destination and continue it until your return. Sounds easy too, except that this agent may have undersirable side effects in some people, like nausea and various sensitivity reactions.

Why No Treatment May Be the Best Treatment

What causes travelers' diarrhea, and are all these things we do to prevent and treat it really good for us? Most cases are caused by an ordinarily harmless bug called *E. coli* (although there are forms of this organism that are virulent). *Turista* is not life-threatening, just a nuisance for a few days. Of course, in some people—the elderly or the chronically ill—even mild diarrhea can be serious if it persists. But for the rest of us, it is not. There is a growing number of doctors who believe that the drugs that kill the relatively benign *E.* *coli* organisms also eradicate many of the other bacteria that normally live in the healthy bowel and whose function it is to protect us against more serious infection. The ecology of the bowel is much like that of the forest. When we take any antibiotic to eliminate the *E. coli* in order to prevent simple diarrhea, we may facilitate the growth of more sinister agents, which can give us dysentery or amebiasis. The latter are more serious illnesses, more persistent and harder to treat. So, maybe you ought to think twice about trying to prevent travelers' diarrhea with drugs. Take some gamma globulin against hepatitis before you leave, be very careful about what you eat and drink, keep your fingers crossed, and your hands clean. Quite frankly, that's what I do.

When Diarrhea May Actually Be Good for You

Suppose that you do get diarrhea on one of your vacations. The tendency is immediately to take something to stop it, like Kaopectate, Lomotil, Immodium or another obstipating drug. Believe it or not, that may not be the right thing to do either. Diarrhea is, after all, nature's way to rid your bowel of an irritant or some other infectious material. If you suppress the diarrhea, these agents are retained. So, the current attitude of some doctors is to let the diarrhea run its course (so to speak) for a few days. Naturally, if it persists, that is another matter.

When you return from a trip anywhere and have *chronic* diarrhea, don't keep dosing yourself with home remedies and over-the-counter obstipants. See your doctor and have him analyze your stool in order to identify the specific agent (which may be a bacterium or a parasite) that is giving you the symptoms. There are cures for every infection that you may pick up along the way. But diagnosis comes first.

Inflammatory Bowel Disease—Ulcerative Colitis and Crohn's Disease

The intestinal tract has three major divisions; an upper portion consisting of the esophagus, stomach and small bowel; a middle section, the large bowel; and a terminal portion, the rectum and anus. The suffix *itis* means "inflammation." Thus, inflammation of stomach lining is called *gastritis,* and of the duodenum, *duodenitis*. When the large bowel, or colon, is involved, you have *colitis*. There are two major forms of inflammation of the bowel, ulcerative colitis and Crohn's disease. Together, they account for several thousand new cases every year in the United States. Their cause is unknown. You should know about these two conditions, because they are common, their respective treatments may be very different (and are changing), and their long-term outlook is also dissimilar.

Crohn's Disease—A Normal Sigmoidoscopy Is Not Enough

Crohn's disease is an inflammation predominantly of the large bowel (but not infrequently portions of the small intestine too) which involves the full thickness of the gut. (Ulcerative colitis, on the other hand, involves mostly the lining and rarely goes through and through.) We see it most commonly in persons between twenty and forty years of age. Because it affects all layers of the bowel, it often penetrates the wall causing adhesions and tracts involving other intestinal structures, the bladder and even the skin. You should know about it, because—unlike ulcerative colitis, which, as you will see later, often has an explosive onset—Crohn's disease may smolder for a long time before ever being recognized. In fact, it takes the average patient five years before he consults a doctor about it. The chronic fatigue, anemia, aching belly, and loss of appetite of Crohn's disease are often blamed on the irritable bowel, while the "belly-ache" in a child is attributed to an attention-seeking device.

When the doctor is finally consulted and he does a sigmoidoscopy, it may be normal, because that instrument reaches only twelve inches up the bowel, and this disease is usually situated higher up than that. *The diagnosis of Crohn's disease requires a barium X ray; a negative sigmoidoscopy does not exclude it.* If your doctor insists on taking a look, he will need to perform colonoscopy, which, because it involves a thinner, flexible instrument, can go much higher.

Ulcerative Colitis—The Contrast with Crohn's

Symptoms of *ulcerative colitis* appear at about the same time as do those of Crohn's disease, but the former disorder has some very interesting racial and religious predilections. For example, if you are Jewish, your chances of getting it are two to four times greater than those of the rest of the population; if you are white, your vulnerability is four times that of nonwhites—and don't ask me why. It also seems to hit certain families more than others, and more women have it than men.

Ulcerative colitis will probably impel you to see your doctor sooner than you would if you had Crohn's disease. What brings you to him first is some pus or blood in the stool. The diarrhea typical of ulcerative colitis doesn't usually set in until later. The severity of the symptoms is often a harbinger of whether the disease will become a serious threat to you, or just annoying. In most people, they are mild. In contrast to Crohn's disease, the trouble is usually much lower in the bowel, so that the sigmoidoscope is often the best way to make the diagnosis (even though the barium X ray also has to be done). But remember, if you are having *acute* symptoms— with fevers, blood or pus in the stool, and abdominal pain, the barium enema, sigmoidoscopy or colonoscopy may be hazardous. Wait until you have responded to palliative measures, and *then* have the tests done.

Treating Inflammatory Bowel Disease

Once the diagnosis of ulcerative colitis or Crohn's disease has been made, there are medications that will give you relief. Lomotil and other obstipating agents help to control diarrhea, but they do nothing to influence the underlying disease processes. Azulfidine (sulfasalazine), a combination of sulfa and aspirin, also reduces symptoms, but it may have unpleasant side effects. Interestingly, it was first developed in 1942, in the hope (not substantiated) that it would help patients with rheumatoid arthritis. By accident, however, it was noted that in some patients, who had ulcerative colitis as well as rheumatoid arthritis, the bowel symptoms improved. Since then, Azulfidine has remained an effective treatment for that disease.

When symptoms are severe in both ulcerative colitis and Crohn's disease, cortisone-type drugs become necessary. In the former, we try it in enema form first. If that doesn't work, the cortisone is given by mouth. As many as 90 percent of patients will improve on this therapy, after which the dosage of steroids is gradually reduced and Azulfidine is resumed. In many cases of Crohn's disease, maintenance cortisone therapy is required. When that fails, surgery becomes necessary, as happens in about 60 percent of cases after five years. The sad part is that there is recurrence in the majority of these patients a few years after surgery.

Unlike the irritable bowel or diverticulosis, diet does not appear to play an important role in the management of inflammatory bowel disease.

Patients with Crohn's disease may suffer serious complications, such as perforation of the bowel and mechanical obstruction. The most dreaded risk of ulcerative colitis, on the other hand, is cancer. In fact, one third of the deaths from ulcerative colitis are due to cancer. The longer you have the disease in its continuously active form and the more extensive it is, the more likely you are to develop a malignant tumor of the bowel.

The question (for which there is no easy answer) naturally arises as to whether the involved portion of bowel in ulcerative colitis should be removed *before* cancer develops. Statistically, total removal of the bowel becomes necessary in about 25 percent of patients with ulcerative colitis in the first five years of their disease. If this operation is recommended to you for whatever reason—because of bleeding, adhesions or an abscess, get another opinion from a competent gastroenterologist. There are many specialists who now feel that such surgery is often unnecessary and that intensive medical treatment should be tried somewhat longer.

But if surgery does become necessary, depending on which part and how much of the bowel is removed, you may end up with a colostomy or ileostomy, and provided with a pouch which sits on the outside of your abdomen and through which you move your bowels. There's no reason to get unduly depressed about it. The pouches these days are plastic, nonodorous and very easy to use. They are clean, flat, adherent to the skin and are no longer a social disaster.

It's Probably Not a Matter of Personality

It is almost always assumed that patients with colitis have some kind of personality or behavior problem. There are still doctors who will straightaway send you into psychotherapy. There are even stereotype personality descriptions of persons with colitis. They are said to be intelligent, to suppress their anxieties and conflicts, and to be very passive. They "let go," so to speak, with their bowels. The fact is that recent observations have not substantiated a psychological basis for colitis. For example, it does not explain the racial differences in the disease described earlier, nor why it may be found in the course of routine proctoscopy among persons with no symptoms at all. So, if you are referred to a psychiatrist *pro forma*, simply because you have colitis, think twist about going.

KEY FACTS TO REMEMBER

Gas, cramps, indigestion, constipation and diarrhea plague most of us some time or other, depending on what we eat and where we've been traveling. In many cases these complaints are "functional"—i.e., without underlying bowel disease. But frequently, a cause for the symptoms can be found and treated.

Most bowel symptoms are due to diets lacking in bulk and fiber. Others are due to unsuspected food "allergies," notably to milk and milk products, or gluten (rye derivatives).

Diverticulitis is a common condition, probably due to our diet and the way in which our foods are processed. We used to treat it with a low-residue diet. We now know that roughage is what is needed.

Most cases of *travelers' diarrhea* are due to an otherwise harmless bacteria. Left alone, the symptoms usually run their course without complications. The overenthusiastic use of antibiotics and antidiarrheals may do more harm than good.

Inflammatory disease of the bowel encompasses two different disorders called ulcerative colitis and Crohn's disease. The latter is an inflammation of the full thickness of the wall of the large bowel; the former affects only the lining of the gut. Ulcerative colitis can almost always be diagnosed by looking into the bowel (sigmoidoscopy), while the diagnosis of Crohn's disease usually requires an X ray. Diet is not an important factor in management, but there are several drugs, including cortisone, that may alleviate symptoms. The question of surgery in both these diseases is of great importance and should be considered only in consultation with experienced gastroenterologists. Since severe, long-standing ulcerative colitis may become cancerous, the question of prophylactic removal of the affected bowel is one that should be made only after the input of expert opinions.

25

The Prostate Gland—
From Infection to Tumor

An Educated Finger

In *The Complete Medical Exam* I discussed the anatomy of the prostate gland, its function (to provide nourishment for the sperm and fluid in which they can travel), and the various tests that we perform to check its status. You should suspect a developing problem when the force of your urinary stream is reduced, when you have trouble starting it and dribble when you finish, and when you find yourself getting up several times a night to empty your bladder. Your doctor's educated finger is the simplest way to confirm these suspicions.

How It Acts Up

You can develop several kinds of prostate trouble. The normal-sized gland can become infected or inflamed (*prostatitis*), at any time during adult life (but more commonly as you grow older). It also enlarges with the passing years. Or, it can develop a malignant tumor (that likelihood too increases with age). In fact, when we examine tissue from a "benignly" enlarged prostate removed from a man in his seventies or eighties, we often find tiny islands of malignancy. These went unnoticed and undiagnosed.

Diagnosing Prostate Infection

Occasionally, the prostate becomes congested or infected if you have had too much sexual activity—or not enough. Whatever the cause, when you have prostatitis, you urinate frequently and experience discomfort in the lower back and genital areas doing it. Also, when you have to "go," you really need to get there quick. (We call that "urgency.")

And when you actually pass the urine, it burns. You also find that you have to get up at night for no apparent reason (you haven't been taking a lot of liquor, wine or other fluids at bedtime). You may or may not have any fever. The urinalysis usually, but not always, shows evidence of infection and may reveal a little blood, particularly as you finish voiding. When your doctor does a rectal exam and fingers the prostate he will find it boggy—you will find it tender. When he massages the gland, pus cells are forced out and will then appear in the urine. The doctor will then "culture" the specimen—that is, incubate it to see what organisms, if any, grow out. But, very often (in contrast to kidney infections), no bacteria are identified in prostate "infections." If there was any blood in the specimen, a portion of it will also surely be sent for a Pap test to exclude the possibility of a malignancy.

How It's Treated

There is no problem in treating prostatitis. You will be given an appropriate antibiotic, told to drink plenty of fluids (nonalcoholic) and take hot baths. You will soon feel better. But if you don't, and the infections keep recurring, ask to see a urologist. There may be some special reason why you are having the trouble, over and above simple infection.

With regard to antibiotics, be sure to tell your doctor if you are allergic to the penicillin family of drugs, the sulfas or tetracycline, because these are the agents most widely used in treating urinary-tract infections.

The Big Prostate, and Why It Makes You "Go" So Often

Urine made in the kidney is delivered via a long duct called a ureter (there is one for each kidney) to the bladder, where it is stored. After a certain amount of urine has accumulated in the bladder, the wall of that organ is stretched, signaling you that it's time to "go." Urine then leaves the bladder through another duct called the urethra. When the prostate gland enlarges, it compresses the urethra, causing obstruction to the outflow of urine. The stream becomes narrow, you end up dribbling and develop the other symptoms of prostatism. Urine backing up into the bladder, whence it came, distends it like a balloon. Because of the obstruction of the urethra caused by the large prostate, a greater pressure is required for the urine to be passed. As a result, there is always some left in the bladder ("residual urine"). The bladder dilates progressively to accommodate the extra volume of urine. Finally, when it can no longer dilate, it overflows, forcing you to the toilet—fast. The residual urine remaining in the bladder stagnates and becomes a fertile breeding area for any bacteria that happen to be around. This leads to the infection so common in prostatism.

At Some Point It Needs to Come Out

There is really only one way to treat an enlarged prostate—surgical removal. When to operate depends not only on your symptoms but on certain objective information as well. You will need to have an intravenous pyelogram (IVP); dye is injected into a vein in your arm into the bloodstream to the kidney, then to the urinary bladder and out through the penis. This contrast material shows up both kidneys (telling us whether or not they are enlarged), as well as the ureters which carry the urine from the kidney to the bladder (indicating any obstruction there). Also, when you are finished voiding and think your bladder is completely empty, the IVP reveals whether there is, in fact, any urine left behind. A large amount of residual urine in the bladder usually indicates that you are likely to develop acute and total urinary obstruction and, thus, require surgery.

But even when the residual volume is not all that large, you may be left enervated from getting up every hour or two during the night. So many men with this problem are always tired only for want of a good night's sleep. Before you consider surgery, ask your urologist about a drug called *dibenzyline*. (If you have a heart condition, be sure to tell the doctor

about it. Being a urologist, he may not be aware of it.)
It frequently reduces the number of times you have to empty
your bladder.

Of Prostates and Hernias

Suppose that you suddenly notice in your groin a lump
that is diagnosed as a hernia. If you are fifty years or older,
that may be due to an enlarged prostate, which has made you
strain when passing urine. So, if you come to your doctor
expecting to be sent home for a hernia repair and he tells you
to have your prostate gland fixed first, he is probably right.
Puzzled, you are likely to go for an unnecessary second
opinion.

Roto-Rooter Surgery

Once the decision to operate is made, you should know
that there are two different ways to do it. In the *transurethral*
approach, an instrument is inserted through the penis like a
Roto-Rooter and the enlarged prostate is literally scraped out
or "shaved." This approach is easier, safer, takes less time and
is preferred, especially if you are old, have heart disease or
are otherwise a poor surgical risk. But it can't always be done,
especially if the prostate is very large. Also, after several
years, the gland, which was not completely removed in the
first place (but merely reamed out), may grow back, making a
repeat operation necessary.

The second technique involves an incision in the lower
abdomen, and cutting the prostate gland away under direct
vision. If you have been told that you need a prostatectomy
and there is any question about how it should be done, get a
second opinion.

Cancer of the Prostate

Cancer of the prostate is usually detected during a rectal
exam. Your doctor will note that portions of the gland feel
hard and irregular. A needle biopsy, done by a urologist, is
necessary to confirm the diagnosis (just as a lump in the
breast is almost always biopsied before any treatment decision is made). A prostate biopsy is fairly simple. The needle is
introduced from the outside, between the scrotum and the

rectum, directly into the suspicious area. A core of tissue is obtained and looked at under a microscope.

Treatment, discussed in greater detail in the section on Cancer, will depend on whether the malignancy has spread, either within the prostate or to distant tissues like bone and lungs.

KEY FACTS TO REMEMBER

The prostate gland may become infected, enlarged or cancerous. Most infections are easily treated with antibiotics, but if they recur, you should consult a urologist to determine the reason(s). The basic treatment for an enlarged prostate causing symptoms is surgical removal. Surgery can be done in two ways, one of which is simpler and safer than the other. Before having such surgery, it may be wise to consult a second urologist. Cancer of the prostate, which is discussed elsewhere, may be treated surgically, by radiation, with hormones, or by benign neglect, depending on the stage of the disease.

26

Hemorrhoids—No Laughing Matter

When in the Seat of Power

We all know what varicose veins in the legs look like. They are dilated, enlarged and sometimes painful vascular cords. Hemorrhoids are the same kind of varicose veins, situated inside or outside of the anus. Although they are not life-threatening, they are uncomfortable and troublesome. Occurring in the seat of power, they have on occasion affected the course of history. It is said that Napoleon changed his battle plans for Waterloo when he couldn't sit on his horse one day. President Carter's bout with hemorrhoids, on the other hand, made headlines, not history. Anyone suffering an acute attack of hemorrhoids will not find puns and flippant comments at all funny.

Ads in subways and buses constantly remind us that hemorrhoids are very common. By middle age, at least 50 percent of all people have them. They may be internal or external. They can result from any condition that increases pressure on the veins of the anus and rectum. Chronic constipation, straining at stool, a tumor in the pelvis or abdomen, and pregnancy are the most common causes. You can reduce the risk of getting hemorrhoids by eating plenty of roughage and fiber, avoiding constipation, not straining at stool, and fostering regular bowel habits.

Engorged, hemorrhoidal veins may be painful. Inflamed clots frequently form within these dilated blood vessels, just as they do in thrombophlebitis of the legs. But unlike the latter situation, there is no risk here of the clot traveling anywhere else in the body. You merely suffer from local pain and bleeding.

Hemorrhoids, however small or painless, can lead to complications. There is the possibility that chronic, insidious bleeding will cause anemia and weakness. Moreover, when the bleeding is detected, there is always the danger of attributing it to the obvious hemorrhoids and overlooking another, more ominous and simultaneous cause of the blood loss—a cancer higher up in the bowel. *Never be lulled into a false sense of security when you see blood in your stool simply because you know that you have hemorrhoids*. Everyone with "bleeding" piles should have a proctoscopy at least once. If you are young, and the bleeding is clearly hemorrhoidal, that is enough. But if you are over fifty, and the source of the bleeding is not all that apparent, you should also have a barium enema, thus laying to rest the possibility of a tumor. That is not to say that every time your hemorrhoids bleed, you have to hurry over for a complete gastrointestinal workup. Just once—that's all. I can remember several cases in which I found chemical evidence of blood on a routine stool analysis and was tempted to attribute the finding to "obvious" hemorrhoids, only to discover a cancer or polyp in subsequent testing.

Preparation "This and That"

How should bleeding, painful hemorrhoids be treated? Stool softeners and roughage in the diet are helpful—as is the bidet, found in most European countries; there is nothing like sitting in one and bathing the inflamed area with the soothing warm water. Since you are not likely to have a bidet, you will have to settle for just sitting in a warm tub for twenty to thirty minutes a couple of times a day.

Creams and ointments that contain a local anesthetic, like benzocaine and novocaine, will often ease the pain. Or, you can insert a rectal suppository or foam that may contain small amounts of cortisone to reduce inflammation and swelling. And, in most cases, such local measures are all you need.

Never rub the hemorrhoids with dry tissue after a bowel movement. Use lubricated or moistened pads. And don't dally on the toilet.

Occasionally, hemorrhoidal bleeding and pain persist and require more definitive treatment. I remember during my internship days assisting in several hemorrhoid operations. They were brutal and bloody, and they kept you in the hospital a week or more. We used to give patients large doses of pain-killing narcotics, which also left them constipated, so that they wouldn't move their bowels and thus further irritate the operated area. Such procedures are infrequently necessary or done anymore. If it is proposed to you, double-check with an expert, irreverently referred to in the profession as a "rear admiral."

The Rubber Band

If you are told you need an operation—any operation—to fix your hemorrhoids, ask about the "rubber band" treatment. This technique simply involves tying the dilated veins with a rubber band. It is performed in the doctor's office; it does not require anesthesia; it shrinks the hemorrhoid by cutting off its blood supply. Dilating the anus may also yield good results. If your doctor doesn't know about it or demurs, consult a proctologist or rectal surgeon.

Another (not so hot) way to approach the problem without surgery is to freeze the hemorrhoids—cryosurgery. It is not as effective as the "rubber band" which most proctologists prefer.

Many doctors still inject the hemorrhoid directly when possible. But if it can be injected, it can be tied off, and you are better off with the latter.

KEY FACTS TO REMEMBER

Hemorrhoids ("piles") are dilated, inflamed varicose veins in the anus; they usually result from chronic constipation and multiple pregnancies. Unlike such veins elsewhere, notably the legs, they are rarely dangerous, but they can cause much pain and bleeding.

A diet containing roughage and fiber, together with healthy bowel habits are the best protection against developing hemorrhoids.

Never automatically attribute blood in the stool to hemorrhoids, even if you have them. This may divert attention from a tumor in the bowel.

Treatment of bleeding or painful hemorrhoids may consist of ointments and suppositories, injections, tying off the engorged veins with the rubber-band technique, or surgery. Which course to follow may require the opinion of an expert in the field.

27

Cancer—New Horizons, New Hope and More Options

How to Approach It?

Books and articles about cancer deal with the subject in a variety of ways. They may focus on its *causation*. What role do viruses, personality, genetics and pollution play? The "epidemiology" of cancer is of great interest to society. We are concerned with the safety of our environment—what we eat (does increased fat in the diet really cause more cancer of the bowel, breast and prostate?), drink (do artificial sweeteners increase the risk of cancer in humans as well as in rats?), and breathe (do cigarettes really play so important a role in cancer of the lung and of the cervix, of all places?). We are concerned about the additives in our cosmetics, our clothes, and even our children's toys. Hardly a week goes by without reports claiming that some substance—a medication, food or pollutant—is carcinogenic.

Then there is the matter of cancer *diagnosis*—how to detect it early enough to cure it. There are books dealing with the *treatment* of cancer—X ray, surgery, drugs and immunotherapy. There are texts discussing the *psychology* of the cancer patient—how to cope with it yourself and how to help others do so. There are even volumes now on the management of terminal cancer cases when cure and remission are no longer possible.

It Boils Down to Early Diagnosis and Treatment

It is not possible for me to cover in depth all the ramifications of cancer in one chapter. But I do want to present to you some basic facts about the modern approach to the treatment of malignant disease. Above all, I want you to know why and where to get proper care early, if you should be unfortunate enough to face the specter of this disease yourself. In cancer, *time and the correct diagnosis are of the essence*.

Lesson Number One

As a result of recent and continuing advances in the field, several kinds of cancer, if discovered in time, are now curable. A larger percentage than ever are manageable—that is, the duration of comfortable survival is significantly prolonged. For these reasons, perhaps more than in any other field of medicine, *it is extremely important to get the best and most up-to-date opinion from an expert in the field about how to treat any malignancy* as soon as it is discovered.

It's Better to Know

Many people skip over any article dealing with "cancer." There are those who won't even utter the word, a kind of superstitious denial mechanism. Healthy persons would rather not get involved with it for fear of spoiling their luck. Those who suspect or are afraid that they may have cancer but are not really sure, don't want to read anything that might confirm it for them. In other words, they believe that what they don't know won't hurt them—a poor policy that can end in disaster.

Not All Tumors Are Cancerous

The word *tumor* simply means "growth." Some growths are benign. They hardly ever kill. Removing them at any stage of their development usually results in complete cure. Others, however, are malignant and will eventually kill. But even many of the latter, if detected before they have spread, can be cured, or at least controlled, for long periods of time. Finally, there are still some cancers that continue to resist all the currently available forms of therapy, no matter how early we find them. Fortunately, their numbers are decreasing.

Pessimism Is Often Unwarranted

There are still too many patients (and doctors) who are not attuned to the times, and who remain unrealistically pessimistic when dealing with cancer. Families of a loved one so stricken will plead for nothing vigorous, "heroic" or experimental to be done. Patients in good health want me to sign notarized promises that, if they develop cancer, I will hasten the end. Not long ago I discovered lung cancer in a woman in her early eighties. She was coughing, had chest pain and was short of breath. The family made it clear to me that they wanted her given no therapy whatsoever. "Just let her die as soon as possible." I explained that while there was nothing that would cure their mother, we could make her more comfortable in the time she had left. But that would require treatment, in this instance, radiation. (X-ray techniques are now so sophisticated that very substantial doses can be administered with minimal or no side effects.) I hoped that this might shrink the tumor and decrease the obstruction to the air passages—which was causing most of the symptoms. The family agreed, albeit reluctantly. My patient did rather well for the next seven months. She was more comfortable, required fewer narcotics and was able to enjoy her family, particularly her grandchildren, a little longer. Furthermore, she remained at home, where she was happier than she would have been in hospital, and where she did not dissipate her life's savings.

What Is the Truth?

The other question raised by this woman's family was what to tell her about her disease. She was intelligent enough so that I would lose my credibility with her if I did not tell her the truth. But does truth demand using the word "cancer," a term synonymous with pain, suffering and death?

In this case, I informed my patient that she had a *tumor* that would be treated vigorously by every means available and appropriate, and that we would hope for the best. That reassurance was enough for her, as it is for most patients. And the truth is that chemotherapy, radiation, surgery and other forms of therapy often will buy time and comfort and cure. No doctor can tell for certain how long a patient will live, nor can anyone predict what advances will be made during the time that has been "bought."

"But Should I Settle My Affairs?"

That raises the question of giving a patient enough information so that he can "settle his affairs." In these days of complicated tax and estate laws, it is often vital that certain legal aspects be attended to—in fairness both to the patient and to the surviving next of kin. In my experience, that can be handled in an effective, sympathetic way, without removing all hope—by stressing that just as healthy persons should have their wills and business affairs in order, so should one who is sick, regardless of the disease or prognosis. Most cancer patients get the message and act on it, without asking the doctor to spell out all the grim details. There is an art to doing it. Make sure, if a loved one of yours is involved, that the doctor running the case knows how to handle that aspect of it. Rehearse exactly what the patient will be told. If it comes out harshly or insensitively, have someone else do it. Also make sure about the consistency of the presentation by all concerned.

It's a Very Big Field—and There's Much to Know

The quality of life for however long a cancer patient survives will depend very much on the kind of medical care he gets and the attitude of his physician and loved ones. *If you are told that you have cancer, regardless of its type or location, no matter what outlook you are given, you must get an opinion from an expert oncologist.* Your family doctor, internist, and even *one* cancer specialist may not be enough. Knowledge in this field is changing from day to day. Your doctor may not know of some very recent breakthrough, especially if he is not a specialist, and sometimes even if he is. There are several subdivisions in the field of oncology itself. Some institutions and physicians are expert in treating cancer of the bone, or the blood (leukemia), the breast, prostate or lungs. No one oncologist knows everything about every area.

And None of Them Died

I could fill this book with accounts of how important it is to be sure that you are getting the best treatment available. One involves a relative of mine. About ten years ago, while in his early seventies, he was found to have a malignant condition called *mycosis fungoides*. This is a form of cancer that manifests itself initially as a skin rash. His internist, a competent clinician, called to tell me he had reviewed the current literature and could find no specific effective treatment for this disorder. Such cases, he said, survive for an average of "a couple of years." But he assured me that he would do everything to make the patient comfortable and would not "prolong his agony."

I discussed the problem with several colleagues working in this field, and they referred me to an oncologist in Philadelphia specializing in *mycosis fungoides*. I sent the patient to him. He was treated for ten days with immunotherapy and chemotherapy which were new at that time. After a few weeks, the skin lesions disappeared and the patient was cured. He died years later in his eighties from heart disease.

In another instance, a friend living in a large city called to tell me that his eleven-year-old son had just been found to have Ewing's sarcoma (a highly malignant tumor of bone) in the leg. Local specialists were pessimistic about the child's chances for survival and recommended immediate amputation. Again, I made inquiries and learned that there was a team at New York's Sloan-Kettering Memorial Hospital especially interested in this particular tumor and working on a novel treatment approach. The boy was taken there forthwith and thoroughly studied. These doctors did not think amputation was at all necessary. Instead, they removed only a small piece of bone containing the cancer, and began therapy with drugs and radiation. They have given the boy a 75-80 percent chance of cure, and they don't think that the leg will ever have to come off. The specialists who had seen him first were competent. They simply did not have the expertise for this particular tumor.

I know many women who, with advanced cancer of the breast, had been "given up." Years later they were still alive and comfortable as a result of new treatment for that disease.

Doctors Vary in Knowledge and Expertise

One shouldn't approach cancer with kid gloves. This is a disease in which your life is on the line. Given that diagnosis, regardless of the pessimistic or nihilistic attitude of friends, family or physician, you must immediately obtain an opinion from a qualified oncologist. Call the National Cancer Institute in Bethesda or the American Cancer Society. Or ask your doctor to do so. Tell them what kind of cancer you have and ask where they recommend you go for specialized treatment.

On the basis of such inquiries for my patients, I have sent them to various centers throughout this country, each particularly expert in a specific type of tumor—Sloan-Kettering Memorial Hospital in New York; the M. D. Anderson Hospital in Houston, Texas; the Mayo Clinic in Rochester, Minnesota; Stanford University in Palo Alto, California; Roswell Park in Buffalo, New York; the Sidney Farber Cancer Center in Boston; New York Hospital-Cornell Medical Center and the Mt. Sinai Hospital, in New York.

The Local Cancer Specialist

There are many expert oncologists who, practicing in smaller communities, do not yet have access to every new piece of equipment or medication. The good ones will make sure that somehow you get it, since most smaller hospitals have some tie-ins with nearby larger centers. So, living away from the medical mainstream does not necessarily mean that you are deprived of the benefits of the knowledge explosion in this field. The key is your ability to discuss with your own doctor the need for consultation—and his willingness to cooperate.

The Magnitude of the Problem

Almost 800,000 new cases of cancer are now diagnosed every year in the United States. Of these, some 400,000 die. One in three will be alive in five years. These figures do not include the many thousands of innocuous cases of localized skin cancer, which are easily cured just by their removal. Nor does it embrace the 40,000 women who each year are found to have the very earliest incidence of cancer in the Pap test, and who also are cured by surgery.

The Breakdown

Among the 800,000 new cases of "real" cancer each year, 183,000 are in the digestive system, 112,000 in the lungs alone, about 18,000 in bone and skin (of which almost 14,000 are the malignant melanomas, among the most highly and rapidly fatal of all cancers), 107,000 breast cancers, some 130,000 malignancies of the genital organs (comprised of 60,000 cancers of the prostate, 53,000 of the uterus and 17,000 of the ovaries), 45,000 cases of cancer of the urinary tract (broken down roughly into 30,000 in the bladder and 15,000 in the kidney), 11,000 brain malignancies, and about 9,000 cancers of the hormonal glands, mostly thyroid. In addition to these tumors of "solid" organs, there are some 21,000 cases every year of blood cancer (leukemia) and about 38,000 cases of lymphoma (tumors of the lymph glands). These data all add up to the fact that cancer is the second-leading cause of death, outranked only by diseases of the heart and circulation.

So much for the statistics of cancer. But what *is* cancer?

The Cancer Process

The millions of cells that comprise a given organ of the body normally grow in an orderly fashion. When the tissue becomes cancerous, these cells, previously so well behaved, suddenly begin to multiply wildly, totally out of control. As the cancer expands and extends, it presses the life out of surrounding organs and structures. In the lungs, for example, a malignancy might start as a tiny nubbin. The wildly growing cells eventually spread out every which way, blocking the air passages and invading blood vessels, which they then use as a conduit to all parts of the body. Wherever they lodge, they resume their crazy growth. In so doing, they choke off and replace the normal components of whatever organ they strike.

When cancer develops among the red blood cells (polycythemia vera) or white blood cells (leukemia), they multiply and spread into the lymph glands, bone marrow, liver and spleen, interfering with normal blood function and formation.

Why Do the Cancer Cells Go Crazy?

What causes a cell that has previously been well balanced suddenly to lose control is the key question to which nobody really has the answer. Is a virus responsible? Probably, in certain types. Is the trigger some chemical irritant in the environment, like asbestos or tobacco smoke or X rays or uranium? It no doubt is in some instances. Is it some other air pollutant, an additive in our food, a hormone that we are taking for one reason or another? Possibly. It may be any of these, or even a combination of all. No one knows for sure. And there is a host of other unanswered questions. For example, why do Egyptians have so much bladder cancer? Why does it strike the Chinese in the esophagus so often? Why do the Japanese have so great a predisposition to cancer of the stomach? Why is there so much cancer of the liver in Africa? Why did one community in New Jersey recently report an unusual number of cases of leukemia? What is going on in the genes of one family I know in which the maternal grandmother, mother and two daughters all had breast cancer?

First You've Got to Make Sure

So much for speculation about the cause. Suppose, then, that you are told you have cancer. It may have been found in a routine physical exam; in a chest X ray, during a proctoscopy, or in a blood test taken because you were a little more tired than usual. Before proceeding any further, *you must have the diagnosis confirmed*. Regardless of the tissue or organ involved, have another expert evaluate the evidence.

Staging and Searching

If the diagnosis of cancer is certain, a specialist should then "stage" the disease—that is, determine how "wild" the cells are and to what extent they have already spread. This means looking elsewhere in the body, away from the original site, for evidence of tumor activity. Such spread, when it occurs, is called *metastasis*, or *metastatic disease*.

The search for metastases involves blood tests and examining literally every part of the body by means of conventional X rays, radioactive scans, sonograms or a CT (computerized tomography) scan. The number and extent of the diagnostic tests required will depend on which organ was primarily involved. Cancers in different tissues spread predictably to favored sites.

The way the cancer is going to be treated and the outlook for your recovery will depend on whether it is still localized—that is, remains where it began—or there is demonstrable evidence of spread. If it is still localized, cure is possible, usually with surgery, radiation or both. (By cure, I mean that you are finished with it; it will not recur.) On the other hand, if the cancer has already spread, chances of cure are reduced, but effective control may still be possible for varying lengths of time.

While surgery and radiation traditionally afford the best chance for obtaining a cure, some cancers are now also being effectively controlled by chemotherapy—that is, drugs that are toxic to the cancer, but do not destroy healthy tissue. But before any course of treatment is selected, there should be consultation with an expert oncologist.

Radiation—How and Why It Works

It is ironic that despite all the adverse publicity concerning the cancer risk of excessive and unnecessary radiation, it is one of the most effective ways to treat many malignancies. When trying to cure a disease that may kill in a matter of months, there is not much point to wondering about possible adverse effects fifteen or twenty years later.

Radiation therapy (radiotherapy) can be administered to vulnerable or radiosensitive tumors either by powerful X-ray equipment or by radioactive materials like cobalt or radium, which emit gamma rays similar to X rays. These penetrate the wildly growing cells, altering the genetic substance within them, preventing their multiplication and ultimately destroying them. When the tumor is small enough, sufficiently localized, and "radio sensitive," such treatment is sometimes as effective as surgery. But when the mass of cancerous tissue is large, some cells survive the onslaught of radiotherapy. Those that do so then continue to multiply, requiring more and more radiation to effect control.

The equipment originally available for the X-ray therapy for cancer was primitive by today's standards. We were unable to focus on the small area we wanted to destroy, and thus normal tissues were also damaged by the treatment. In order to direct enough radiation into the cancerous material, we had to administer so much that it made the patient sick and nauseated. Side effects were frequently worse than symptoms of the disease itself. Today, however, there are linear accelerators and cobalt generators that can deliver powerful, concentrated radiation, pinpointed to and penetrating limited areas of the body without even burning the overlying skin.

Radiation is useful in the treatment of virtually every kind of cancer—in the brain, lungs, uterus, skin, prostate, bladder and other areas. It is especially useful when the tumor is deep and intertwined with other tissue, so that it is difficult or impossible to remove surgically, or where the risk of operation is great, as in elderly or debilitated patients.

Chemotherapy—Eliminating the Stragglers

Since it is always possible that some residual microscopic cancer cells have been left behind after either radiation or surgery, we now add chemotherapy and/or immunotherapy, just to be sure. Such "adjuvant" therapy is like an insurance policy against any remaining tumor tissue, even if none is apparent to the naked eye.

The concept of chemotherapy originated in 1941, when it was observed that the administration of female hormones caused regression of prostate cancer. Hormones were subsequently tried in the management of breast cancer, and here too an effect was noted. In 1943, nitrogen mustard was found to have definite activity against certain lymph-gland tumors. In 1947 it was demonstrated that other drugs produced short remissions in some forms of childhood luekemia.

In the forty years since these first observations we have identified several tumors that can be not only controlled but even cured with chemotherapy. These include Hodgkin's disease, Wilms's tumor in children, certain forms of leukemia and other lymph-gland malignancies. So this is no time to have a negative attitude toward cancer.

Combination Therapy—A Job for a Pro

Chemotherapy interferes with the multiplication (or division) of abnormal cancer cells. Although it can cure some malignancies, more commonly its net effect is to control them, that is, hold them in check. To understand how it does so, you must know a little about cell biology. There are different stages in the life cycle of every living cell. First, there is the phase during which DNA is synthesized. This is followed by a "resting" period, and then by the stage of "mitosis," during which the cell divides. The approximately thirty different anticancer drugs in current use act at different times in this cell cycle. Some are more effective during DNA synthesis, others during mitosis, while still others destroy the cell only when it is resting. Since the cells in any tumor mass are in various phases at any given time, administering a single drug will affect only a portion of the tumor, leaving intact all those cells in a different stage of biologic activity. But to cure cancer, *every* abnormal cell must be destroyed, for even if only one remains, it has the potential to continue the malignant process and ultimately kill the patient. For this reason, the experienced cancer specialist uses *combinations* of anticancer agents, to cover as much of the cells' life cycle, and thus kill as many cells as possible in any one treatment.

There are four main categories of drugs available for cancer chemotherapy. These include: (a) *antimetabolites* (example: 5-FU, 6-MP, methotrexate). They act in an interesting way. They are actually poisons but chemically they resemble nutrients or vitamins. The cancer cell gobbles them up, but then dies because the antimetabolites interfere with vital cellular processes; (b) *antibiotics* (bleomycin, Andriamycin) which interfere with the cancer cell's ability to make protein; (c) *alkylating agents* (Cytoxan, L-PAM, Myleran) which act on cell division described above; (d) *steroid hormones* which probably prevent the function of the cancer cell's enzyme systems. As you can see, when used in combination, these agents can hit hard at the malignant cell in a variety of ways.

An important drawback of chemotherapy is that it not only destroys malignant cells, but also may hurt normal ones as well. Treatment, therefore, is administered in cycles, so that normal cells (which recover from injury more quickly than do sick cancer cells) can bounce back, before the abnormal ones have gotten over the effects of the medication, thus permitting another treatment course to be started safely. Knowing which combination of drugs to use against a specific tumor and in what dosage requires skill and experience. For that reason, in cancer chemotherapy, you should always have an expert involved.

Coping with Side Effects

The side effects of chemotherapy are myriad and they vary in severity and duration. The most common are nausea and vomiting, rashes, loss of hair, disturbances of heart rhythm, damage to the heart, or interference with bone-marrow function (so that the numbers of red cells, white cells and platelets are reduced). Unfortunately, such side effects become intolerable in a significant percentage of cases.

If you develop severe reactions and are advised to terminate or reduce treatment substantially, ask for a second opinion from an experienced chemotherapist. Side effects can frequently be controlled by various ingenious techniques. Here is a case in point. There is an anticancer drug called Adriamycin, which, though effective, often causes severe hair loss. Some very observant nurses working in a tumor clinic found that when they applied ice packs to the scalp at the time of the administration of the drug (it is given by vein), the loss of hair was minimized. Today, patients receiving Adriamycin treatment sit around with ice packs on their heads. The cold application constricts the local blood vessels so that less blood, and hence less Adriamycin is delivered to the area. This is undesirable, of course, when the tumor that is being treated is situated in the head.

Marijuana also reduces the severity of nausea and vomiting, sometimes permitting chemotherapy to be continued in greater comfort. For this reason, it is now legally available for cancer patients in several states and is supplied by the National Cancer Institute.

Frequently, certain elements within the blood, like platelets, white cells or red cells, are destroyed by chemotherapy. When that happens, other drugs can be substituted and treatment continued.

Treating Cancer in the Test Tube

There is an experimental technique in the administration of chemotherapy now being evaluated of which you should be aware. Normally, the oncologist selects the drug with which to treat you on the basis of the size of the cancer, its location and its "stage." His choice is based on the track record of that agent in similar cancers in which it has been used. But the fact that it worked in other patients doesn't necessarily mean that it is going to be effective in your case. An analogy may be made in the way we manage infections. There is a process called "culture and sensitivity," to determine the best antibiotic against a given bacterium. For example, when you have a sore throat, we swab it and incubate the material in a series of test tubes. To each of these we add a different antibiotic and later look at the results. Where the antibiotic has destroyed the organism, the test tube is clean, with no evidence of bacterial growth. Where it was ineffective, the infection continues rampant in the culture medium.

What has all this got to do with cancer? A similar technique has been developed at the University of Arizona. A small piece of tumor, a sliver, is taken from the patient, and its cells are grown in the laboratory. Then, various anticancer drugs are applied to them, just as antibiotics are administered to bacteria. The effect of each agent is assessed outside the body. If this technique proves to be reliable it will, in the future, spare a great deal of time, money, inconvenience, side effects and even danger to cancer patients by allowing the best drug to be given first, without speculation, trial and error.

Immunotherapy—Dealing with the Breakdown in Law and Order

When you are given a protective vaccine against some infection or other, your body manufactures specific antibodies against the dead organisms in the vaccine. Your immune, or protective, system doesn't distinguish between live and dead enemies; they are all treated alike. The vaccine causes complex biological defenses to be mobilized and ready so that, should the *live* pneumonia, smallpox or whooping-cough agent ever strike, your body will be able to ward it off. In other words, it bolsters your immunity. Many scientists believe that cancer represents a breakdown in the body's defense or immune system and that immunotherapy restores that capability.

The efficacy of the immune system diminishes with age. Indeed, with some exceptions, cancer is basically a disease of the elderly. It would, therefore, seem logical to try to enhance resistance to cancer, just as we do against infection. To that end, the effectiveness of several anticancer vaccines is now being studied. For example, BCG vaccine, used to confer immunity against tuberculosis, is effective in bladder cancer. Some investigators speculated that malignant melanoma, the particularly lethal form of skin cancer, and certain leukemias might possibly be controlled for longer periods of time by adding BCG to chemotherapy and other measures. Unlike bladder cancer, I don't think this has worked out very well. Other drugs that enhance immune function may have a beneficial effect on cancer of the breast. *Immune stimulation*, though it may not cure the malignancy, may prolong remission and survival when used together with other forms of therapy.

Different Forms of Immunotherapy

There are several different forms of immunotherapy currently available. The first is called *active, nonspecific* immunotherapy, in which some "messenger of immunity" like interferon (an antiviral protein) or a vaccine (like BCG) enhances the immune response. In *active, specific* immunotherapy, extracts of your own tumor cells are reinjected into your body to boost your immunity to your own cancer. Another approach called *adaptive* immunotherapy involves the administration of substances (immune RNA, thymosin) derived from defense cells (lymphocytes) in the body. Then, there is *passive* immunotherapy in which antibodies from animal sources or from patients who had a cancer identical to yours and from which they were cured, are injected to act against your tumor cells. Finally, there is *local* immunotherapy, in which agents are inoculated directly into the tumor. Thus far, the most successful among these five approaches have been *active, non-specific* immunotherapy and *local* immunotherapy.

Interferon—An Exciting Promise?

You may very well have been reading about interferon recently, the "hottest" new anticancer product now in research. It is an antiviral protein that we have known about for a long time, but which, until quite recently, was thought to have potential only against viral infections.

Interferons (there are more than one) are made by many different kinds of cells in response to attack by a virus. Once formed, interferon circulates in the bloodstream, stimulating cells everywhere to develop resistance to the virus. In other words, it mobilizes the body defenses against attack. There is now some evidence that interferon may work not only against viruses but against some cancer cells as well. Much more experience with this agent will be necessary to determine how effective it really is, in what dosage, administered for how long, and in combination with what other forms of therapy.

Interferon was given in 1971, by Dr. Hans Strander in Stockholm, to several patients with an almost universally fatal cancer of the bone (osteosarcoma). He reported impressive results. The number of patients to whom it has been given has thus far been very limited. However, more efficient techniques for the mass production of interferon, by means of "gene-splicing," are ongoing. The human interferon gene is "spliced" into bacteria, so that these organisms can then produce virtually unlimited amounts of the pure substance. There will soon be enough pure interferon to permit the systematic study of its effects in every malignancy and in viral diseases as well.

Feeding the Cancer

Patients with advanced cancer lose weight and are gaunt, pale and fragile. I have always wondered how a cancer, sometimes smaller than one's thumb, can wreak such havoc on the rest of the body. I am not sure that anybody understands how such malnutrition is caused by cancer. Some of it is, of course, due to poor appetite, resulting from the disease itself or from its treatment. But the cancer itself must also produce some substance, not as yet isolated, that is responsible for this wasting.

Hyperalimentation is a new approach to the management of cancer that focuses on nutrition. If your physician has not proposed it, ask him about it. Hyperalimentation involves the intravenous administration of vitamins, minerals and other nutrients, and can provide a cancer patient with as many as 4,000 calories a day. Such enhanced nutrition may possibly increase the effectiveness of other forms of therapy and lead to prolonged survival (despite the fact those extra calories are also feeding the tumor).

Laetrile—Remember Krebiozen?

Chances are that you will find very little if anything about *Laetrile* in the standard textbooks of medicine, even those dealing with cancer. The medical profession has taken a very defensive position in dealing with a question that simply cannot be ignored. There are, after all, at least fifty thousand people (that we know about) with cancer who are now taking Laetrile in the United States. It has been legalized in at least seventeen states, where anybody who demands it can get it. Public testimonials by cancer patients who have been "successfully" treated with Laetrile reach the layman every day, and he is first puzzled, then hostile, because of the implacable opposition of "organized" medicine. The "establishment" has a genuine feeling that the public is being duped and that the proponents of Laetrile are more interested in exploiting its economic potential than in establishing its scientific credibility.

Most doctors, including me, are convinced that Laetrile is totally inefective and often dangerous. When used in those forms of cancer for which there is good treatment (and the number is growing every day), we believe that to give Laetrile instead is indefensible.

Laetrile is not inert. Its active substance is cyanide which, according to the manufacturers, kills malignant cells but spares healthy ones. However, in experiments, rats receiving it in high dosages have died—and so have some patients. So taking Laetrile is not like eating apricots, from which it is derived.

Despite the fact that there have already been numerous studies showing that Laetrile is of no use whatsoever, its makers are still not satisfied. They insist that no one has yet shown, *beyond any doubt*, that it is ineffective. I'm not sure they will *ever* be satisfied.

Cancer of the Lung

This year, 115,000 new lung cancers will be diagnosed in the United States and 105,000 of us will die from it. It remains the leading cause of cancer deaths among men. As compared with forty years ago, twenty times the number of people now die from this disease. Nor is treatment very successful. Despite all we can do, only 8 percent of men and 12 percent of women with lung cancer will be alive five years after the disease has been discovered. Although lung cancer still strikes men more frequently than women, and absolute numbers are increasing for both sexes, the male-female difference is narrowing as more and more women use cigarettes. Indeed, lung cancer in women is said to be approaching epidemic proportions.

You Can Be Too Rich or Too Thin

A few years ago, a fifty-year-old woman consulted me because she was troubled by palpitations. As happens so often, these "extra beats" were especially frequent after drinking too much coffee, taking an extra martini, or smoking cigarettes. I was able to persuade her to switch to decaffeinated coffee and cut down on the alcohol, but she simply would not do anything about the thirty or forty cigarettes she was smoking every day. "It's not really a habit," she told me. "I can quit anytime, but if I do, I'm afraid I'll gain weight." That was her excuse.

I continued to warn her about the relationship of tobacco, heart disease and lung cancer, but without success. She continued to smoke—and endured not only her heart pounding but her "morning cough" as well. She used a mouth wash to mask the tobacco breath and wore nail polish to cover the nicotine stains. In her mind, these were only minor inconveniences one had to pay as the price of remaining elegantly thin.

One day, while on a tour abroad, she contracted "pneumonia." After treatment with appropriate antibiotics, she improved. When she returned home, we checked on the status of her infection. A chest X ray revealed cancer of the lung. (Lung cancers frequently resemble pneumonia initially, because of the obstruction and infection associated with the tumor.)

Despite all our efforts—surgery, radiation, chemotherapy and immunotherapy—she died two years later.

Prevention and Early Detection

This story highlights two very important points: (a) that the outlook in lung cancer is still bleak; and (b) that tobacco plays an important role in the causation of most cases. At the present time, the only hope for successful treatment lies in early detection. Those at highest risk are smokers of more than one pack a day and certain industrial workers. The recommendation of the American Cancer Society notwithstanding, I advise annual chest X rays for such persons. In 1980 alone, in my own practice, I found two silent cancers of the lung early enough to be cured by surgery. These two patients are thankful I did the routine chest film. Early detection and removal may result in up to 25 percent survival for five years, and even a complete cure in some cases. Elimination of tobacco from our society would significantly reduce the incidence of this dreaded affliction.

Will Surgery Really Help?

Although the only chance for cure in cancer of the lung is its early removal, if an operation is suggested to you, get another opinion. It may be too late for surgery, and an operation may only add unnecessary pain and suffering. The conventional chest X ray cannot always be depended on to provide the information whether surgery can, in fact, help you. Your doctor will want to perform a radioactive scan, which may indicate whether the tumor is confined to one portion of the lung (and is curable) or has already spread within it (too late). There is also the mediastinoscope, an instrument that is passed into the space between the lungs and permits the surgeon to search for additional evidence of inoperability. The CT scan, in expert hands, can also reveal important information about the nature of a lung tumor and the extent to which it has grown.

Vaccine Against Cancer

Finally you should know about a most interesting development. A vaccine has been produced that can apparently *prevent* lung cancer in animals. It is now being tested in persons who are especially vulnerable to cancer of the lung—

middle-aged men who smoke two or more packs of cigarettes per day and/or those who work in the uranium or asbestos industries, or coke ovens. One thousand people given the vaccine will be examined over a five-year period, at the end of which we shall know how effectively it prevents cancer in humans.

Curiously enough, although this vaccine is basically for *prevention* and not for cure of lung cancer, it may nevertheless prolong survival in those who already have it. Fifty-two persons with lung cancer in whom the tumor was small and localized, with no evidence of spread, were studied. Half were treated with surgery alone; the others were also given the vaccine after the operation. Three years later, 95 percent of the patients who had received the vaccine were alive, as compared with only 51 percent of those who were treated without it. At four years, there was 80 percent survival in the vaccine group as compared to 49 percent treated with surgery alone. Although this work is still a big "maybe" and it is too early even to justify much optimism, it gives you some idea of what is on the horizon.

Cancer of the Kidney—A Bad One to Have

The only hope for curing cancer of the kidney is to discover it very, very early. That is often difficult, because this particular malignancy remains "silent" for so long. The experience of one patient highlights that fact. A musician, he was on a ship to South America, where he was scheduled to perform. While at sea, some twenty-four hours from port, he suddenly found himself unable to pass his urine. The ship's surgeon passed a tube (catheter) into the bladder, drained the obstructed urine, and left the catheter in place. The cause of the trouble was a big prostate that needed immediate removal. My patient canceled his performance and took the next plane back to New York. He was immediately admitted to the hospital for the necessary prostate surgery.

But before prostate surgery, certain routine tests and X rays are almost always done. These include an intravenous pyelogram which, in this case, indicated an abnormality in the right kidney. A sonogram (sound waves directed at the mass) indicated that the shadow in question was solid tissue and not a cyst. Cysts of the kidney (sacs containing fluid) are almost always benign, while solid masses are usually malignant. What was to have been a simple prostate operation ended in an exploratory procedure of the kidney, as a result of which cancer of that organ was found. Happily, it had not yet spread. The kidney was removed, and six years later my patient remains perfectly well.

When cancer of the kidney is not found accidentally, as it was in this case, it usually makes its presence known through blood in the urine. The only treatment for renal cancer is surgical removal. Although chemotherapy is also administered, that is done more out of desperation than out of hope. To date, the cure rate and even the incidence of response are very low, because by the time the affected kidney has been removed, the cancer has usually already spread.

There is some promising work now in progress suggesting that immune RNA may have an antitumor effect. So, if you have cancer of the kidney, before accepting a pessimistic outlook, get a second opinion from a cancer specialist. As always, check with the National Cancer Institute or the American Cancer Society about any new progress in this field.

Testicular Cancer, Formerly Fatal—Now Curable

Testicular cancer is the fourth-leading cause of death from malignancy among young men, but there has been dramatic progress in its treatment.

Although testicular tumors are very highly radio-sensitive and can often be cured with radiation alone, surgery is usually also required. But the big breakthrough is the high percentage of cures with chemotherapy, especially when radiation and surgery have not been completely successful. Combinations of such drugs as bleomycin, cisplatinum and vinblastine have been very effective *after the testicular cancer has already metastasized*.

So, if you develop a testicular malignancy, ask to be referred to a major cancer center and inquire whether you are a candidate for this chemotherapy, in addition to whatever radiation and/or surgery are administered.

Bladder Cancer

Cancer of the bladder strikes about 35,000 people a year and kills about 10,000. It is most commonly found in men between the ages of sixty-five and seventy. The few women who do get it are likely to be even older. Its incidence is increasing in most of the world by 3 or 4 percent a year, and equally so in both sexes, except in the United States. Here it is becoming somewhat more frequent in men, while the incidence in women has declined by 25 percent in the last twenty-five years. Smoking and industrialization are thought to have some role in its causation.

It's Rarely Silent

There is nothing vague or subtle about cancer of the bladder. Unlike many other neoplasms (the medical term for cancer) that remain undiagnosed for months because their only symptoms are nonspecific, like fatigue or insidious weight loss, bladder cancer declares itself early, usually with the appearance of blood in the urine or a change in voiding habits. Since these symptoms may be due to several other causes, your doctor will first do a Pap test on the urine when you report a bloody urine, looking for tumor cells there. Then, an IVP (kidney and bladder X ray after injection of dye) will be performed, followed by cystoscopy, in which the urologist will actually look into the bladder through an illuminated scope. He will biopsy whatever growths he sees and then cauterize them, that is, burn them away with an electrical current. That may be all that is necessary if the cancer was detected early enough. Even so, you will have to come back at appropriate intervals (the usual schedule is every three months for the first year, then every four to six months therafter) to make sure that the cancer has not started up again. If it has, it will simply be burned away again. The cure rate of such bladder cancers is about 70 percent. I know many men who have been coming into the hospital twice a year for at least fifteen years for repeated electrosurgical removal of their bladder cancers. Except for the cost, inconvenience and discomfort, they have been able to lead normal lives in every other respect. I have already mentioned earlier the effectiveness of BCG vaccine instilled directly into the bladder in such cases. Ask your urologist about it.

When the Cancer Is Advanced

When the cancer is so deeply embedded in the bladder that cautery alone will not remove it, you will need a major operation to remove the entire bladder and almost all the tissue around it. Without your bladder, you will now pass your urine through a small tube emerging from your abdomen. Although the penis is intact, sexual function is compromised because of all the surgery done in the pelvic area. A major recent development in the treatment of advanced bladder cancer is a drug called *cisplatin* which prolongs survival in as many as one third of all patients treated.

Early Detection—Key to Survival

The key to successful management of cancer of the bladder, as in so many other locations, is early detection. *Never ignore blood in the urine*. You may get the providential warning only once.

Cancer of the Breast

Cancer of the breast is the most prevalent malignancy in women, there being some 110,000 new cases and 36,000 deaths every year in the United States alone (as of 1982). In recent years we have acquired a greater understanding of how the disease spreads and the best means available to treat it. In the following pages you will see why it is important to get a second opinion after one doctor's evaluation of a lump in your breast.

Exit the Traditional Radical Mastectomy

In the past, any woman unfortunate enough to develop breast cancer almost routinely underwent an extensive operation (radical mastectomy) in which not only the breast itself was removed, but muscles, nerves and fatty tissue all the way into the armpit were also dissected. Such surgery resulted in disfigurement, frequently left the patient feeling depressed and sexually inadequate, sometimes threatened marital relationships, and often left the woman with pain, stiffness and swelling in the arm on the affected side.

The rationale for this extensive procedure was the belief that cancer of the breast usually spreads at least early on, by direct extension, encroaching gradually on adjoining tissues. If a lump was found in the breast, it seemed logical that the best way to contain it was prophylactically to cut away as much of the surrounding structures as possible—all the lymph glands from the breast to the armpit, the pectoral (chest-wall) muscles and connective tissue—to make sure that the most advanced part of the tumor was excised. If at the time of operation, the cancer was found to have already involved the lymph glands, radiation therapy was administered.

But Was It Really Necessary?

Over a forty-year span, however, as we looked at the results of such extensive surgery, we realized that it did not yield any appreciable reduction in the death rate from breast cancer. Doctors then began to wonder whether the radical mastectomy, with all its adverse physical and emotional consequences, was worth the price. Might less drastic surgical procedures be at least as effective in coping with the problem?

You Think You're Cured—and Then Suddenly . . .

There are several important new facts that have now become apparent. The first is that the spread of breast cancer is not primarily by extension, as we once thought. What happens is that in even the smallest cancers, microscopic cells can migrate to various parts of the body, not necessarily by direct extension toward the lymph glands, but through the bloodstream and lymphatic channels in the area of the lump itself. Some of the cancer cells that disseminate in this way are probably destroyed by the body's defense mechanisms, but some are not, and theoretically it takes only one to perpetuate the cancer at another site. This seeding of malignant cells (metastasis) to distant parts of the body, such as the lung, bones or brain, may be followed by a silent interval of several years, during which time these microscopic foci, with their ominous potential, lie dormant. Then suddenly, five, ten or even fifteen years later, long after the patient was considered cured, she (and occasionally *he*, for we develop breast cancer too) develops bone pain, or finds a lump somewhere. We never really understood until fairly recently the mechanism of this unexpected recurrence. We now know that it is due to the *early* spread of tumor cells, a phenomenon which is not prevented by the radical mastectomy, which may therefore be likened to locking the barn door after the horses have gone. Why then remove all that tissue—muscle, sinew and fat—when the malignant cells may have already escaped from the primary tumor by another route?

The Modified Radical Mastectomy—Is It Enough?

This appreciation of how cancer of the breast spreads has led to a modification in treatment. First and most important, extensive surgery is not always necessary. For some patients, instead of the radical mastectomy, "simple" mastectomy, that is, removal of the affected breast, or "lumpectomy" (simple removal of the visible portions of the tumor with a little more tissue around it to spare) may suffice. Or, you will probably need a *modified* radical mastectomy, in which only the breast and any involved lymph glands are excised. A major advantage of these lesser operations is that they permit reconstruction of the breast so that it can assume an almost normal appearance. (More about that later.) Some oncologists then follow-up with radiation to the affected breast. Others, a distinct minority, even recommend no more than "lumpectomy" a simple mastectomy followed by "definitive" radiation.

Surgery Alone Is Not Always Enough

Although it is still too early to be sure, the statistics so far suggest that these more limited approaches (sometimes followed by irradiation) carry with them the same cure and relapse rate as the more aggressive surgery. One other observation of critical importance is that follow-up (adjuvant) chemotherapy with anticancer drugs and/or hormones, after the visible tumor has been removed, is effective in delaying the appearance of any metastases that may have already taken place. Whatever the treatment, the main determinant of your future outlook with breast cancer is how many glands turn out to be involved in your armpit. If the malignancy has gone that far, chances of being free of the disease in ten years are only 25 percent.

Planning the Biopsy

When a lump is discovered in your breast, your doctor will usually perform a biopsy to determine whether it is malignant. That sometimes can be done by freezing the area locally and sucking out the contents with a needle. But more commonly you are taken to the operating room and anesthetized while a piece of tissue from the growth is sent for analysis. If the pathologist reports back that the tumor is malignant, the surgeon will usually want to proceed with the surgery then and there. Should you give him carte blanche to do so?

The Meaning of Informed Consent

The law states that no patient should have *any* operation unless he or she (or a legal representative) understands what is going to be done—and agrees to the procedure in writing. That is especially pertinent in breast surgery. If a breast biopsy reveals a malignancy, you have two alternatives with regard to the next step. The first—and the one that I usually recommend—is to request the surgeon *not* to proceed with the operation. The next day you, your husband and your surgeon can discuss the nature of the surgical approach that he proposes. That may be a good time to get a second opinion. This field is changing so radically and opinions are so divergent that you may benefit from another competent viewpoint. The disadvantage of this approach is that you end up with two operations (and two anesthetics) instead of one. Some women prefer to settle it all beforehand. Whichever course you choose, your consent to surgery should be fully informed.

Aside from giving you some time to think it over, delaying your final decision has other advantages. The analysis of the tissue removed is more accurate when studied with conventional staining techniques than in the frozen section done at the time of biopsy while the surgeon waits with scalpel poised; also, a malignant tumor can be more accurately "staged"—that is, the extent and degree of its spread can be more carefully assessed. If it is determined, after such careful workup, that other sites are already involved, there is much less reason to do extensive local surgery in the breast.

The Importance of Chemotherapy

Researchers in several countries are currently assessing the effect of different combinations of anticancer drugs for breast tumors, and the results reported so far are most encouraging. In the months and years to come, much of these data will be refined and we will know statistically which treatment is best.

Will You Need Hormones Too?

Another important observation affecting treatment of breast cancer involves "estrogen receptors." The cancerous breast tissue itself is tested to determine whether it accepts, or "binds," estrogens. If it does, then the patient may respond better after surgery to hormones and go into a remission that may last for many months. (Such estrogen binders respond particularly in pre-menopausal women to *antiestrogen* therapy [Tamoxifen].)

If the cancer does not have estrogen binding sites, then chemotherapy is likely to be of greater benefit than hormones. So, we can now predict, with reasonable accuracy, who is apt to respond to which treatment and why.

When the Cancer Is Advanced

When breast cancer has spread throughout the body, even if it is of the positive estrogen-receptor type, it may be too late for hormones alone. Your doctor may now recommend removal or destruction of the pituitary gland (in the brain) or the adrenals, which are located atop the kidneys or ovaries. Before you agree to these measures, always ask for another opinion from a specialist in breast cancer to determine whether such therapy is really necessary.

The Role of Immunotherapy in Breast Cancer

As I indicated earlier, cells may escape from the cancer and lie dormant in various parts of the body for months or years, waiting for the right moment to resume their explosive growth. Some of these are destroyed by the body's immune mechanism before they begin to multiply. Those that remain perpetuate the disease. So it stands to reason that anything we can do to help the body cope with these malignant cells may improve the outlook. There is evidence in several different cancers, including that of the breast, that enhancement of immune capability may be of help even *after* spread has occurred.

A Second Look at Mammography

When and how often should a woman have mammography? Some years ago, after Mrs. Gerald Ford and Mrs. Nelson Rockefeller were found to have breast cancer, there was a stampede for mammography in the United States. The demand was so great that patients sometimes waited weeks for an appointment. Since then, we have taken a hard second look at this procedure, because it does involve radiation, and the less you get of that, the better. Although the newer X ray equipment does reduce exposure somewhat, it does not eliminate it.

I believe a base-line mammogram should be obtained between thirty-five and forty years of age. Thereafter, most doctors now agree that it is a good idea and worth the small risk to have a mammogram done every year or two in the following situations: If you are over fifty years of age; if your breasts are large and difficult to examine, so that they may conceal small cancers, even from the fingers of an experienced doctor; if you have had cancer of one breast and are therefore more vulnerable to developing it in the other; if there is a strong family history of the disease—as, for example, when your mother or sister has had breast cancer.

Removing the Cancer-Prone Breast

When should a high-risk patient have a breast removed *before* the cancer actually develops? Take, for example, a woman I know. She is thirty-two years old. Her mother had cancer in both breasts. Last year, a sister was found to have a malignant tumor of the breast which spread rapidly and for which she is now being treated. My patient is terrified—and who can blame her? To make matters worse, she has cysts in both breasts which require biopsy and mammograms at regular intervals. In such a case, it is not unreasonable to consider prophylactic removal of her breast tissue, a procedure called *subcutaneous mastectomy*. The skin and only a minimal amount of breast tissue are retained, and after the reconstruction process the breasts are usually almost normal to touch and appearance. Some doctors query whether the operation is worthwhile in view of the fact that we cannot remove all of the potentially malignant tissue, leaving some 15 percent behind. Your decision is as good as anyone's. What you should do is really up to you, but you should be aware of this preventive option.

The "Lumpy Breast" Diet

An interesting bit of news comes to mind which may interest women with benign lumpy breasts. According to one recent report, abstinence from coffee, tea and cola drinks seemed to result in their disappearance. If your breasts are lumpy, why not follow such a diet for about four weeks and see what happens? If it works, please let me know.

In a more recent development, one observer claims success in treating lumpy, painful breasts (which incidentally are associated with a higher incidence of cancer of that organ) with 600 units of Vitamin E daily.

Gynecological Cancers

This year in the United States we expect to detect about 75,000 new cases of ovarian and uterine cancer. Some 22,000 women will die from these malignancies, 50 percent of them from cancer of the ovary (11,100).

Is Your Life Worth $2,000,000—to You?

Not too long ago, to save even a single life, regardless of cost, was paramount. That was in the days of cheap energy and the promise of an increasing standard of living for everyone. All that has changed. We are now preoccupied with *efficiency* of medical care. The major concern of politicians, health administrators, insurance actuaries and, yes, even some doctors today is *cost effectiveness*. Their argument goes something like this. About 50,000 proctoscopies must be done to detect just one curable cancer of the bowel or rectum. Since each proctoscopy costs $25 or $30, we are spending almost $2,000,000 to save one life—and in their view, that is simply not worth it. They hold that the money would have had a greater impact on the health of more people were it spent in some other way. In today's system of medical practice, we still have the choice of practicing preventive medicine. In the future, when almost inevitably someone other than the patient will be picking up the tab, the decision about having the $2,000,000 proctoscopy that may save your life may no longer be up to you.

Logic of the "Minimalists"

Some health "economists" have gone even further with this "logic." They claim there is no use taking even a routine chest X ray, because, if we find a lung cancer, it is too late to do anything about it anyway in *most* instances. The "minimalists," as they've been called, also don't think we should bother taking an electrocardiogram to detect heart disease in someone without symptoms, because "what difference will that make?"

With respect to gynecological cancers, these same "experts" feel that the Pap test (which involves scraping the cervix to look for early cancer cells) constitutes an unnecessary expense. According to them, such early localized malignancies don't often spread, in which event surgery subjects the patient to a greater risk than does the cancer itself. They would have us wait until the cancer begins to bleed, since it *usually* can still be cured at that time.

I don't believe any of this, and neither should you. The fact is that the death rate from cancer of the uterus has dropped to one third of what it was forty years ago. I think that is due to earlier detection, resulting from the widespread use of the Pap test. (Some gynecologists believe that circumcision has something to do with it too, since mates of circumcised men have less cancer of the cervix than those of uncircumcised males. The foreskin may harbor a virus or other agent responsible for inducing cervical cancer.)

Cancer of the Uterus

Uterine cancer may involve either the main portion or "body" of that organ, the lining of its walls (the endometrium, which is shed every month during your period), or its "neck" (the cervix).

Estrogens, Cancer and the Hot Flush

Many postmenopausal women depend on estrogens to alleviate the troublesome hot flushes of the menopause. These hormones also appear to make them look younger, render the skin less dry and wrinkled, and the vaginal vault moist enough to permit intercourse without pain and bleeding.

Telling such ladies that estrogens may give them endometrial cancer is depressing news. Yet, the data suggesting an association between estrogen and such cancer cannot be ignored. The higher the dose and the longer you take the drug, the greater the risk appears to be. These data should, however, be viewed in perspective. Among the 400,000 deaths from cancer each year in the United States, only 3,300 are attributable to endometrial malignancy. So, I recommend the following: If you still have your uterus, don't take estrogens unless you really have to; and never only for cosmetic reasons. However, if you are suffering from troublesome hot flushes, try the estrogens, but be sure to see your gynecologist at least every six months and stop the hormone as soon as you can. If you have had spontaneous bone fractures because of a lack of calcium, there is some evidence that estrogens can help you (especially if you became menopausal after your ovaries were surgically removed). But they may also be of benefit even after a natural menopause. In either event, take them for no longer than three years, during which time your gynecologist should be looking at regular intervals for any evidence of cancer. After that, they are probably of much less help, as far as preventing bone fractures is concerned, and may expose you to an unnecessary risk.

Treating Cancer of the Uterus

How a uterine cancer is treated depends on its stage when found, whether the tumor is still localized or has already spread. Before committing yourself to any therapeutic plan, always first confirm the diagnosis with another gynecologist. I have seen several patients whose "cancer" turned out to be benign after review by someone else. Even if it is malignant, chances for cure are as high as 75 percent, especially if it is still confined to the pelvis.

Whenever possible, the entire tumor should be removed.

If it is either too advanced for that, or not completely accessible to operation, radiation will have to be used. Finally, chemotherapy with several agents in combination—drugs like Cyclophosphamide, Bleomycin, 5FU, Doxorubicin and Methotrexate, as well as certain hormones, are also available and sometimes, but not often, slow down tumor growth and prolong life.

Ovarian Malignancy—The Second-Leading Cause of Cancer Deaths in Women

The incidence of ovarian cancer, second only to malignancy of the breast, is increasing very rapidly, and nobody really knows why. It has been suggested that cosmetic talc in powders, deodorants, soaps, textiles, and on condoms and diaphragms may be responsible in some cases. Dusting babies with talcum powder after the diaper has been removed (or when the baby puts some on her diaphragm after she is grown up) may introduce these particles into the genital tract and cause cancer formation. Interesting! Who would have thought...?

Treatment of ovarian cancer is not as effective as therapy for cancer of the uterus. The patient usually responds for a year or two, but is not cured nearly as often. As in uterine malignancy, the best chance lies in complete surgical removal. Even if the tumor has spread elsewhere in the body, the surgeon should still remove as much of it as possible. Ask for a second opinion if you are advised that, because the tumor has spread, it is too late to operate. The mainstay of subsequent treatment is combined chemotherapy and radiation, although unfortunately, ovarian cancers are not often sensitive to radiation.

Cancer of the Digestive Tract

The digestive tract starts in the mouth and ends at the anus—and any part of it is vulnerable to cancer. The incidence, as well as the location, of such malignancies varies from country to country. For example, in China, there is much cancer of the esophagus, while in Japan the big killer is cancer of the stomach.

The most important cancer in the United States is that of the lung, but when you put them all together, malignancies of the digestive organs account for the highest number of cancer deaths in the United States. There are about 183,000 new cases every year, and 112,000 deaths. Some of these tumors are more deadly than others, the worst ones being esophageal, pancreatic and liver. By the time a cancer is recognized in any of these organs, it is often too late. By contrast, if you are alert to the danger signals of cancer of the bowel, early diagnosis and surgery will result in cure in some 52 percent of cases. So, if you have an unexplained pain in your belly, find blood in your stool, or notice a change in your bowel habits (sudden constipation alternating with diarrhea or the appearance of narrow, ribbonlike movements) have yourself checked right away. There are some sensitive new diagnostic techniques like the body scanner and ultrasonography, as well as conventional X rays, which can detect many of these cancers in time.

Surgery Is the Key

The key to the treatment of intestinal cancer is surgery. Complete removal of the malignant growth offers the best chance for cure. One of my patients, who lived abroad, consulted me because of bloody diarrhea, which developed after he had eaten some "bad roast beef" somewhere in the Far East. I found nothing abnormal in a complete physical examination—and that included a careful rectal probe. In pursuing the history in greater detail, however, I learned that these symptoms had appeared in the preceding months. I then aranged for a sigmoidoscopy to be done. This didn't appeal to the patient (it never does—to anyone) but he went through with it anyway. We found a cancer of the lower bowel, situated just beyond the reach of my examining finger (that is why the rectal exam was normal). The rest of the story has a happy ending. At surgery the cancer was found not to have spread. The patient made an uneventful recovery and is alive and well ten years later.

But Radiation May Be Necessary

Radiation therapy becomes necessary when an intestinal cancer is too extensive to eradicate at operation. Unlike its effect on malignancies of the prostate and bladder, radiation is rarely curative in the bowel, but it may prolong life and render the patient more comfortable in some cases, especially when combined with chemotherapy.

Frequently, the surgery that can cure you may necessitate a colostomy, that is, an opening of the bowel externally through the abdominal wall. Patients dread this prospect and some even tell me that they would rather be dead. That attitude is so foolish these days, when colostomy bags are odor-free, lie flat on the abdomen and are quite easy to manage. Patients who wear them soon adjust very well and lead virtually normal lives. Colostomy is a small price to pay for a cancer cure.

There is no definite evidence to date that giving chemotherapy after a tumor has been completely removed makes any difference to the subsequent course, but, I think that it's a good idea to do so anyway. If just a few cells have been left behind, chemotherapy may possibly eradicate them. So, if you are told that you don't need any further treatment after a malignant tumor of the bowel has been removed, get a second opinion from a cancer specialist.

Cancer of the Prostate

There are about 66,000 new cases and 22,000 deaths from cancer of the prostate every year in the United States alone. For some reason, it affects blacks more commonly than whites. Equally perplexing is the fact that it is uncommon in Japan. Would that we understood the genetic or environmental factors that give Japanese men so much cancer in the stomach and so little in the prostate.

How It's Discovered

The news that you have prostate cancer may very likely come as a surprise to you. It's often discovered in the following way: You notice some trouble passing your urine; it takes longer to start voiding, the stream is narrow and you "dribble" when you should have finished; you also have to get up several times at night. But everyone knows that that is what happens to many men as they get older, so there is nothing about these symptoms that would make you suspect you have cancer.

When you start having to "go" more frequently during the day too, you decide to consult your urologist. He first examines your prostate with his finger in the course of a rectal examination. He finds it enlarged, but doesn't feel any growth to worry about. He then has you undergo an intravenous pyelogram (a dye is injected into your vein, and an X ray is then taken that outlines the kidneys and bladder), which tells him how much urine you are retaining in your bladder after you think you have emptied it. The bigger the prostate, the more residual urine you have. The urologist concludes that you need an operation, and you agree.

Surprise, Surprise!

After the gland is removed, the pathologist has a surprise for you. He reports that he has found a small area of cancer, very deep in your prostate. Fortunately, it is surrounded or walled-in by completely normal tissue. At that point, it is at what we call Stage A. Such islands of cancer are frequently found in older men, and they are nothing to worry about. Under the microscope, such a cancer almost always appears well *differentiated*, that is, the cells, though malignant, are fairly orderly in appearance. If a number of such cancer "islands" are present, you will likely be advised to have a "radical prostatectomy," that is, get the whole gland out, because of the possibility that there may be some cancer cells left in the remaining tissue. That is good advice. If you are not given it, get a second opinion. Failure to clean out all the cancer leaves you one chance in five of developing a serious prostate malignancy within two years.

"Silent" Prostate Cancer

Your prostate cancer may also be detected during a routine checkup. A careful doctor will always do a rectal examination, regardless of symptoms, at least once a year on every male patient forty-five or older. At that time, if you have a "silent" prostate cancer, one that is not giving you any symptoms, he may find a suspicious area that feels irregular and harder than the rest of the prostate. A "needle biopsy" must then be done. This is a fairly easy procedure in which a needle is introduced from the outside (through the skin) into the gland. The only problem here is that occasionally the needle may miss the cancer, especially if it is a small one. Before undergoing such a biopsy, however, you might ask the doctor to try a course of antibiotics first. Occasionally, chronic infection can cause a little swelling that feels like a cancer. If, after a couple of weeks, the suspicious area does not disappear, then you must have the biopsy, and two weeks is not going to make any difference in the outlook.

If the biopsy confirms the presence of cancer, you are in what we call Stage B, defined as a cancer large enough to feel, but still within the gland and not yet spread. At this point, your best chance for cure is surgery. And that is what most doctors will recommend. You may, however, be offered radiation if you are very old or considered to be a poor operative risk. *If you are advised against surgery for any reason at this point, get a second opinion from another urologist.*

In some centers, Stage-B cancer of the prostate is also treated with surgically implanted pellets of radioactive iodine in the gland to reduce the likelihood of recurrence. Ask your urologist about the necessity or desirability of this technique in your case.

Now You're in Real Trouble

Suppose that, in the course of the rectal examination, your doctor finds a tumor not only in your prostate but also in neighboring tissue (local extension). If it has not yet spread to your bones, liver or lungs, you are now in Stage C of the disease. At this point, as much of the prostate and tumor tissue as possible is removed, especially if the enlarged gland is causing obstruction to urine outflow. But since it is now virtually impossible to remove the entire cancer, surgery at this point is "palliative," rather than curative. Radiation may now be advisable, to destroy as many of the remaining cancer cells as possible.

New X-ray techniques like the linear accelerator make it possible to pinpoint high doses of radiation to the affected area and so control the disease for years. Another method of delivering radiation is by implanting radioactive iodine seeds locally as is done in Stage B. This requires a long and difficult operation, but the malignant tissue can be radiated very accurately, since the radioactive material is placed directly into it under direct vision. If radiation is suggested, ask your doctor about this particular technique. It is a sophisticated procedure, which should only be done by an experienced surgeon. Such radioactive pellet implantation is usually reserved to cure cancers in Stages A and B, or smaller ones in Stage C. If it is not recommended for you, ask for another opinion.

Most doctors do not prescribe additional female hormones or "anti-male" hormones at this stage, unless radiation is unsuccessful.

Advanced Prostate Cancer

That brings us to Stage-D cancer of the prostate. You probably got that far without warning, by avoiding a checkup, when earlier Stages B and C might have been detected (and more successfully treated). If it is any comfort to you, prostate malignancy presents at this stage in at least 50 percent of patients. What started off as a "silent" nodule has now spread to the lymph glands and other organs in your body—that is, it has metastasized. You will know that has happened because of bone pain, usually in the spine.

When you finally show up in his office with Stage-D cancer, the doctor will feel a rock-hard prostate gland, very irregular and diffusely enlarged. Blood tests will indicate the presence of enzymes that have seeped from the cancerous bones (elevated acid phosphatase) while X rays and radioactive scans of the skeleton will confirm the spread of the cancer.

You are now in serious trouble, but all is not yet lost. At this point, it is usually too late for surgery unless the gland is so big that it obstructs your urinary outflow. But if you are voiding satisfactorily and are advised to have an operation, get another opinion from another urologist. You probably don't need surgery, and removing some of the tissue will not make one iota of difference in the long run. At this stage, you still have a 70–80 percent chance of improvement. Your pain can be lessened, and the rate of spread of the malignancy can be slowed, but not cured. Such palliation can be achieved either with hormones (estrogens) or by having your testicles removed. In either event, forget about having any more erections. Your main objective now is survival and freedom from suffering.

When a Man Needs a Woman's Hormones

If you are given estrogens for advanced prostate cancer, take the smallest amount necessary, because cardiovascular complications (clots in various blood vessels) may develop at higher dosages. And remember, you need surgical removal of the testes (orchiectomy) *or* hormones. There is no evidence that doing both is any better than either alone.

Little Plastic Balls

Many men are psychologically distraught when their testes are removed—at any age. To help them cope, at least in the locker room, the surgeons can insert little plastic balls or even some of your own tissues from elsewhere in the body into the scrotal sacs to create the appearance and feel of normality.

There are many studies currently being conducted to determine whether chemotherapy is useful in cancer of the prostate. To my knowledge, there is no effective combination of drugs now available for that purpose.

Cancer of the Glands and Blood

No discussion of cancer is complete without mention of the lymphomas (tumors of the lymph glands) and leukemias (which strike the bone marrow and the blood), a special group of malignancies that affect all age groups and both sexes.

Lymphomas

Lymph nodes, or glands, are collections of tissue found throughout the body. Their function is the regional defense of the area in which they are situated. They filter fluid passing through them, removing harmful bacteria and entrapping any circulating tumor cells that may happen by. Normally, when not inflamed, infected or infiltrated by cancer cells, lymph glands cannot be felt. Any gland you or your doctor can detect is, by definition then, already enlarged. When lymph glands are diseased by infection, they are usually swollen and tender. When malignant, however, they are, as a rule, harder and almost painless.

Lymphomas are tumors (of which Hodgkin's disease is one type) in which the cells within the lymph glands, normally very orderly and well behaved, become malignant. The disease process usually involves most of the glandular system, so that enlarged lymph nodes can be felt in many areas of the body. Untreated, lymphomas are ultimately fatal.

Cancer specialists classify the lymphomas into various categories, which need not concern us here. Suffice it to say that about 65,000 such cancers appear every year in the United States, and result in about 21,000 deaths—a serious business.

When I was graduated from medical school, these disorders were virtually always fatal. Today, Hodgkin's disease, once lethal, can be cured, in 80 percent of cases, and modern treatment can induce long remissions and cures in several of the other lymphomas.

Your lymphoma may be discovered in the following way: While shaving, or putting on your makeup or deodorant one day, you may find a swollen gland somewhere, usually in the neck or armpit. It is painless and feels hard and rubbery. You probably won't tell your doctor about this finding, because it doesn't really bother you and you know that most swollen glands are harmless and will soon disappear. You may then notice that when you have a cocktail, the gland aches a little. (Alcohol-induced pain is characteristic of some lymphomas, and we don't know why.) A few weeks later, the gland is larger, and you find another one nearby. You decide to see the doctor.

He will need to do a biopsy to establish the diagnosis of lymphoma. But some infections mimic cancer cells under the microscope and are not always interpreted correctly. So, at this point, as in all cancers, before any treatment is instituted, get a second opinion.

The basic therapy of localized lymphomas, when only a single gland or one area is involved, is radiation. The new high-powered mega-voltage machines are able to pinpoint delivery of the rays and focus a very high concentration to the specific target without unduly injuring adjacent healthy tissue. Make sure, again, that the facility where you are receiving this treatment has the most modern equipment available. A second opinion from a qualified radiotherapist can assure you of that.

After radiation, some patients are given chemotherapy. One currently used combination in Hodgkin's disease consists of nitrogen mustard, vincristine, procarbazine and prednisone. Chemotherapy and/or radiation can effect a cure in most cases of Hodgkin's disease and will control and sometimes cure other lymphomas as well. In addition to chemotherapy there is new work with concomitant immunotherapy. Results, however, are still inconclusive at this time with respect to this form of treatment.

The Leukemias

The prefix *leuk* means white; *emia* refers to blood. So *leukemia* means "white blood." The term embraces a group of malignant diseases in which the white corpuscles, normally numbering from 6,000 to 10,000 per cubic centimeter of blood, go "crazy"—values as high as 50,000 to 100,000 or more are found. When we look at them under the microscope, not only do we see too many, but they look very abnormal too. There are 22,000 new cases every year and about 16,000 deaths.

As you know, white blood cells are made in the bone marrow, and are normally released fully matured into the bloodstream at a controlled rate. In leukemia, the process controlling the growth of these cells and the rate at which they are fed into the blood breaks down. As a result, immature blood cells, not fully formed, are released prematurely into the circulation. One of the main functions of the white blood cells is to counter infection. But that is a "man's job" (for mature cells), which the juvenile ones can't perform. (All they do is clog the circulation, invade other organs of the body, and finally cause death.) As these immature white cells pack the marrow, they replace other elements that should be formed there—elements that have important roles to play. For example, the platelets are responsible for normal clotting; the red cells carry oxygen. So, in leukemic patients we find anemia (not enough red cells) and hemorrhage (due to platelet deficiency). Also, infections are rampant in leukemic patients, because the abnormal white cells can't cope with bacterial invasion as do their healthy counterparts.

No Longer Always Fatal, but Be Good to Your Brothers and Sisters

Not so many years ago, leukemia was uniformly fatal. Today, however, it is curable in about 55 percent of children. But that requires treatment planned and executed by highly skilled specialists. Management consists of chemotherapy, radiation and perhaps immunotherapy. In special circumstances, after destroying the leukemia cells, we now even transplant normal bone marrow into leukemic patients, if compatible donors (almost always brothers or sisters) can be found.

While the outlook for adults with acute leukemia is not as good as for children (the cure rate is only 15 percent), they often sustain long remissions with the same kinds of treatment. As I have repeatedly said in these pages, it is critical to buy time, because nobody knows what new therapy will bring as early as tomorrow—especially in the field of leukemia.

KEY FACTS TO REMEMBER

The news about cancer is both good and bad. The good news is the fact that improved methods of diagnosis and treatment have resulted in increasing numbers of cures and more prolonged survival. The bad news is that with a few exceptions, the over-all incidence of cancer is increasing.

The major facts to remember about cancer generally are:

1. Whenever the diagnosis of cancer is made, it should be confirmed by an expert specializing in the field (oncologist) before further steps are taken.

2. Not all cancers are fatal, and not all tumors are malignant.

3. Early diagnosis and treatment are critical.

4. Techniques of managing and controlling cancer are changing rapidly; therefore, your doctor must constantly be aware of what is new and available and so should you. Major approaches to the treatment of most cancers consist of surgery, irradiation, chemotherapy and immunotherapy. The rule of thumb to follow is that a cancer should be completely removed surgically whenever possible. The decision to use other forms of treatment in addition to, or in place of, surgery

is based on many considerations and should be made by experts in the field.

Cancer of the Lung

Cancer of the lung is the leading cause of cancer deaths in the United States. Though still more common in men, its prevalence in women is increasing in epidemic numbers, presumably due to changing smoking habits and environmental pollution. Although a small number of cases, if detected early enough, can be cured, for the most part, cancer of the lung remains incurable. A vaccine, for prevention and treatment, is now under study.

Cancer of the Kidney

Cancer of the kidney, except when detected very early, is highly malignant and usually refractory to all treatment.

Cancer of the Testes

Testicular cancer, formerly fatal, is now frequently curable by a combination of surgery, chemotherapy and radiation.

Cancer of the Bladder

Bladder cancer usually declares itself by the appearance of blood in the urine. It is basically a disease of males. Treatment consists of cauterizing the tumor where possible, or instilling BCG vaccine into the bladder followed by a search at regular intervals for evidence of recurrence. However, when the malignancy is advanced, complete excision of the bladder itself is usually required.

Cancer of the Breast

Cancer of the breast is the most prevalent malignancy in women. The traditional radical mastectomy is much less frequently done now, having been replaced by the "modified radical" in which only the breast and involved lymph glands are removed. Muscles, tendons and connective tissues are spared. There are doctors who limit the surgery to excision of the cancer itself. A few depend solely on radiation. Whichever of these approaches is suggested for you, always ask for a second opinion.

Since breast cancer spreads not only by direct extension to neighboring tissues, but also via blood and lymph channels to distant sites, surgery should almost always be followed by chemotherapy and/or hormones and, in some cases, immunotherapy. The best combination of drugs should be decided in consultation with an expert oncologist.

Mammography should be done routinely for patients over the age of fifty. In younger women, it is required only when there is particular vulnerability to the disease, as might be evidenced by a strong family history or a history of cancer in the other breast.

Cancer of the Uterus

Cancer of the uterus is a common form of malignancy, whose risk is thought to be increased by the use of female hormones (estrogen). These should never be taken without the explicit knowledge and consent of your gynecologist. If estrogens are required for whatever reason, routine pelvic exams should be done every six months. Cancer of the uterus is best treated with surgery and radiation.

Cancer of the Ovary

Cancer of the ovary is an important cause of cancer deaths in women, second only to breast cancer. Treatment is basically surgical, followed by chemotherapy and radiation.

Cancer of the Digestive Tract

Cancer of the digestive tract, in aggregate, is the most important malignancy today. Wherever it strikes, gastrointestinal cancer should be surgically removed, when possible. Follow-up chemotherapy and radiation may prevent subsequent recurrence and increase the chances of cure.

Cancer of the Prostate

Cancer of the prostate is a very common disease of older men. The early forms are often accidentally discovered, easily removed and curable. Although the outlook is less good for cure, after local extension or distant spread has occurred, prolonged survival is still frequently possible. Treatment consists of surgery, when possible, followed by radiation (external or by means of implanted radioactive-iodine seeds) and hormone therapy. An alternative to the latter is removal of the testes.

Lymphomas and Leukemias

Lymphomas and leukemias are malignancies of the lymph glands, blood-forming tissues and blood constituents. Once uniformly fatal, several types are now curable, including certain childhood leukemias and Hodgkin's disease. The mainstays of treatment are chemotherapy and radiation.

28

Arthritis—Avoiding a Laissez-Faire Approach

Common, Costly and Chronic

You are not likely to take arthritis seriously or consider it a very important disease unless you actually suffer from it yourself. It is not as dramatic as a stroke, as threatening as a heart attack, or as devastating as cancer. What's more, joint aches and pains are so common, they are often lumped into the "arthritis" category and taken for granted as the inevitable result of the wear and tear of living. In actual fact, however, more than twenty million people in the United States have arthritis that is troublesome enough to require medical care. Nor is this a disease of old age. Ten percent of all those *disabled* by arthritis are under forty-five years of age. To paraphrase Winston Churchill, "Never have so many suffered so much for so long" as do these patients. Over and above the pain it causes, arthritis also exacts an enormous economic toll. Absence from work and loss of productivity due to this group of disorders costs this nation billions of dollars annually.

Because of its chronicity, too many patients with arthritis do not take advantage of newer concepts, drugs and treatments which can make life lots more bearable, if not actually cure the disorder.

Arthritis means "inflammation of a joint" (from *arthron*, Greek for "joint," and-*itis*, medical suffix, derived from the

373

Latin and meaning "inflammatory disease"). Used alone, it is not a specific diagnosis, because the causes and anatomical locations of such inflammation are legion. Those causes include simple wear and tear (osteoarthritis); infection (gonorrhea); a generalized disease (rheumatoid arthritis), which involves, in addition to the joints, many other systems in the body (the heart, arteries, muscles and other internal organs); and a disorder of the joints traditionally attributed to "high living" (gout). Each of these forms of "arthritis" requires different treatment and has a different outlook. So, if you are told, with a shrug of the shoulders, that "all you have is arthritis," make sure that you understand precisely what kind it is and are convinced that everything possible is being done to help you. If you are in doubt, see a rheumatologist—he's an internist with special training and expertise in the various types of arthritis.

Rheumatoid Arthritis—The Worst Kind

Rheumatoid arthritis (RA) is usually the worst kind you can have. It is three times more common in women than in men and strikes most frequently between the ages of twenty-five and fifty. Although RA can involve many different joints of the body, it usually is most apparent in the small ones, like in the fingers. It is generally symmetrical—that is, affects both sides of the body. Joints are swollen, stiff, painful and warm to the touch. In most patients, attacks are mild, and there are periods of remission during which symptoms are either slight or absent. Such letup occurs frequently and may persist for months. In other instances, the disease may progress relentlessly to the crippling stage. Because this is a generalized disease striking other organs of the body as well as the joints, you feel pretty miserable with it. You have no energy, tire easily, your appetite is poor, you lose weight and may run a low-grade fever.

Treatment of rheumatoid arthritis must be aggressive and have as its major goals relief of joint pain and swelling and prevention of joint deformity and destruction.

Helpful Medications

The most useful drug to try first is aspirin. But you will have to take it in large doses—twelve or more a day—to have it do the job. Aspirin is irritating to the gastrointestinal tract, and you may end up bleeding from the stomach or bowel if you take such large doses for any length of time. So, if you have ever had a peptic ulcer, make sure to tell your doctor. Also, ask for several of those Hemoccult cards to facilitate checking for blood in the stool. Every few weeks, you smear a tiny film of stool on a card and mail it to the laboratory, where it is tested for any chemical evidence of blood. Continue to do this as long as you take large doses of aspirin. Important bleeding in the gut is not always visible to the naked eye.

Most patients tolerate aspirin in one form or another, but you may require the coated preparation that is much less irritating to the gut. But always remember to report any "indigestion" or bleeding immediately.

Aspirin alone is often all you will need if your rheumatoid arthritis is mild. Since symptoms are usually worse in the morning, so that you awake with pain and stiffness of the joints, take "time-release" or long-acting aspirin at bedtime, so it will be working when you get up.

Despite the veneration in which aspirin is held (and for good reason), there has been a good deal of active research to produce salicylate drugs that create less gastric irritation. There are now on the market two such preparations that I have found as effective as aspirin. They are marketed in the United States as Disalcid and Trilisate. Their advantage lies in the fact that they need only be taken two or three times a day, rather than every two or three hours.

When Salicylates Aren't Enough

When salicylates either don't work or are not well tolerated, another group of drugs is available for control of the symptoms of RA. Though neither more potent nor better than aspirin, they are different and often give good results when aspirin does not. They go under such trade names as Indocin, Motrin, Naprosyn, Tolectin, Nalfon, Feldene and Clinoril. None is the "magic bullet" of rheumatoid arthritis, all the flamboyant advertising notwithstanding. They may cause gastric irritation much as aspirin does. There is no evidence that using them in combination is any more effective than prescribing them singly. The response of any given patient to any one of these drugs is unpredictable. You may benefit from one and not from the other and it's often a matter of potluck.

The Next Level of Treatment

If these fairly nontoxic preparations don't give you relief, you will have to move on to a drug like phenylbutazone (Azolid, Butazolidin). However, in most situations, this preparation should not be taken for more than five or six consecutive days, because, in a small number of patients, prolonged use can seriously damage the bone marrow. Incidentally, there is nothing to prevent you from taking aspirin with any of the drugs mentioned above. Occasionally, it is more effective in combination with another preparation.

Make Sure You Don't Get Hooked

An important principle for you to follow, especially in the early stages of RA, is to avoid taking narcotics for pain relief. None of the drugs mentioned above will make an addict out of you, but I know of several tragic cases of patients with rheumatoid arthritis who, racked with pain, pleaded, cajoled, insisted and finally persuaded the doctors to give them codeine, Dilaudid, Demerol, Talwin, Percodan, or other "controlled" substances. If you use them regularly, you may well get "hooked." That may not be an important consideration in late-stage cancer; but in RA, after the disease goes into remission, you may have a drug problem on your hands for the rest of your life.

Beware of the Rip-Off Artists

Suppose you have tried all the above medications without success. At this point, it is easy to fall prey to forms of quackery. Some of it is innocuous, like the copper bracelet, to which I have no real objection. (Although some patients swear it works, I know of no scientific evidence to prove it.) Since it is decorative, and the worst it can do is give you a green wrist from the oxidation of the copper, by all means wear it if you think it helps.

While copper bracelets are harmless, the same can't be said for some of the "arthritis clinics" that operate barely within the law. Here you will be given combinations of drugs which, at best, don't help, and frequently are dangerous. Or you go on a nutrition binge. No "special" diet I know is likely to make one whit of difference to your disease. (Just be sure to eat balanced and nutritious meals containing plenty of protein and food rich in iron.)

The Gold Rush

If none of the medication mentioned thus far has helped, instead of looking for a miracle, you should consider gold therapy. Even though injectable gold for rheumatoid arthritis was first used in France fifty years ago, it has remained fairly controversial to this day. Most rheumatologists, however, believe that properly administered, gold will bring on a complete remission or significantly improve 50–60 percent of patients. The full course of treatment takes up to twenty weeks. Although not without risk, gold therapy should be tried if your symptoms are progressive and severe. But remember, not every doctor is experienced with this technique. If yours isn't, ask him to recommend a rheumatologist. Because of its potential toxicity, the administration of gold is not something to be taken casually, either by you or your doctor.

If you continue to suffer even after a course of gold therapy, the next step may be antimalarial drugs (Chloroquin, Hydroxychloroquin), which in some cases have a salutary effect on rheumatoid arthritis. They are not very popular because of the frequency with which they damage the eyes. Think twice before accepting this treatment.

If antimalarials don't help either, or you decide not to use them, you have yet another option—a drug called Penicillamine (don't confuse it with penicillin, of which it is a synthetic relative). Penicillamine is not an antibiotic; it is, like gold, a potent chemical with potentially serious side effects. It controls symptoms in some patients with rheumatoid arthritis, but it should be administered only by experienced specialists. If you are given Penicillamine, don't expect immediate results; it may take as long as two or three months before you begin to respond. During the entire time you are on the drug, you have to be watched very carefully for toxicity. Experts in its use tell me that only one patient in four is able to tolerate it, the major problems being kidney trouble, rashes and gastrointestinal symptoms. If you have a preexisting kidney condition, chances are that you will not be eligible for this therapy.

When Penicillamine works, it not only acts on the joints,

but attacks the underlying disease process too, so that you will feel a whole lot better generally, with less fever, improvement of appetite and a sense of well-being. We are not quite certain about how it works. Perhaps it enhances the body's own defense mechanism, the so-called immune system.

The Ubiquitous Immune System

A word about the *immune system* here. When you are infected by a bug or virus of some kind, the body develops antibodies to neutralize or destroy the invader. But sometimes this defense mechanism gets all mixed up. It forgets who's who and what's what, and begins to attack the body itself instead of, or in addition to, the "enemy." In the case of rheumatoid arthritis, healthy joints become its target. The rationale for treating rheumatoid arthritis with "immunosuppressant" drugs is to tone down such inappropriate actions. Sometimes, these measures are effective. The trouble is that when we suppress the aspect of the immune system that has gone wrong, we also impair its other vital mechanisms that protect against real threats to the body. So use of immunosuppressive agents can be hazardous in that, while they improve symptoms of rheumatoid arthritis, they may also lower natural protection against other disease. For that reason, anyone taking these drugs must be monitored very closely for evidence of other trouble.

The Hazards of Steroids

You and your doctor should try to resist the temptation of trying steroid (cortisone) drugs in rheumatoid arthritis. Their long-term use in large doses (and we usually have to use progressively larger amounts to obtain the same effect) can produce threatening or otherwise undesirable complications. Cortisone repeatedly injected into a joint may eventually cause its destruction, just as surely as will the disease itself. The temporary benefit of oral steroids is short-lived and you usually pay heavily for it. You become more vulnerable to infection, you may develop a peptic ulcer, your bones may lose their calcium and become so thin that they fracture spontaneously, you may develop diabetes or high blood pressure. But despite the dangers and drawbacks, there *are* special circumstances when severe complications of arthritis, such as inflammation of the blood vessels in the heart, brain or liver, make the use of these hormones necessary. Even so, consult with a rheumatologist before deciding to take them.

The Unfortunate Few

Remember that, despite all our efforts, a substantial number of patients with RA do progress to the crippling stage of the disease. In that case, long-term management involves more than pills and injections. While drugs help to control pain, we must address ourselves to the mechanics of the joints themselves. Adequate rest is essential, but too much will eventually leave them rigid and immobile. You will have to apply heat liberally, because that increases the range of joint motion. Supervised exercises prescribed by professional physiotherapists or experts in rehabilitative medicine may prevent loss of motion and strengthen the muscles around the joints. You may require specially fitted splints to prevent deformity. The most important part of physiotherapy is a home exercise program and that is basically your own responsibility.

When to Call the Surgeon

In special circumstances, surgical removal of the lining of the diseased joint may reduce pain and slow the progress of RA. But it takes a skilled rheumatologist to know when to call for the surgeon. Occasionally, pain is so severe in the moving joint that you may have to undergo a fusion operation. Here we deliberately sacrifice joint mobility for comfort. You may even be a candidate for complete joint replacement. These are all decisions that must be made from time to time in the management of your disease, and should not await arbitrarily set appointments at six- or eight-month intervals.

Little Tips Can Help Big Medications

Many patients with rheumatoid arthritis are able to lead productive lives. A wise, experienced doctor can give you useful little tips in addition to big medicines. For example, there is the question of sexual activity. Your doctor should instruct you in coital positions that are comfortable enough to make sexual relations enjoyable. I remember one woman in her late forties who had moderately severe rheumatoid arthritis. There were many days when she felt "lousy," with a low-grade fever, pain and stiffness of the joints and beginning deformity of her hands and knees. She was extremely depressed, for which she was given various mood-elevating drugs. It took just a few minutes talking together for me to discover that her depression was due not only to the pain, but also to the fact that she believed she was sexually undesirable to her husband. So she withdrew from any sexual relationship, not wishing to "force herself" on him in this "deformed and ugly state." The fact was that he loved her and, despite her arthritis, wanted her. *He* did not wish to force himself upon *her* for fear of aggravating her symptoms. When it was all straightened out, she no longer needed the antidepressants and adopted a more realistic outlook on her disease. The final result was a beneficial effect not only on her emotions, but also on her underlying illness.

The treatment of arthritis is changing rapidly. Keep in touch with the Arthritis Foundation, which has branches in most large metropolitan areas. To find the one nearest you, write to the Arthritis Foundation, 3400 Peachtree Road, N.E., Atlanta, Georgia 30326. They will send you all the latest literature and tell you where to find the special counseling services that can help you live with this disease.

Osteoarthritis

Let us assume that you have consulted the doctor about pain, stiffness and a little swelling of some of your joints. You are worried about the possibility of unrelenting or progressive deformity. But the doctor tells you that you have *osteoarthritis*, the noncrippling disease and not rheumatoid arthritis. (He will probably have taken some X rays, which help to differentiate the two, as well as some blood tests.) Unlike rheumatoid arthritis, which is a generalized disease, osteoarthritis affects only the joints.

Even in Dinosaurs

Osteoarthritis is not a new disease of civilization. We see evidence of it in dinosaur skeletons representing life 200,000,000 years ago as well as in the bones of Neanderthal man 40,000 years ago. Most doctors refer to osteoarthritis as "degenerative" (as opposed to "infectious" or "inflammatory" joint disease), because it is believed to result from simple wear and tear on the joints over the years. So, you would expect to find this form of arthritis predominantly in athletes, parachutists and others who impose repeated, abnormal strain on their joints. But while Sandy Koufax had osteoarthritis in his arm and Joe Namath is said to suffer from arthritis of his knees, they aren't the only ones who get it. Many who lead "ordinary" lives also develop osteoarthritis.

Controlling Pain

Even though osteoarthritis is not usually as crippling as rheumatoid arthritis, you should not be satisfied with a treatment program limited to a few aspirins and nothing more, if that leaves you in chronic pain. Make sure that your doctor is aggressive about and interested in the management of your problems.

The mainstay of pain control, as in RA, is aspirin. Here too you may need a lot of them—six, eight, ten or more a day—and you must be constantly alert to the risk of gastric irritation or ulceration. If you now have, or ever have had, a peptic ulcer, aspirin in such large doses may constitute a problem. As mentioned earlier, there are several new salicylates, like Trilisate, that are as effective as aspirin, and since they need be taken only twice a day may irritate the stomach lining less.

Many of the newer "nonsteroidal" anti-inflammatory drugs like Indocin, Motrin or Naprosyn, discussed earlier in reference to rheumatoid arthritis, are also useful in osteoarthritis. Physiotherapy and occasional injection of small amounts of cortisone into the affected joint can be useful. Again, try to avoid oral medication containing cortisone or narcotics for relief of pain. If you are given any, get another opinion from a rheumatologist.

My Own Nonoperation

Not too long ago I had a firsthand experience that highlights the need for a good second opinion. I began to notice pain whenever I rotated my right wrist. I consulted a very good orthopedic surgeon, who first splinted the wrist. After ten days, all I had to show for my effort was a stiff joint. The pain persisted. My doctor then suggested a surgical procedure to excise one of the small wrist bones that he firmly believed was giving me all the trouble. I was about to submit; but, since I practice what I preach, I discussed the matter with another colleague. He was very much opposed to surgery and referred me to a physiatrist (that's an M.D. who specializes in physical and rehabilitation medicine) who also thought that surgery was unnecessary. He recommended exercises to stretch the tendon in my wrist. I performed them faithfully for a week. He then injected the joint with a tiny amount of steroid. That cured me—at least my wrist has been free of pain for the past three years. So, even in a matter as relatively trivial as a little arthritis of the wrist, a second opinion spared me the pain and cost of an unnecessary operation.

Mechanical Measures

In addition to injecting something into a joint to obtain relief, you may also benefit from the *removal* of fluid that has accumulated in it (for example, "water on the knee"). Physiotherapy too can yield very gratifying results in osteoarthritis. Unfortunately, it is very much underutilized, largely because it is time-consuming and there are not enough well-trained people around to treat everybody who needs it (about 50 percent of the population over fifty is troubled by some form of osteoarthritis). As in rheumatoid arthritis, physical measures must be tempered with daily rest periods. When weight-bearing joints are involved, a cane, crutch or other support may be helpful during the acute phase.

Doctors often don't have the time to discuss with you the details of your life style. So many symptoms can be minimized by avoiding unnecessary stair climbing, wearing proper shoes to correct the line of weight bearing, advice on posture, and enforced weight loss in the obese. (The heavier you are, the greater the stress on your weight-bearing joints.) When you have pain in a limb or a joint, you tend to favor it. This results in the muscles around the affected joint becoming thin or, as doctors refer to it, atrophied. Also, remember that osteoarthritis can produce pain at a distance from the actual site of involvement. For example, the bony spurs that develop when you have arthritis in the spine may press on nerves that emerge from it to go to other parts of the body. So, if you have arthritis of the neck, you may awaken one morning with chest pain and think you have had a heart attack. Under these circumstances, traction (which eases the pressure on the affected nerve) or even a soft, fitted collar can be of help.

Physiotherapy for Spasm Control

Much of the discomfort that you experience when your spine or shoulders are involved by osteoarthritis is due to spasm of the muscles in the affected area. Muscles are nature's splints. If you have arthritis in the bones of your spine, the muscles in the area become tense and rigid in order to prevent the bones from moving too much. But in so doing, the muscles themselves become painful, and you end up with a "bad back." So, good physiotherapy to relax the muscles prescribed by somebody who understands the relationship between joint and muscle structure and function can be enormously helpful. I have known many patients who were spared disc surgery by an intensive program of physiotherapy. *Whenever surgery is recommended for osteoarthritis, make sure that you have exhausted all the nonsurgical alternatives* (exercise, heat, bracing and drugs for pain relief).

Reassurance Is Not Enough

If your osteoarthritis is severe, you need proper treatment. Reassurance that you are not going to be crippled is not enough. Moreover, some cases do indeed end up with deformities. If that happens, you may ultimately require braces or an operation either to stabilize or replace the involved joint.

The most important breakthrough in this area has been the ability of surgeons to replace a painful, deformed hip. Patients who only a few years ago would have been virtually crippled are now leading normal lives because of this incredible surgical procedure. So, if you have been limping along with pain because of arthritis of the hip and are living on pain killers, ask whether you are a candidate for *total hip replacement*. The risk is very small when the operation is done by an experienced team.

We are now able to replace not only hips, but knees, elbows and other joints as well. These other procedures are, however, not yet as well developed as is that for the hip.

As remarkable as the joint-replacement technique is, always get a second opinion whenever it is recommended. First, to make sure that it is needed, and then to determine whether the surgical team that is doing it is sufficiently experienced.

No discussion of arthritis (osteo or RA) these days is complete without a reference to DMSO. Is it a wonder drug, or a nostrum? Thousands of Americans are using it, and the literature on the subject is replete with anecdotal accounts of how great it is. Jim Jones, an Atlanta Falcon quarterback says having his shoulder rubbed with DMSO made it possible for him to throw a football. It is approved for use in the Soviet Union (it was first synthesized by a Russian chemist over 100 years ago). In this country, vets may use it for muscle and joint sprain in horses. Physicians, thus far, are only allowed to prescribe it for an inflamed urinary bladder in humans—not for joint pain.

DMSO was originally (and still is) used as an industrial solvent. It was first reported to have potential medical application in 1964. And since then, the controversy has raged—does it or doesn't it help joint pain? Part of the problem of assessing it objectively has been due to the fact that one can't do a double-blind study on it—the kind where two identical preparations are administered, one of which is inert (placebo) and neither the patient nor the treating doctor knows who's getting what. You see, DMSO, when rubbed into and absorbed by the skin gives an unmistakeable garlic-like odor to the breath, and so a "double-blind" is not really possible.

You would think some pharmaceutical company would be eager to test it once and for all. Not a single one is willing to do so. I'm not sure why. Do you think it could possibly be because DMSO is not patentable?

So what's the bottom line? Should one use it or not? I can't advise you to take any drug which is not approved by the FDA. But if you do get hold of any, and decide to try it, make sure it's pure. It's so well absorbed, it can also permit any contaminants present in the ointment to enter the body!

Gout—The Rich Man's Disease?

No one with gout is amused by the traditional cartoons depicting that disease—the corpulent man with bulbous nose, who has obviously indulged to excess, sitting with outstretched leg while a valet ministers to his acutely inflamed big toe. Although this disorder may be precipitated in vulnerable subjects by prolonged, excessive use of alcohol, overweight and diets rich in animal organs (liver, brain, pancreas, kidney) it also plagues those who are moderate both in their incomes and life styles—men much more often than women.

Fact and Fantasy

What is fact and what is fantasy in this disease? Gout has very little to do with diet. It results from an impairment in the way the body handles certain chemical processes. This results in too much *uric acid* in the body, either because it is excessively produced or not eliminated properly. Gout develops when uric-acid crystals form in the joints and inflame them. The most commonly affected site is the big toe, but gout can involve other joints—the knee, elbow, wrist, heel and so on. The attack is occasionally mild, but more often so exquisitely painful that you cannot bear even the slightest pressure, such as a bed sheet, on the affected area.

A Tricky Diagnosis

The diagnosis of gout is not always easy to make, and may be confused with several conditions ranging from gonorrhea to osteoarthritis, all of which may cause a joint to become inflamed. What further complicates the picture is the fact that the uric-acid level in the blood is not always elevated. One of my patients was a seventy-eight-year-old man whose knees (both of them) were acutely swollen. It is unusual for gout to strike two joints at the same time. The fact that the uric-acid level was normal also made the diagnosis of gout unlikely. It looked just like acute osteoarthritis. Aspirin was of no help; neither were Motrin and Clinoril. He had too much pain to do any exercise. Because he was so uncomfortable, I admitted him to the hospital with the diagnosis of "arthritis of unknown origin." It was only when we withdrew some of the fluid from the swollen joint, analyzed it under the microscope and actually saw the urate crystals in the fluid, that we were able to confirm the diagnosis of gout.

Over the years, we have learned how more effectively to prevent and treat gouty arthritis. You should be aware of this new knowledge, because the manner in which the acute attack is handled is important to your comfort. Modern therapy may eliminate recurrences in most patients, often permitting them to eat and drink what they like.

When the Cure Is Worse than the Disease

The specific medicine for the acute attack of gout is called colchicine. (Not so long ago this was the only drug we had for that purpose.) It is used in the following way. When the pain starts, colchicine is given every hour until either relief is obtained or you are so sick from the treatment that it has to be stopped. The abdominal cramps, diarrhea, nausea and pain in the belly from colchicine are almost as bad as the symptoms of gout itself. Most patients have to be pushed to the limits of tolerance to colchicine before they obtain relief from the pain. There are among my colleagues some old-timers who still use this treatment. It is effective, mind you, and it has the advantage of being diagnostic as well. In other words, if you suddenly develop acute pain in a joint and neither you nor your doctor are sure what kind of arthritis it is, relief with colchicine is virtually certain evidence that it is gout, for it does not influence the pain from any other form of arthritis.

But, in my opinion, once the diagnosis of gout is established colchicine is no longer the best drug to use. Most doctors now prefer Indocin, an anti-inflammatory agent that has fewer side effects than colchicine, but which can irritate an empty stomach. If you have severe coronary artery disease, Indocin, according to a recent study, may be harmful. Phenylbutazone (marketed as Butazolidin or Azolid) is equally effective, but carries with it the risk of dangerous injury to the bone marrow if taken for more than a few days.

How to Prevent Recurrences

When the acute attack is over, you and your doctor should decide what to do to prevent a recurrence. Most patients don't like to take medication indefinitely, but that is what you will have to do if you are vulnerable to gout. Simply changing your life style is no guarantee against future attacks. For example, even if you lose weight, watch your diet and abstain from alcohol, the risk of acute gout is somewhat reduced, but not eliminated. Interestingly enough, if you follow the currently fashionable high-protein, low-carbohydrate diets in order to reduce, you may actually precipitate an attack. This happens as the result of a chemical change called *ketosis*. When women, who normally have a much lesser incidence of gout than do men, go on one of these high-protein mixtures, their natural protection or resistance to the disease is compromised, and they sometimes end up with gout.

Gout and Alcohol

Should patients with gout ever drink? In moderation, alcohol is not likely to give you any trouble. But if you are a heavy drinker, even if you take prophylactic medications, your life is likely to be punctuated by attacks of gout.

So, by all means try to lose weight, reduce alcohol intake, and avoid excessive amounts of foods rich in *purines* (animal organs), but don't count on these measures alone to keep you gout-free. You will likely need preventive maintenance medication in addition. Those most widely used include *allopurinol* (marketed as Zyloprim in the United States, Zyloric in Europe), Benemid or Anturane. Zyloprim prevents gout by decreasing the amount of uric acid the body produces; Benemid doesn't interfere with the manufacture of uric acid, but increases its excretion in the urine. Since it is urate crystals (derived from elevated uric-acid blood levels) that sit down in the joints and inflame them, you end up with fewer, if any, attacks of gout using either drug. Anturane (sulfinpyrazone) resembles allopurinol in its actions. In addition, it interferes with blood clotting and has recently been found to be protective in heart-attack patients, in whom it apparently reduces the likelihood of subsequent sudden death.

Water Pills and Gout

There are many thousands of patients who regularly take "water pills" for one reason or another—high blood pressure, heart failure or retention of fluid due to severe liver or kidney disease. Virtually all diuretics increase the uric-acid level. If they are prescribed for you, and you have had problems with gout in the past you should, in addition, take allopurinol or one of the other preventives.

The Bad Back

A "bad back" may be due to several different causes. It may result from a deformity present at birth, an infectious disease eroding the bone structure, decreased calcium content of bone because of an abnormality in the way your body absorbs or handles this mineral (especially common in postmenopausal women), an old injury that has caused disruption in the normal alignment of the bones in the spinal column, or the common, garden variety of "arthritis." Whatever the reason, you end up with chronic back pain. Because the bad back is so common, those who suffer from it tend to accept it as inevitable and just "live with it." Either that, or they become so desperate that they submit to management that is too aggressive—ranging from heavy braces to unnecessary surgical procedures.

Whom to See First—and Last

At the first sign of back trouble, see your internist. The problem may not even be orthopedic. It may, for example, be due to your kidneys. Only when other medical causes have been excluded should you consult an orthopedist or rheumatologist. If it is confirmed that you have a "bad back" due to strain or arthritis, go to a physiatrist. Many general hospitals now have departments of physiatry, or rehabilitation medicine, where patients can be given significant relief of symptoms by learning exercise programs that can later be performed at home.

There's a Lot That Can Be Done

There are many ways to obtain relief of back pain due to orthopedic causes or arthritis. These include a judicious balance between rest and specific, appropriate exercises (depending on the muscle groups involved), heat therapy, novocaine injections, splinting or bracing, properly fitting shoes, correction of posture, physiotherapy, medication and, finally, but only as a last resort, surgery. Unfortunately, too few internists or family practitioners have the time, patience, interest, facilities or skill to treat a back problem and to stay with it. Orthopedic surgeons are busy setting broken bones and dealing with other *acute* surgical problems, and are not usually enthusiastic about embarking on a long program of supportive measures for the patient with backache. (Even massage parlors don't have the back as their major priority; they address themselves primarily to your other needs and wants.)

When It's a Disc

Discs are the pads between the spinal bones, and they cushion the friction between those bones. When they wear out or are displaced, the nerves that leave the spinal cord on their way to parts of the body are impinged upon. When a nerve is thus compromised, the muscle groups it supplies are weakened, and the irritation of the nerve itself produces pain. The most common example of symptoms from such nerve pressure is sciatica, in which the sciatic nerve emerging from the lower spine is damaged by spurs from the vertebrae themselves or by a displaced disc.

If the disc is causing sufficient pressure on one or more nerves in your back, so that there is muscle weakness or loss of sensation, then surgery may be required.

The Controversial Alternative to Disc Surgery

The surgical approach to a displaced disc is to remove it. But in recent years, an alternative to this procedure has been introduced; it involves the injection of a material called chymopapain (derived from the carica papaya) into the disc space. Chymopapain is an enzyme that digests protein. When injected into the damaged disc, it dissolves some of it, thus reducing the pressure on the nerve roots responsible for the pain and weakness. Since disc disease is very common (almost 250,000 patients a year undergo surgery in the United States alone), it would indeed be useful to be able to avoid surgery by means of such an injection.

But Is It Safe and Effective?

Until recently, use of chymopapain was permitted in only two states, Illinois and Indiana, but the original manufacturer was not even distributing the drug at all commercially in the United States. Now, however, the drug is being manufactured by several companies and is legally available in Texas where it is being used in Dallas and Houston. Furthermore, the original manufacturer has been granted permission to conduct widespread trials in centers throughout the United States in order to evaluate the efficacy of this therapy. In addition to these recent developments in the United States, chymopapain has remained a routine alternative to surgery in in other countries, like Canada and Russia. The reasons for the original ban by the FDA related to sensitivity reactions reported after the injection of the substance and to the fact that it has not been proved effective. Its advocates—and there are many—say that new purification techniques have eliminated these adverse effects and that the drug's effectiveness has been demonstrated.

The Epidural Injection for Sciatica

If you have severe sciatica due to disc disease in your lower spine, and conservative measures, like heat, rest and appropriate exercise, have all failed, there is a 50 percent chance of improvement for at least one year by having an injection (epidural) of cortisone into the area where the nerve leaves the spinal cord. Cortisone works by reducing inflammation and swelling of the irritated nerve. This treatment, which has been the subject of many favorable reports, is worth inquiring about too. If your own doctor has no experience with it, ask him if he knows of someone who does.

Little Old Ladies in Pain

We focus so much on arthritis, muscle spasm and injury as causes of backache that we tend to forget one very important group of people who suddenly and for no apparent reason develop such problems. These are the "little old ladies" among us. How do they get that way? As they approach the sixties, their bones begin to thin due to a lack of calcium. We tend to think of bone as biologically dead (until we break one), very much like nails or hair we can cut without pain (until, of course, the nails break and the hair begins to fall out). The truth is that bones are dynamic, living parts of the body. After a break, the first evidence of its adaptation is the formation of a callus in a few days. This is essentially a patch that forms over the break. The bone musters all its resources to grow very rapidly in the injured area, coating and "welding" it with new bone.

Continual stress and strain on the skeleton result in adaptation. That is why a child's posture will determine the mold of his skeleton later in life. Adaptation is the result of two simultaneous on-going processes within the bone. One is *formation* of new bone, responsive to and dependent on the demands of the skeleton; the other is bone *resorption*. If the bone simply kept making new calcium without reabsorbing any, we would all grow to be as big as dinosaurs. This constant turnover—formation of new bone and reabsorption of old bone—normally occurs at approximately the same rate. This balance is maintained by several hormones, one of which is produced by the parathyroid—a tiny set of glands behind the thyroid. They can't ever be felt by the doctor, because they are too small and too deep within the neck. We check their function by means of blood tests. When a tumor of the parathyroid develops, calcium metabolism is affected with resultant changes in bone metabolism.

After the Menopause

After the menopause, the calcium content of bone is decreased for reasons that we really don't understand, and the bone becomes brittle—a phenomenon called *osteoporosis*. This thinning of the bone in women is almost universal after the menopause and accounts for the large number of hip fractures older females suffer after a trivial fall. In any event, the "little old lady," now lacking in calcium, suddenly develops severe pain in the back for little or no apparent reason. Occasionally, it happens after a bumpy car ride, stepping down hard because of a missed stair or some other jolt, causing the fracture of a vertebra in the spinal column. Whatever the mechanism, the symptoms lead to a vicious circle. The pain keeps the patient in bed. But that causes the skeleton to lose even more calcium, and more fractures may ensue, even after something as minor as a vigorous cough. (That is one of the reasons for having you up early and exercising after an illness or operation, in order to prevent demineralization of the skeleton; another is to prevent blood clotting.)

When the vertebrae fracture, they become compressed and so our female patient does, in fact, become shorter. The term "little old ladies" then derives from the fact that osteoporosis occurs primarily in older women, after the menopause, as a result of compression fractures that shorten the spine and reduce height. The spontaneously fractured bones in the spine, as they heal, may also become distorted. The result is that many of these elderly women develop back deformities, leading to the term "widow's hump" or "dowager's hump."

How Useful (and Safe) Are Estrogens?

Estrogens are popular in the treatment and prevention of osteoporosis. The logic for this therapy goes something like this: Since osteoporosis occurs most commonly in postmenopausal women and since the menopause is obviously associated with a decrease in female hormones (estrogens), let us replace what is missing. Another theory is that since *male* hormone stimulates growth of body tissue, let us also give these little old ladies some male hormone too. Have them take lots and lots of calcium as well, together with fluoride and other minerals. All this therapeutic enthusiasm raises the further question of how much of what we do helps and how much hurts.

Several widely used approaches to the treatment of osteoporosis are controversial and possibly harmful. Most doctors feel that estrogens improve osteoporosis, just as they do the "hot flushes" of the menopause. Presumably, they decrease the reabsorption of bone and thus result in a decrease in the number and rate of fractures. Given these observations, what do we do with the fact that the estrogens are also associated with an eightfold increase in cancer of the uterus? Should women with osteoporosis take this hormone anyway, despite that risk? Personally, I believe that if your bones are breaking all over the place, you have very little choice. You must take the estrogen, but if you do, you should have regular gynecological exams and Pap tests every six months, and report any vaginal bleeding immediately to your doctor.

If, however, you have but a single fracture after a fall and an X ray happens to show some thinning of the bone, which is not otherwise giving you any problem, I think it is not prudent to take estrogens. If you are prescribed estrogen under these circumstances, you might ask your doctor about the risks involved and perhaps get a second opinion, especially if the hormone is making your breasts swell or giving you renewed "periods."

Male Hormones for Women?

What about giving male hormones to osteoporotic women? The evidence favoring it is much less convincing than that for estrogens. In addition to putting hair on your face and endowing you with other male characteristics, male hormones taken by mouth can also hurt your liver. So, whether in combination with estrogens or alone, male hormones really have no place in the treatment of osteoporosis. You should get a second opinion if you are told to take them.

If you think that calcium supplements are useful in osteoporosis—since, after all, that is what the bone is lacking—you are absolutely right. But, although we associate calcium with milk, that is not a particularly good way to take it. The best source is in simple calcium carbonate tablets. Many patients ask for the calcium to be given intravenously. There is no need to do that either. In osteoporosis a little Vitamin D—and I emphasize *little*—is also useful, as is sodium fluoride supplement by mouth.

KEY FACTS TO REMEMBER

Arthritis or "inflammation of the joints" is not a single disease, but one that may be due to several different causes—infectious, chemical, traumatic, mechanical and "unexplained." So, always find out what kind of "arthritis" you have.

Rheumatoid arthritis (RA) is the worst type. Although it is often mild, chronic and insidious, it may be painful, progressive and crippling. It is a generalized disease of the body which makes itself most apparent in the joints, but affects internal organs as well. Treatment goals should be directed at pain control and prevention of joint deformity and destruction.

The most useful medications in the treatment of RA are salicylates (aspirin) or some of the newer antiarthritis drugs, gold, Penicillamine and, in resistant cases, steroids. Physiotherapy is extremely important and, in some cases, surgical correction of the joints becomes necessary.

Osteoarthritis is the wear-and-tear form of arthritis. It is not usually as crippling or debilitating as rheumatoid arthritis, but it also requires adequate control of pain, physiotherapy and, when the joint is severely damaged, as may occur in the hip, surgical replacement.

Gout is a disease of metabolism that affects various joints, classically the big toe. It can now be prevented by maintenance medication and the acute attack itself can be treated effectively. Severe dietary restrictions are no longer required, as a rule.

The *bad back* is usually due to arthritis, bone deformity or muscle spasm. It can often be managed by heat, rest, analgesics and exercise but occasionally disc surgery is required. An alternative to operation, the injection of an enzyme called chymopapain into the disc space is still a matter of controversy.

Osteoporosis, or thinning of the bones, is a frequent cause of fracture in women who are beyond the menopause and are calcium deficient. The management of this disorder involves supplementing the diet with calcium and administering estrogens under careful control. Male hormones are probably of no use in these cases.

Reflections

The Wary Patient

Public education about medicine is a good thing. Understanding the nature of a disease and what its treatment is all about, helps us to take better care of ourselves, and in many cases provides the motivation to follow doctors' orders more intelligently, conscientiously and effectively. But a little knowledge can also create problems, especially when it leads you to suspect that your doctor may not be up to date, or that his treatment is not accepted by some of his colleagues. But remember that, no matter what your doctor tells you about almost anything, if you look hard enough, you can always find an opposing view—one that you would prefer to hear. The medical establishment does not speak with one voice on many fundamental medical questions—cholesterol, hysterectomies, coronary-bypass surgery, and literally hundreds of other practical matters. Becoming aware of the "facts" of medicine also means exposure to its "controversies"—something that patients don't always appreciate and with which they are not always able to cope.

When Doctors Disagree

Disagreement among scientists is not new, but in the past, when doctors argued at their conventions, the door to the public was closed—and locked. Outsiders were not privy to these family disputes. Most doctors felt that laymen had no business being there. When there was a security lapse and an unauthorized reporter managed to "sneak" in to a convention, medical jargon, like the unintelligible Latin prescription, shielded the profession against his prying. Part of this attitude by "organized medicine" was admittedly sheer arrogance, but there was also the fear that "civilians" might misunderstand and, therefore, distort the meaning of the technical deliberations.

How times have changed! Now the Bernsteins and Woodwards are everywhere. Science reporters—astute, enthusiastic and well trained—are not only allowed into medical conferences, they are actually invited. And they work fast. Whereas it takes months for an important piece of news to reach the doctor in the medical journals, the very next day's media carry the story worldwide.

When What You Read or Hear Is Wrong

How do doctors feel about this widespread availability of medical information? We have learned to live with it, but not always happily. It is confusing enough for us when conflicting data appear in the scientific literature, but all hell breaks loose when these reports are carried in the lay press before we have heard about them or had an opportunity to evaluate and discuss them among ourselves. Suppose, for example, while casually browsing through your morning newspaper, you read that a pill your doctor prescribed is bad for you. This report may, of course, be correct, but it may also turn out to be either wrong, or valid only in certain circumstances. I remember three of my own patients with severe angina pectoris, in hospital and awaiting bypass surgery, reading in the newspaper that according to a Veterans Administration study the procedure was of no benefit. Those conclusions were subsequently disputed and largely rejected, but not before one patient had me cancel his operation, and the other two were wheeled to surgery not with the hope and optimism so important when one is sick, but feeling like sheep being led to slaughter. (Tragically, the man who backed out died three weeks later. The other two are fine.)

So the medical profession is in constant competition with *Time*, *Newsweek*, the *National Enquirer*, TV and Walter Cronkite, a contest the doctor doesn't always win.

Yesterday's Remedy—Today's Poison

Don't let your confidence in your doctor be shaken by the fact that his (or her) advice seems always to be changing.

Do you remember when the best treatment for a heart attack was prolonged bed rest, followed by forced retirement from work? Available knowledge *at that time* suggested that was the best thing for you to do. Today we have you virtually dancing with the nurse in the Coronary Care Unit as soon as your chest pain subsides, and then sign you up for a vigorous physical rehabilitation program after you return to your job. That is because we now know that such activity is good for you.

Yale Versus Johns Hopkins

Your doctor is not to blame for all this confusion. Like you, he is buffeted by the changing winds of new scientific information. Consider estrogens discussed earlier. A group of medical scientists from Yale University recently claimed that all previous studies linking estrogens to cancer were in error, that there was no association between the two. So, the conscientious, up-to-date physician dutifully notified his hormone-deprived patients that they could safely resume their medication. For a few weeks, pharmacies across the land did a booming trade in female hormones. But just as the last hot flush disappeared, the same journal carried a later report from Johns Hopkins Medical School, an equally hallowed institution, refuting the Yale Group. So back to the telephone we went, to retract last month's advice.

So you now know what treatment options you have, at least for the specific symptoms and diseases discussed in the preceding pages. That does not mean that you must challenge *any* advice your doctor gives you. You should, however, be able and willing to discuss alternative approaches that appeal to you. Remember, too, that simply because your own doctor favors a specific course of action with which some other physician disagrees, he is not necessarily wrong. There is usually more than one way to skin a cat in medicine.

The best recourse for you, the patient, is to try to keep abreast of those advances in medicine of particular relevance to you—not in a posture of challenge, criticism or suspicion, but with the spirit of partnership, which is what the good patient-doctor relationship is all about.

Index

ABOUT THE AUTHOR

ISADORE ROSENFELD, M.D., a cardiologist, is Clinical Professor of Medicine at The New York Hospital—Cornell Medical Center. In addition to his private practice and his teaching and research activities, he also serves as a consultant to the National Institutes of Health in the areas of arteriosclerosis, high blood pressure, and sudden death. He is the author of *The Complete Medical Exam*, the coauthor of a textbook on cardiology, and a prolific contributor to the scientific literature. Dr. Rosenfeld lives in Westchester County, New York, with his wife and four children.

SLIM DOWN!
STAY HEALTHY!

These bestselling Bantam books can help

THE PRITIKIN · PERMANENT WEIGHT LOSS MANUAL
by Nathan Pritikin
> *Over two months on the New York Times*
> *Bestselling List*

Here is a lower-calorie version of the bestselling PRITIKIN PROGRAM FOR DIET AND EXERCISE that can help you achieve weight loss safely, painlessly and permanently while you eat all day long. Included is a 14-day menu plan based on four different calorie intake levels, over 200 delicious recipes such as Stuffed Breast of Chicken with Lemon-Wine Sauce and Crab Crepes, a practical exercise program and a program to maintain your slimmed-down weight permanently. (#20494-7 · $3.95)

DIET FOR LIFE
by Francine Prince

You can lose 8 pounds in 14 days with bestselling author Francine Prince's quick and easy-to-follow plan for weight loss and a healthier, more invigorating life. This time-tested program will help you win the fight against nutrition-related diseases such as heart attack, hypertension, and diabetes without drugs and will help you to reduce to your ideal weight—and stay there—while savoring over 100 nutritious and high-energy recipes. (#20484-X · $3.50)

SECOND OPINION
by Isadore Rosenfeld, M.D.

"One of the best books I have ever read on medical problems. You simply must get it."—Ann Landers

Whether a disorder is life-threatening, chronic and painful, annoying or merely embarrassing, there are usually several different ways it can be treated. In this invaluable guide, completely expanded and updated for this first paperback edition, Dr. Rosenfeld offers detailed information on why, when and where to ask for a second opinion—and how you can possibly avoid unnecessary surgery. (*On sale May 15, 1982* • #20562-5 • *$3.95*)

BOSTON UNIVERSITY MEDICAL CENTER'S HEART RISK BOOK
by Aram V. Chobanian, M.D. and Lorraine Loviglio

Medical research now identifies crucial elements which can result in heart disease. Here—in an easy-to-follow, heavily illustrated guide—are the clear, practical steps you can take to identify and overcome heart risk factors which can effect your life, the life of your spouse and the lives of your children. What are the potential heart risk factors of high blood pressure, cholesterol and smoking? In this book a leading authority at a leading medical center gives the answers and shows you how to help prevent heart attack before it happens. (*On sale May 15, 1982* • #20669-9 • *$2.50*)